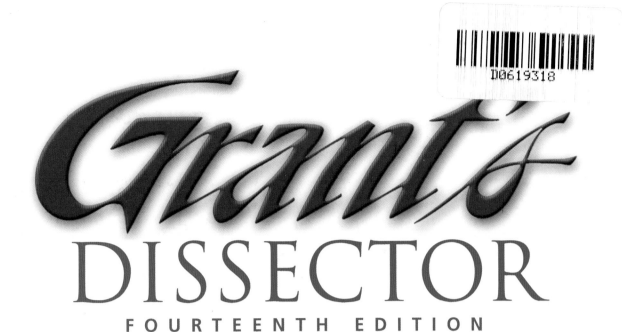

Grant's
DISSECTOR

FOURTEENTH EDITION

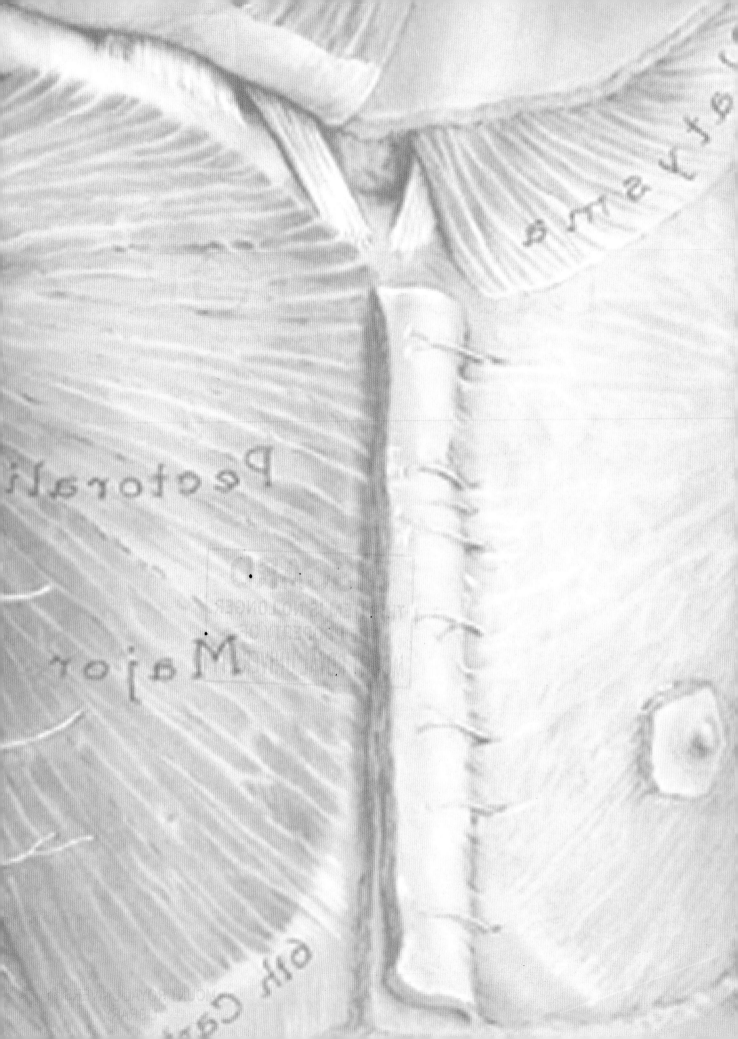

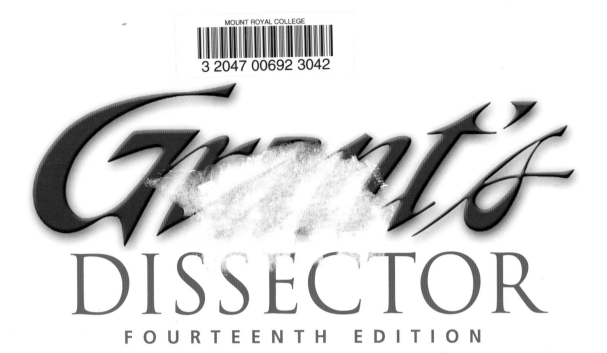

Grant's DISSECTOR

FOURTEENTH EDITION

PATRICK W. TANK, PH.D.

Director, Division of Anatomical Education
Department of Neurobiology and Developmental Sciences
University of Arkansas for Medical Sciences
Little Rock, Arkansas

 Wolters Kluwer | Lippincott Williams & Wilkins
Health

Philadelphia • Baltimore • New York • London
Buenos Aires • Hong Kong • Sydney • Tokyo

Acquisitions Editor: Crystal Taylor
Managing Editor: Stacey L. Sebring
Marketing Manager: Valerie Sanders
Production Editor: Julie Montalbano
Designer: Doug Smock
Compositor: Maryland Composition, Inc.

14th Edition

By J.C.B. Grant and H.A. Cates:
First Edition, 1940
Second Edition, 1945
Third Edition, 1948
Fourth Edition, 1953

By J.C.B. Grant:
Fifth Edition, 1959
Sixth Edition, 1967

By E.K. Sauerland:
Seventh Edition, 1974
Eighth Edition, 1978
Ninth Edition, 1984
Tenth Edition, 1991
Eleventh Edition, 1994
Twelfth Edition, 1999

By P.W. Tank:
Thirteenth Edition, 2005

Library of Congress Cataloging-in-Publication Data

Tank, Patrick W., 1950-
  Grant's dissector.—14th ed. / Patrick W. Tank.
     p. ; cm.
  Includes index.
  ISBN 978-0-7817-7431-4
  1. Human dissection—Laboratory manuals. I. Grant, J. C. Boileau (John Charles Boileau), 1886–1973. II. Title. III. Title: Dissector.
  [DNLM: 1. Dissection—Laboratory Manuals. QS 130 T165g 2009]
  QM34.G75 2009
  611--dc22

                                                            2007042161

DISCLAIMER

Care has been taken to confirm the accuracy of the information present and to describe generally accepted practices. However, the authors, editors, and publisher are not responsible for errors or omissions or for any consequences from application of the information in this book and make no warranty, expressed or implied, with respect to the currency, completeness, or accuracy of the contents of the publication. Application of this information in a particular situation remains the professional responsibility of the practitioner; the clinical treatments described and recommended may not be considered absolute and universal recommendations.

The authors, editors, and publisher have exerted every effort to ensure that drug selection and dosage set forth in this text are in accordance with the current recommendations and practice at the time of publication. However, in view of ongoing research, changes in government regulations, and the constant flow of information relating to drug therapy and drug reactions, the reader is urged to check the package insert for each drug for any change in indications and dosage and for added warnings and precautions. This is particularly important when the recommended agent is a new or infrequently employed drug.

Some drugs and medical devices presented in this publication have Food and Drug Administration (FDA) clearance for limited use in restricted research settings. It is the responsibility of the health care provider to ascertain the FDA status of each drug or device planned for use in their clinical practice.

To purchase additional copies of this book, call our customer service department at **(800) 638-3030** or fax orders to **(301) 223-2320**. International customers should call **(301) 223-2300**.

Visit Lippincott Williams & Wilkins on the Internet: http://www.lww.com. Lippincott Williams & Wilkins customer service representatives are available from 8:30 am to 6:00 pm, EST.

To Suzanne

Grant's Dissector was originally designed as an instruction manual for dissection by the regional approach. The 14th edition continues this tradition. It has been rewritten to make the dissection instructions more concise and more appropriate to today's gross anatomy curriculum. The student is encouraged to rely upon *Grant's Dissector* for dissection instructions and to use a textbook such as *Clinically Oriented Anatomy* and a quality atlas such as *Grant's Atlas* to provide anatomical details.

CHANGES TO DISSECTION ORDER

In addition to refining the dissector's content and adding new figures to each chapter, the order of dissection has been modified in the 14th edition:

* Dissection of the pectoral region has been moved from the thorax chapter to the upper limb chapter.
* Dissection of the testis has been moved from the abdomen chapter to the pelvis and perineum chapter.
* The head and neck chapter has been reorganized so that neck dissections will be completed before proceeding to the head dissections.

These changes were made in response to user requests. They will make the dissector more usable in traditional dissection courses as well as in dissection courses that accompany a systems-oriented curriculum.

OTHER KEY FEATURES

Each chapter in the 14th edition is consistently organized. Each chapter begins with a brief study of **surface anatomy**. Then, **osteology** is presented in a concise way to provide the student with important foundation structures that will aid in localization of soft tissue structures. Each dissection unit begins with a section called **"Dissection Overview."** This section is a thumbnail sketch of what is to be accomplished during the dissection session. In the section entitled **"Dissection Instructions,"** the student is led though the dissection in a logical sequence by use of a series of numbered steps. The numbering sequence allows the student to return quickly to the appropriate place on the page to get the next dissection instruction. Each dissection concludes with a section called **"Dissection Review."** The dissection review is a numbered list of tasks that illustrate the important features of the dissection and encourage the synthesis of information.

Over 40 new illustrations appear in the 14th edition of *Grant's Dissector*. Many of these new illustrations are replacements for existing illustrations and are intended to clarify the intent of the original drawing. The illustrations included in the 14th edition are not intended to take the place of atlas figures, and the dissection instructions contain references to appropriate illustrations in the leading anatomical atlases:

* *Grant's Atlas of Anatomy*, 12th edition, by Anne Agur and Arthur Dalley
* *Lippincott Williams & Wilkins Atlas of Anatomy*, 1st ed., by Patrick W. Tank and Thomas R. Gest
* *Atlas of Human Anatomy*, 4th edition, by Frank H. Netter and a team of consulting editors (Jennifer Brueckner, Stephen Carmichael, Thomas Gest, Noelle Granger, John Hansen, and Anil Walji)
* *Anatomy: A Regional Atlas of the Human Body*, 5th edition, by Carmine Clemente
* *Color Atlas of Anatomy: A Photographic Study of the Human Body*, 6th edition, by Johannes Rohen, Chirhiro Yokochi, and Lutjen-Drecoll

The changes described above are intended to increase the adaptability of *Grant's Dissector* to a variety of dissection needs. Since the chapters are written to stand alone, the dissection sequence can be modified or regional units may be eliminated with a minimum amount of effort. This flexibility is intended to make *Grant's Dissector* the obvious choice to support comprehensive dissection in a changing curricular environment.

CONTENTS

7 THE HEAD AND NECK

FIGURE CREDITS

CHAPTER 1

Modified from Agur A. *Grant's Atlas of Anatomy*, 9E. Baltimore: Lippincott Williams & Wilkins, 1991. Figures 1.05, 1.06.

Modified from Tank P, Gest T. *Lippincott Williams & Wilkins Atlas of Anatomy*. Baltimore: Lippincott Williams & Wilkins, 2009. Figure 1.09.

From Basmajian JV. *Grant's Method of Anatomy*, 11E. Baltimore: Williams & Wilkins, 1989. Figure 1.11.

Modified from Woodburne RT, Burkel WE. *Essentials of Human Anatomy*, 9E. Oxford University Press, 1994. Figure 1.17.

CHAPTER 2

Modified from Netter F. *Netter's Atlas of Human Anatomy*, 3E. Carlstadt, NJ: Icon Learning System, 2002. Figures 2.05, 2.16, 2.21, 2.33, 2.36, 2.37.

Modified from Tank P, Gest T. *Lippincott Williams & Wilkins Atlas of Anatomy*. Baltimore: Lippincott Williams & Wilkins, 2009. Figure 2.07.

CHAPTER 3

Modified from Woodburne RT, Burkel WE. *Essentials of Human Anatomy*, 9E. Oxford University Press, 1994. Figure 3.01.

Modified from Tank P, Gest T. *Lippincott Williams & Wilkins Atlas of Anatomy*. Baltimore: Lippincott Williams & Wilkins, 2009. Figure 3.12a.

Modified from Clemente CD. *Anatomy Dissector*. Baltimore: Lippincott Williams & Wilkins, 2002. Figure 3.14.

Modified from Netter F. *Netter's Atlas of Human Anatomy*, 3E. Carlstadt, NJ: Icon Learning System, 2002. Figures 3.21, 3.22.

CHAPTER 4

Modified from Tank P, Gest T. *Lippincott Williams & Wilkins Atlas of Anatomy*. Baltimore: Lippincott Williams & Wilkins, 2009. Figures 4.17, 4.18, 4.30, 4.31, 4.33, 4.34, 4.35.

Modified from Agur A, Dalley AF. Grant's Atlas of Anatomy, 11E. Baltimore: Lippincott Williams & Wilkins, 2005. Figures 4.20, 4.40, 4.41, 4.47.

Modified from Moore K, Agur A. *Essential Clinical Anatomy*, 2E. Baltimore: Lippincott Williams & Wilkins, 2002. Figure 4.11.

Modified from Moore K, Dalley AF. *Clinically Oriented Anatomy*, 4E. Baltimore: Lippincott Williams & Wilkins, 1999. Figures 4.22, 4.42.

Modified from Netter F. *Netter's Atlas of Human Anatomy*, 3E. Carlstadt, NJ: Icon Learning System, 2002. Figures 4.06, 4.09, 4.10, 4.12, 4.16.

CHAPTER 5

Modified from Tank P, Gest T. *Lippincott Williams & Wilkins Atlas of Anatomy*. Baltimore: Lippincott Williams & Wilkins, 2009. Figures 5.02, 5.10, 5.18, 5.19, 5.24a, 5.25, 5.31, 5.34, 5.38a.

Modified from Agur A. *Grant's Atlas of Anatomy*, 9E. Baltimore: Lippincott Williams & Wilkins, 1991. Figures 5.12, 5.22, 5.23, 5.28, 5.36, 5.37.

Modified from Clemente CD. *Anatomy Dissector*. Baltimore: Lippincott Williams & Wilkins, 2002. Figures 5.03, 5.20, 5.33.

Modified from Moore K, Agur A. *Essential Clinical Anatomy*, 2E. Baltimore: Lippincott Williams & Wilkins, 2002. Figures 5.11, 5.17.

Modified from Moore K, Dalley AF. *Clinically Oriented Anatomy*, 4E. Baltimore: Lippincott Williams & Wilkins, 1999. Figures 5.13, 5.27, 5.29, 5.30.

CHAPTER 6

Modified from Woodburne RT, Burkel WE. *Essentials of Human Anatomy*, 9e. New York: Oxford University Press, 1994. Figures 6.07, 6.08.

Modified from Tank P, Gest, T. *Lippincott Williams & Wilkins Atlas of Anatomy*. Baltimore: Lippincott Williams & Wilkins, 2009. Figures 6.13, 6.17, 6.22, 6.26ab, 6.27, 6.28, 6.29.

Modified from Netter F. *Netter's Atlas of Human Anatomy*, 3E. Carlstadt, NJ: Icon Learning System, 2002. Figures 6.16, 6.23, 6.24, 6.34.

CHAPTER 7

Modified from Agur A. *Grant's Atlas of Anatomy*, 9E. Baltimore: Lippincott Williams & Wilkins, 1991. Figures 7.14, 7.15, 7.22, 7.44, 7.71, 7.80, 7.93.

Modified from Agur A, Dalley AF. *Grant's Atlas of Anatomy*, 11E, Baltimore: Lippincott Williams & Wilkins, 2005. Figures 7-1, 7-22, 7-24, 7-96.

Modified from Bailey FR. *Bailey's Textbook of Histology*, 16E. Baltimore: Williams & Wilkins, 1978. Figure 7.95.

Modified from Clemente CD. *Anatomy Dissector.* Baltimore: Lippincott Williams & Wilkins, 2002. Figures 7.18, 7.28, 7.48, 7.50, 7.51, 7.59.

Modified from Hansen JT. *Essential Anatomy Dissector,* 2E. Baltimore: Lippincott Williams & Wilkins, 2002. Figure 7.77.

Modified from Moore K, Agur A. *Essential Clinical Anatomy*, 2E. Baltimore: Lippincott Williams & Wilkins, 2002. Figure 7.22.

Modified from Moore K, Dalley AF. *Clinically Oriented Anatomy*, 4E. Baltimore: Lippincott Williams & Wilkins, 1999. Figure 7.81.

Modified from Netter F. *Netter's Atlas of Human Anatomy*, 3E. Carlstadt, NJ: Icon Learning System, 2002, Figures 7.32, 7.63, 7.72, 7.85, 7.98.

Modified from Woodburne RT, Burkel WE. *Essentials of Human Anatomy*, 9E. Oxford University Press, 1994. Figure 7.03.

INTRODUCTION

"The essence of good dissection is to display each structure fully, clearly, and cleanly. This takes time but it is time well spent. No mental picture can ever be obtained if blood vessels and nerves are seen only through a maze of fat and areolar tissue, if muscles are never cleaned to their bony attachments, and if ligaments are left undefined as to their margins, direction of their fibers and attachments. Cleaning a structure, therefore, means much more than the mere recognition of its existence."

— J.C.B. GRANT

Excerpt from the 5th edition of *Grant's Dissector*, 1959

As you undertake the study of human anatomy, it is important to heed the words of Dr. Grant. Clean dissection yields great reward but comes at the expense of time and effort. The time is but brief if weighed against the length of your career during which the gained knowledge will be put to use. If you view the study of anatomy from this perspective, you will be rewarded with the most memorable learning experience of your medical career.

YOUR FIRST PATIENT

The cadaver that will be used for dissection was donated by a person who wished to make a contribution to your education as a physician. It is not possible to put into words the emotions experienced by that individual as he or she made the decision to become a body donor. It goes without saying that the value of the gift that the donor has made to you cannot be measured, and can only be repaid by the proper care and use of the cadaver. The cadaver must be treated with the same respect and dignity that are usually reserved for the living patient.

Upon entering the laboratory, you will find that the cadaver has been embalmed with a strong fixative. The veins are sometimes full of clotted blood and sometimes empty. In some schools, the arteries are injected with red dye. The whole body has been kept moist by wrappings or by submersion under preservative fluid. Dessication of the cadaver will quickly render the specimen useless for study because once a part has been allowed to become dry, it can never be fully restored. Therefore, expose only those parts of the body to be dissected. Inspect every part of the body periodically and moisten the wrappings during each dissection session.

DISSECTION INSTRUMENTS

It is generally true that large dissection equipment (hammers, chisels, saws, etc.) is provided for you but personal dissection instruments must be purchased. The well-equipped dissector should have the following instruments (Fig. I.1):

- **Probe** – the primary dissecting tool, after your fingers. A probe is designed to tear connective tissue and allow the user to feel nerves and vessels before they are damaged.
- **Forceps** – used to lift and hold vessels, nerves, and other structures while blunt dissecting with a probe. Two pairs of forceps are needed. One pair should have tips that are blunt and rounded and the gripping surfaces should be corrugated. The second pair should have teeth (also known as tissue forceps or rat-toothed forceps) for gripping tissue.
- **Scalpel** – primarily used as a skinning tool. Scalpels are not recommended for general dissection because they cut small structures without allowing you to feel them. The scalpel handle should be made of metal (not plastic). The blade should be about 3.5 to 4 cm long. The cutting edge must have some convexity near the point. A sharp blade must be used at all times because no one can do good work with a dull scalpel. Therefore, a sufficient supply of blades will be needed.
- **Scissors** – useful in cutting, blunt dissection, and transection. Two pairs of scissors are recommended: a large, heavy pair of dissecting scissors (about 15 cm in length) and a small pair of scissors with two sharp points for the dissection of delicate structures.
- **Hemostat** – a powerful grasping tool that is helpful in skin removal. The hemostat has two disadvantages: First, it crushes delicate structures. Second, it cannot be repositioned quickly like forceps can, thereby slowing progress.

GLOSSARY OF DISSECTION TERMS

This dissection manual repeatedly uses a number of dissection terms. Before beginning to dissect, learn the meaning of the following:

- **Dissect** – to cut apart. In the context of this dissection manual, the meaning of dissect is to tear apart. The dissection approach throughout this manual is to dissect as much as possible with the fingers, to next use a probe, and to then use scissors. A scalpel is used only as a tool of last resort for crude cuts or to dissect extremely tough connective tissues.

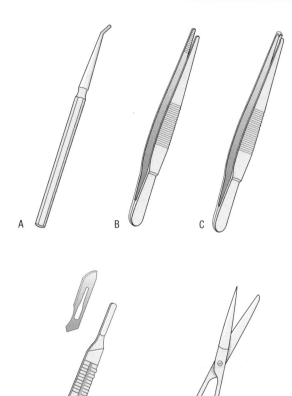

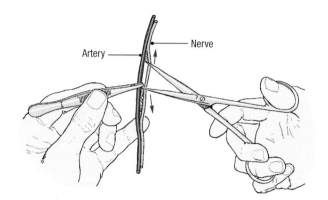

Figure I.2. Scissors technique for separating structures. Closed scissors are inserted between structures, then opened.

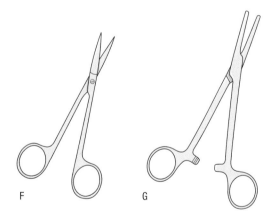

Figure I.1. Personal dissection instruments: **A**. Probe. **B**. Forceps. **C**. Tissue (rat-toothed) forceps. **D**. Scalpel and removable blade. **E**. Large scissors. **F**. Small scissors. **G**. Hemostat.

- **Blunt dissection** – to separate structures with your fingers, a probe, or scissors.
- **Scissors technique** – a method of blunt dissection in which the tips of a closed pair of scissors are inserted into connective tissue and then opened, tearing the connective tissue with the back edge of the tips (Fig. I.2).

The scissors technique is an effective way to dissect vessels and nerves.

- **Sharp dissection** – to dissect by use of a scalpel. Sharp dissection is discouraged and will be recommended only in rare situations.
- **Clean** – to remove fat and connective tissue by means of blunt dissection (preferred) or sharp dissection.
    Clean the border of a muscle – to define the border by using fingers or a probe to break the loose connective tissue that binds the muscle to surrounding structures.
    Clean a nerve – to use a probe (or scissors technique) to break the connective tissue around the nerve for purposes of observing its relationships and branches.
    Clean a vessel – to use a probe (or scissors technique) to strip the fat and connective tissue off the surface of a vessel and its branches to illustrate its relationships.
- **Define** – to use blunt dissection to enhance a structure to better illustrate its relationships. Defining a structure usually involves bluntly dissecting the loose connective tissue away from it by use of a probe.
- **Retract** – to pull a structure to one side to visualize another structure that lies more deeply. Retraction is a temporary displacement and is not intended to harm the retracted structure.
- **Transect** – to cut in two in the transverse plane, as in transection of a muscle belly or tendon.
- **Reflect** – to fold back from a cut edge, as in folding back both halves of a transected muscle. The reflected tissue should remain attached to the specimen.
- **Strip a vein** – to remove the vein and its tributaries from the dissection field so that the artery and related structures can be seen more clearly. Veins are stripped by blunt dissection using a probe.

ANATOMICAL POSITION

Anatomists describe structures with the body in the *anatomical position*. In the anatomical position the person stands erect with the feet together, arms by the sides, and the palms facing forward (Fig. I.3). During dissection, structures are described as though the body were in the anatomical position, even though the cadaver is lying on the dissection table. When encountering a structure during dissection, be aware of its position, its relationship to other structures, its size and shape, its function, its blood supply, and its nerve supply. Learn to give an accurate account of each important structure in an orderly and logical fashion by describing it to your lab partners. Always base your descriptions on the anatomical position.

Before beginning to dissect, consult your textbook for a description of **anatomical planes** and a definition of **terms of relationship and comparison**, **terms of laterality**, and **terms of movement**. These terms form the language of anatomy and it is not possible to understand anatomical descriptions without being able to understand these terms.

ANATOMICAL VARIATION

All bodies have the same basic architectural plan but no two bodies are identical. Minor variations commonly occur and should be expected. You should learn normal (average) anatomy rather than the variation unless specifically instructed to do otherwise. Take time during each dissection period to view several dissections so that you can learn to appreciate anatomical variations.

DAILY DISSECTION ROUTINE

To get the most out of dissection, it is recommended that you establish a routine approach to each day's dissection. Some suggestions are offered:

- **Prepare before lab.** Read the dissection assignment and become familiar with the new vocabulary, the structures to be dissected, and the dissection approach. You must deliberately search for structures and advance preparation will make the exercise go more quickly.
- **Use a good atlas** in the dissection lab. This dissection manual provides references to four atlases to help you quickly find illustrations that support the dissection.
- **Palpate bony landmarks** and use them in the search for soft tissue structures.
- **Remove fat, connective tissue, and smaller veins** to clean up the dissection.
- **Review the completed dissection** at the end of the dissection period and again at the start of the next dissection period. To help you do this, review exercises are included at strategic points in each chapter.
- **Complete each dissection before proceeding to the next** because each new dissection is an extension of the previous dissection.

LAB SAFETY

While in the laboratory, protect your clothing by wearing a long laboratory coat or apron. For sanitary reasons, this outer layer of clothing should not be worn outside of the dissection laboratory. Do not wear sandals or open-toed shoes in the laboratory, as a dropped scalpel can seriously injure your foot. Gloves must be worn to prevent contact with human tissue and fixatives. When cutting bones, wear glasses or goggles to protect your eyes against flying chips.

SKIN REMOVAL

Since skin removal is the first step in dissection, a few suggestions are offered to help you get started. A variable amount of subcutaneous tissue (also called superficial fascia) lies immediately deep to the skin. The subcutaneous tissue contains fat, cutaneous nerves, and superficial blood vessels. Throughout this dissection manual when you are instructed to skin a region, **the skin should be removed and the subcutaneous tissue should be left behind**. Subsequent dissection instructions will be provided for dissection and removal of the subcutaneous tissue.

The thickness of skin varies from region to region. For example, the skin is relatively thin on the anterior surface of the forearm and it is considerably thicker over the back. Generally, skin incisions should not extend into the subcutaneous tissue. To begin skinning, raise the skin at the intersec-

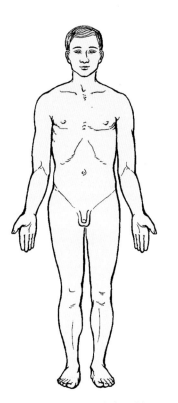

Figure I.3. Anatomical position.

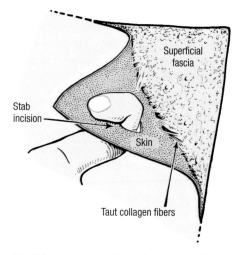

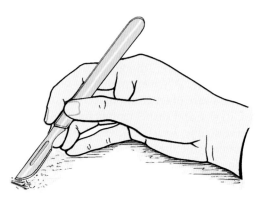

Figure I.5. When dissecting, rest the hand to reduce unsteady movements.

Figure I.4. When removing skin, make a stab incision to help you apply traction. Use the scalpel blade to cut the collagen fibers from the deep surface of the skin where the fibers are taut.

tion of two incision lines by use of toothed forceps and the scalpel blade. Once a skin flap has been raised, place traction on the skin as it is being removed and direct the scalpel blade toward the deep surface of the skin to cut the taut collagen fibers (Fig. I.4). To steady your scalpel hand, rest it against the cadaver and hold the scalpel as you would hold a pencil (Fig. I.5). Make short sweeping motions, and to prevent accidents, do not work too close to your lab partners.

CHAPTER 1

THE BACK

The back region contains the **superficial muscles of the back**, the **intermediate muscles of the back,** and the **deep muscles of the back**. All of these muscles attach to the vertebral column. The vertebral column serves the dual purpose of forming the axis of the body and providing a protective bony covering for the spinal cord.

SURFACE ANATOMY

The surface anatomy of this region may be studied on a living subject or on the cadaver. In the cadaver, fixation may make it difficult to distinguish bone from well-preserved soft tissues. Turn the cadaver to the prone position (face down) and attempt to palpate the following structures (Fig. 1.1): [G 320; L 5; N 152]

- **External occipital protuberance**
- **Superior border of the trapezius muscle**
- **Spinous process of the seventh cervical vertebra (vertebra prominens)**
- **Spine of the scapula** (at vertebral level T3)
- **Acromion of the scapula**
- **Medial (vertebral) border of the scapula**
- **Inferior angle of the scapula** (at vertebral level T7)
- **Spinous processes of thoracic vertebrae**
- **Erector spinae muscle** (most noticeable in the lumbar region)
- **Median furrow**
- **Lateral border of the latissimus dorsi muscle (posterior axillary fold)**
- **Iliac crest** (at vertebral level L4)
- **Posterior superior iliac spine**

SKELETON OF THE BACK

Refer to a skeleton. On the **scapula**, identify (Fig. 1.2): [G 477; L 32; N 421; R 371; C 76]

- **Acromion**
- **Spine**
- **Superior angle**

ATLAS REFERENCES:
G = *Grant's Atlas*, 12th ed., page number
L = *LWW Atlas of Anatomy*, 1st ed., page number
N = *Netter's Atlas*, 4th ed., plate number
R = *Color Atlas of Anatomy*, 6th ed., page number
C = *Clemente's Atlas*, 5th ed., plate number

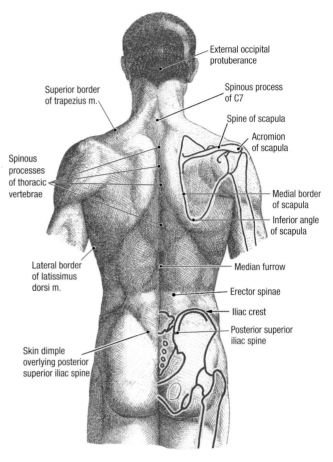

Figure 1.1. Surface anatomy of the back.

- **Medial (vertebral) border**
- **Inferior angle**

On the **ilium**, identify (Fig. 1.2): [G 315; L 5; N 159; R 188; C 265]

- **Iliac crest**
- **Posterior superior iliac spine**

On the **occipital bone**, identify (Fig. 1.2):

- **External occipital protuberance (inion)**
- **Superior nuchal line**

On the **temporal bone**, identify (Fig. 1.2):

- **Mastoid process**

The **vertebral column** (Fig. 1.2) consists of 33 vertebrae: 7 cervical (C), 12 thoracic (T), 5 lumbar (L), 5 sacral

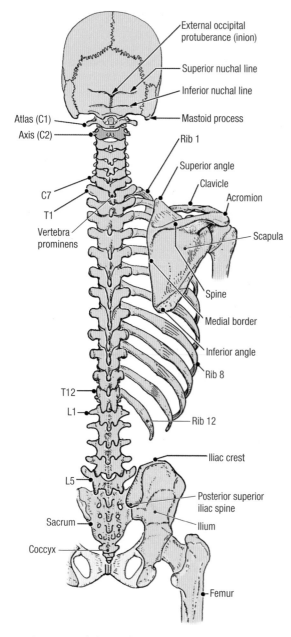

Figure 1.2. Skeleton of the back and vertebral column.

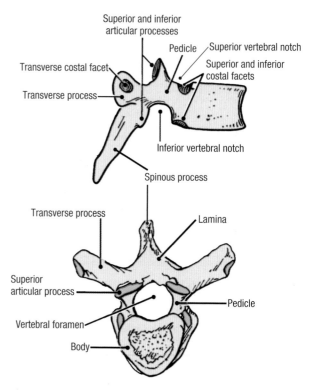

Figure 1.3. Typical thoracic vertebra in lateral and superior view.

- **Transverse process** (2)
- **Transverse costal facet**
- **Spinous process**
- **Articular processes** – superior and inferior
- **Vertebral notches** – superior and inferior
- **Costal facets** – superior and inferior

The spinous process of a thoracic vertebra is long, slender, and directed inferiorly over the spinous process of the vertebra that is inferior to it. Articulation with ribs is a characteristic of thoracic vertebrae. The head of a rib articulates with the bodies of two adjacent vertebrae (Fig. 1.4). The tubercle of a rib articulates with the transverse costal

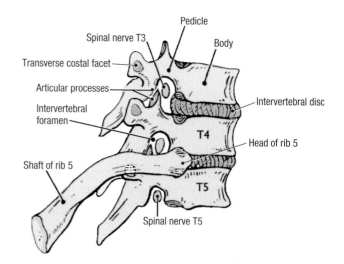

Figure 1.4. Part of the thoracic vertebral column.

(S), and 4 coccygeal (Co). The upper 24 vertebrae (cervical, thoracic, and lumbar) allow flexibility and movement of the vertebral column, whereas the sacral vertebrae are fused to provide rigid support of the pelvic girdle. A typical thoracic vertebra will be described, and the cervical and lumbar vertebrae will be compared to it. [G 288; L 6; N 153; R 193; C 346]

Refer to a disarticulated **thoracic vertebra** and identify (Fig. 1.3): [G 300; L 9; N 154; R 190; C 347]

- **Body**
- **Vertebral arch** – formed by the combination of pedicles and laminae
- **Pedicle** (2)
- **Lamina** (2)
- **Vertebral foramen**

facet of the thoracic vertebra of the same number (i.e., the tubercle of rib 5 articulates with the transverse costal facet of vertebra T5). An **intervertebral disc** and the **articular processes** unite two adjacent vertebrae. The vertebral notches of two adjacent vertebrae combine to form an **intervertebral foramen**. A spinal nerve passes through the intervertebral foramen.

Cervical vertebrae differ from thoracic vertebrae in the following ways (Fig. 1.5): Cervical vertebrae have smaller bodies; larger vertebral foramina; shorter spinous processes, which bifurcate at the tip; and transverse processes that contain a foramen transversarium. On an articulated skeleton, identify the following features common to all cervical vertebrae: [G 294; L 7; N 17; R 190; C 342]

- **Transverse process**
- **Foramen transversarium**
- **Spinous process**

On a skeleton, observe the following features of individual cervical vertebrae:

- **Atlas** (C1) does not have a body.
- **Axis** (C2) has the **dens**, which is the body of C1 that has become fused to C2 during development.
- **Vertebra prominens** (C7) has the most prominent spinous process in the cervical region, hence its name.

Lumbar vertebrae differ from thoracic vertebrae in the following ways (Fig. 1.5): Lumbar vertebrae have larger bodies, have broad spinous processes that project posteriorly, and do not have transverse costal facets for ribs. On a skeleton, observe the lumbar vertebrae and notice that their spines do not overlap like the spines of thoracic vertebrae. [G 302; L 11; N 155; R 190; C 350]

The **sacrum** is formed by five fused vertebrae and it does not have identifiable spines or transverse processes. On the dorsal surface of the sacrum, identify (Fig. 1.6): [G 313; L 12; N 157; R 191; C 353]

- **Median sacral crest**
- **Posterior (dorsal) sacral foramina**
- **Sacral hiatus**

The **coccyx** is a small triangular bone formed by four rudimentary coccygeal vertebrae that are fused together (Fig. 1.6).

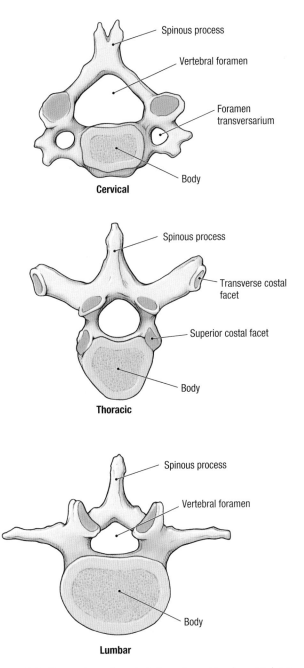

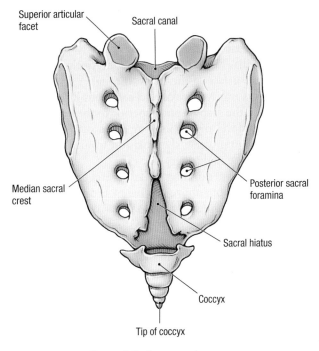

Figure 1.5. Comparison of cervical, thoracic, and lumbar vertebrae.

Figure 1.6. Sacrum and coccyx.

SKIN AND SUPERFICIAL FASCIA

Dissection Overview

The order of dissection will be as follows: The skin will be removed from the back, posterior surface of the neck, and posterior surface of the proximal upper limb. Posterior cutaneous nerves will be studied. The superficial fascia will then be removed.

Dissection Instructions

SKIN INCISIONS

1. Refer to Figure 1.7.
2. Use a scalpel to make a skin incision in the midline from the external occipital protuberance (X) to the tip of the coccyx (S). The skin is approximately 6 mm thick in this region.
3. Make an incision from the tip of the coccyx (S) to the midaxillary line (T). This incision should pass approximately 3 cm inferior to the iliac crest.
4. Make a transverse skin incision from the external occipital protuberance (X) laterally to the base of the mastoid process (M).
5. Make a skin incision along the lateral surface of the neck and superior border of the trapezius muscle (M to B). Extend this incision to point F, about halfway down the arm.
6. At point F, make an incision around the anterior and posterior surfaces of the arm, meeting on the medial side (G). If the upper limb has been dissected previously, this incision has already been made.
7. Make a skin incision that begins at G on the medial surface of the arm and extends superiorly to the axilla. Extend this incision inferiorly along the lateral surface of the trunk, through V to T.
8. Make a transverse skin incision from R to B superior to the scapula and superior to the acromion.
9. At the level of the inferior angle of the scapula, make a transverse skin incision from the midline (U) to the midaxillary line (V).
10. To facilitate skinning, make several parallel transverse incisions above and below the one described in step 9. The strips of skin that result should be about 7.5 cm wide to make skinning easier.
11. Remove the skin from medial to lateral. Detach the skin and place it in the tissue container.

SUPERFICIAL FASCIA

1. In the superficial fascia, locate the **occipital artery** and the **greater occipital nerve** (Fig. 1.8). First, find the occipital artery and then look on its me-

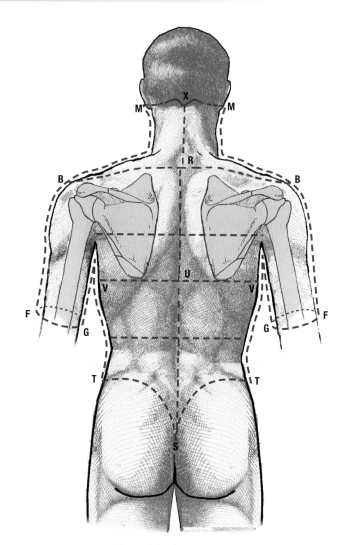

Figure 1.7. Skin incisions.

dial side for the greater occipital nerve. The greater occipital nerve is the dorsal ramus of spinal nerve C2. The greater occipital nerve pierces the **trapezius muscle** about 3 cm inferolateral to the **external occipital protuberance**. The deep fascia in this area is very dense and tough. Therefore, it may be difficult to find the greater occipital nerve, even though it is a large nerve. [G 321; L 16; N 178; R 226; C 338]

2. Read a description of the **dorsal ramus of a spinal nerve**. The **posterior cutaneous branches** of the dorsal rami pierce the trapezius muscle or latissimus dorsi muscle to enter the superficial fascia (Fig. 1.9). To save time, make no deliberate effort to display posterior cutaneous branches of the dorsal rami. [G 20; L 21; N 192; R 229]
3. Reflect the superficial fascia of the back from medial to lateral. Detach the superficial fascia by cutting it along the skin incision lines and place it in the tissue container.

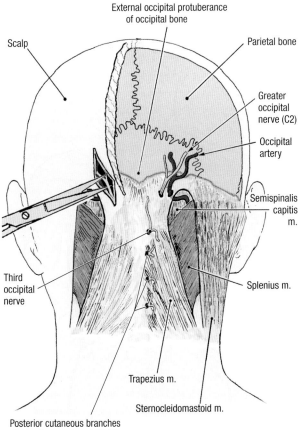

Figure 1.8. Greater occipital nerve and occipital artery.

4. In the neck, reflect the superficial fascia only as far laterally as the superior border of the trapezius muscle. *Do not cut the deep fascia along the superior border of the trapezius muscle.* The accessory nerve is superficial at this location and it is in danger of being cut.

Dissection Review

1. Review the branching pattern of a typical spinal nerve and understand that cutaneous branches of the dorsal rami innervate the skin of the back.
2. Study a dermatome chart and become familiar with the concept of segmental innervation. [G 348; L 27; N 164; C 326]

SUPERFICIAL MUSCLES OF THE BACK

Dissection Overview

The **superficial muscles of the back** are the **trapezius**, **latissimus dorsi**, **rhomboid major**, **rhomboid minor**, and **levator scapulae**.

The order of dissection will be as follows: The superficial surface of the trapezius muscle will be cleaned. The trapezius muscle will be examined and reflected. The latis-

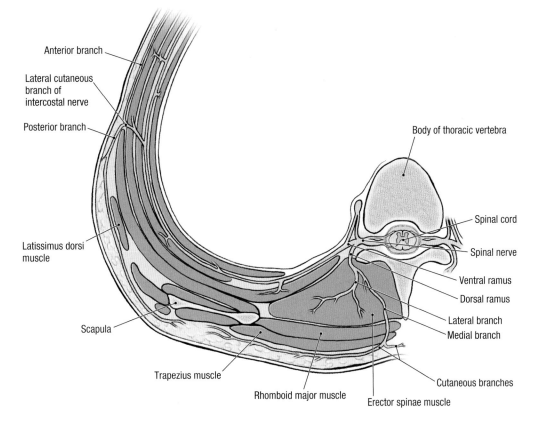

Figure 1.9. Branches of a typical spinal nerve.

simus dorsi muscle will be studied and reflected. The rhomboid major muscle, rhomboid minor muscle, and levator scapulae muscle will be studied. Dissection of the superficial back muscles should be performed bilaterally.

Dissection Instructions

TRAPEZIUS MUSCLE [G 321; L 17; N 174; R 226; C 328]

1. Clean the surface of the **trapezius muscle** (L. *Trapezoides*, an irregular four-sided figure) (Fig. 1.10). *Do not disturb the superior border of the trapezius muscle.* Observe the proximal attachment of the trapezius muscle on the external occipital protuberance, the nuchal ligament, and the spinous processes of vertebrae C7 to T12.

2. Observe the three parts of the trapezius muscle, each of which has a distinctly different action:
   • **Superior part** of the trapezius muscle attaches to the lateral one-third of the clavicle and it elevates the scapula.
   • **Middle part** of the trapezius muscle attaches to the acromion and spine of the scapula and it retracts the scapula.
   • **Inferior part** of the trapezius muscle attaches near the medial end of the spine of the scapula and it depresses the scapula.

3. To reflect the trapezius muscle, insert your fingers deep to the posterolateral border of the muscle (medial to the inferior angle of the scapula). Use your fingers to break the plane of loose connective tissue that lies between the trapezius muscle and the deeper muscles of the back.

4. Use scissors to detach the trapezius muscle from its proximal attachment on the spinous processes and the nuchal ligament (Fig. 1.10, dashed line). Start inferiorly and continue the cut superiorly as far as the external occipital protuberance.

5. Use scissors to make a short transverse cut (2.5 cm) across the superior end of the trapezius muscle to detach it from the superior nuchal line. *Spare the greater occipital nerve, and do not extend the transverse cut beyond the border of the trapezius muscle.*

6. Use scissors to cut the trapezius muscle from its distal attachments on the spine and acromion of the scapula (Fig. 1.10, dashed line). Make this cut very close to the bone. Leave the trapezius muscle attached to the clavicle and cervical fascia.

7. Reflect the trapezius muscle superolaterally. Leave the cervical fascia attached along the superior border of the trapezius muscle to act as a hinge.

8. Study the deep surface of the reflected trapezius muscle. Find the plexus of nerves formed by the **accessory nerve (cranial nerve XI)** and **branches of the ventral rami of spinal nerves C3 and C4**. The accessory nerve provides motor

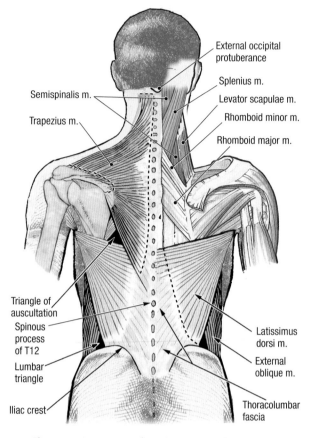

Figure 1.10. How to reflect the muscles of the back.

innervation to the trapezius muscle; the branches of nerves C3 and C4 are sensory (proprioception). The superficial branch of the **transverse cervical artery** accompanies the nerves. Remove the transverse cervical vein to clear the dissection field.

9. The accessory nerve passes through the posterior triangle of the neck. Do not follow the nerve into the posterior triangle at this time. The posterior triangle will be dissected with the neck.

LATISSIMUS DORSI MUSCLE [G 321; L 17; N 174; R 226; C 328]

1. Clean the surface and define the borders of the **latissimus dorsi muscle** (L. *Latissimus*, widest) (Fig. 1.10).

2. The proximal attachments of the latissimus dorsi muscle are the spines of vertebrae T7 to T12, the thoracolumbar fascia, and the iliac crest. The latissimus dorsi muscle also has a proximal attachment to ribs 9 to 12, lateral to their angles.

3. Note that the distal attachment of the latissimus dorsi muscle is the floor of the intertubercular sulcus on the anterior side of the humerus, but do not dissect this attachment. The latissimus dorsi muscle receives the **thoracodorsal nerve and artery** on its anterior surface near its distal attachment.

The distal attachment of the latissimus dorsi muscle, its nerve, and its artery will be dissected with the upper limb.

4. To reflect the latissimus dorsi muscle, insert your fingers deep to the superior border of the muscle (medial to the inferior angle of the scapula), and break the plane of loose connective tissue that lies between it and deeper structures. Raise the latissimus dorsi muscle enough to insert scissors and cut through its proximal attachment on the thoracolumbar fascia (Fig. 1.10, dashed line). Do not cut too close to the lumbar spinous processes.

5. Reflect the latissimus dorsi muscle laterally. Do not disturb its attachment to the ribs. It may also have an attachment to the inferior angle of the scapula. If so, do not disturb its attachment to the inferior angle of the scapula.

RHOMBOID MAJOR AND RHOMBOID MINOR MUSCLES [G 322; L 17; N 177; R 226; C 328]

1. Clean the surface and borders of the **rhomboid (rhomboideus) minor muscle** and the **rhomboid major muscle** (Gr. *Rhombos*, shaped like a kite). Typically, the separation between the rhomboid muscles is not very obvious and the two muscles must be distinguished from each other by using their distal attachments.

2. The proximal attachments of the rhomboid minor muscle are the nuchal ligament and the spinous processes of vertebrae C7 and T1. The distal attachment of the rhomboid minor muscle is the medial border of the scapula at the level of the spine.

3. The proximal attachments of the rhomboid major muscle are the spinous processes of vertebrae T2 to T5. The distal attachment of the rhomboid major muscle is the medial border of the scapula inferior to the spine.

4. The rhomboid muscles retract the scapula, rotate the scapula to depress the glenoid cavity, and hold the scapula close to the thoracic wall.

5. To reflect the rhomboid muscles, insert your fingers deep to the inferior border of the rhomboid major muscle and separate it from deeper muscles.

6. Working from inferior to superior, use scissors to detach the rhomboid major muscle from its proximal attachments on the spinous processes. Continue the cut superiorly and detach the rhomboid minor muscle from its proximal attachments on the spinous processes. Reflect these two muscles laterally.

7. Examine the deep surface of the two rhomboid muscles near their distal attachments on the medial border of the scapula. Use blunt dissection to find the **dorsal scapular nerve** and **dorsal scapular vessels**. Remove the dorsal scapular vein to clear the dissection field. The dorsal scapular nerve and artery course parallel to the medial border of the scapula.

8. The **dorsal scapular artery** may branch directly from the subclavian artery, or it may arise from the transverse cervical artery, in which case it is also called the **deep branch of the transverse cervical artery**.

LEVATOR SCAPULAE MUSCLE [G 322; L 17; N 174; R 222; C 328]

1. Identify the **levator scapulae muscle** (L. *levare*, to raise). At this stage of the dissection, the levator scapulae muscle can be seen only near its distal attachment on the scapula.

2. Note that the proximal attachments of the levator scapulae muscle are the transverse processes of the upper four cervical vertebrae. Do not dissect its proximal attachments.

3. The distal attachment of the levator scapulae muscle is the superior angle of the scapula.

4. The dorsal scapular nerve and artery supply the levator scapulae muscle. The levator scapulae muscle elevates the scapula and rotates the scapula to depress the glenoid cavity.

Dissection Review

1. Replace the superficial muscles of the back in their correct anatomical positions.

2. Use the dissected specimen to review the proximal attachment, distal attachment, action, innervation, and blood supply of each muscle that you have dissected.

3. Review the movements that occur between the scapula and the thoracic wall.

4. Use an illustration to observe the origin of the transverse cervical artery and the origin of the dorsal scapular artery.

5. Observe two triangles associated with the latissimus dorsi muscle: the **triangle of auscultation** and the **lumbar triangle** (Fig. 1.10).

CLINICAL CORRELATION

Triangles of the Back [G 321, 322; L 17; N 254; C 328]

The **triangle of auscultation** is bounded by the latissimus dorsi muscle, the trapezius muscle, and the rhomboid major muscle. Within the triangle of auscultation, intercostal space 6 has no overlying muscles. This area is particularly well suited for auscultation (listening to sounds produced by thoracic organs, particularly the lungs).

The **lumbar triangle** is bounded by the latissimus dorsi muscle, the external oblique muscle, and the iliac crest. The floor of the lumbar triangle is the internal oblique muscle of the abdomen. On rare occasions, the lumbar triangle is the site of a lumbar hernia.

INTERMEDIATE MUSCLES OF THE BACK [G 322; L 17 18; N 174; R 228; C 330]

The **intermediate muscles of the back** are the **serratus posterior superior muscle** and the **serratus posterior inferior muscle**. The serratus posterior superior and inferior muscles are very thin muscles, which may have been accidentally reflected with the rhomboid muscles or the latissimus dorsi muscle. If you do not see the serratus posterior muscles, look for them on the deep surface of the reflected rhomboid muscles or the reflected latissimus dorsi muscle.

1. The proximal attachments of the **serratus posterior superior muscle** are the nuchal ligament and the spinous processes of vertebrae C7 to T3. Its distal attachments are the superior borders of ribs 2 to 5, lateral to their angles.
2. The proximal attachments of the **serratus posterior inferior muscle** are the spinous processes of vertebrae T11 to L2. Its distal attachments are the inferior borders of ribs 9 to 12, lateral to their angles.
3. The serratus posterior muscles are respiratory muscles, and they are innervated by intercostal nerves.

DEEP MUSCLES OF THE BACK

Dissection Overview

The **deep muscles of the back** act on the vertebral column. There are many deep muscles of the back (Fig. 1.11) and only a few will be dissected: **splenius capitis muscle, splenius cervicis muscle, semispinalis capitis muscle,** and **erector spinae muscle**. All of the deep muscles of the back are innervated by dorsal rami of spinal nerves.

The order of dissection will be as follows: The deep muscles of the posterior neck (splenius capitis and cervicis) will be studied and reflected. The semispinalis capitis muscle will be studied. The erector spinae muscle will be dissected and the three columns of muscle that comprise its component parts will be identified.

Dissection Instructions

SPLENIUS MUSCLE [G 323; L 18; N 174; R 226; C 332]

1. Identify the **splenius muscle** (Gr. *splenion*, bandage) (Fig. 1.10). The splenius muscle lies deep to the trapezius muscle. The fibers of the splenius muscle course obliquely across the neck. The proximal attachment of the splenius muscle is the nuchal ligament and the spinous processes of vertebrae C7 to T6.
2. The splenius muscle has two parts that are named according to their distal attachments:
    *   **Splenius capitis muscle** (L. *caput*, head) is attached to the mastoid process of the temporal

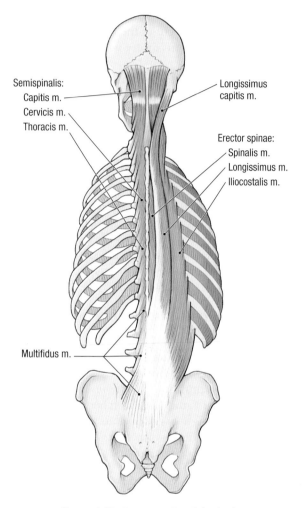

Figure 1.11. Deep muscles of the back.

Semispinalis:
Capitis m.
Cervicis m.
Thoracis m.

Longissimus capitis m.

Erector spinae:
Spinalis m.
Longissimus m.
Iliocostalis m.

Multifidus m.

bone and the superior nuchal line of the occipital bone.
    *   **Splenius cervicis muscle** (L. *cervix*, neck) is attached to the transverse processes of vertebrae C1 to C4.
3. The two parts of the splenius muscle are not easily distinguished at this stage of the dissection. Detach both parts of the splenius muscle from the nuchal ligament and the spinous processes of vertebrae C7 to T6.
4. Reflect the muscles laterally, leaving their distal attachments undisturbed.

ERECTOR SPINAE MUSCLE [G 323; L 18; N 175; R 222; C 333]

1. The **erector spinae muscle** (L. *erector*, one who erects) lies deep to the serratus posterior muscles (Fig. 1.11).
2. Detach both serratus posterior muscles from their proximal attachments on the spinous processes. Reflect the muscles laterally, leaving them attached to the ribs.

3. The erector spinae muscle is composed of three columns of muscle: spinalis, longissimus, and iliocostalis. The intent of this dissection is to identify these three columns of muscle.

4. Use a scalpel to incise the posterior surface of the **thoracolumbar fascia**. Use blunt dissection to remove it from the posterior surface of the erector spinae muscle.

5. Use your fingers to separate the three columns of muscle at midthoracic levels. The columns of the erector spinae muscle are fused to each other at the level of their inferior attachments to the sacrum and ilium.

6. Identify (Fig. 1.11):
   - **Spinalis muscle** – the medial column of the erector spinae muscle. The inferior attachments of the spinalis muscle are on spinous processes. Its superior attachments are also on spinous processes. The spinalis muscle is present at lumbar, thoracic, and cervical vertebral levels.
   - **Longissimus muscle** (L. *longissimus*, the longest) – the intermediate column of the erector spinae muscle. Its inferior attachment is on the sacrum and its superior attachments are the transverse processes of the thoracic and cervical vertebrae. Note that its most superior portion, the **longissimus capitis muscle**, attaches to the mastoid process of the temporal bone.
   - **Iliocostalis muscle** – the lateral column of the erector spinae muscle. Its inferior attachment is the ilium (iliac crest) and its superior attachments are on ribs (L. *costa*, rib).

7. All three columns of the erector spinae muscle extend the vertebral column when both sides work together. If only one side of the erector spinae muscle is active, it bends the vertebral column laterally toward the side that is active.

TRANSVERSOSPINAL GROUP OF MUSCLES [G 326; L 19; N 176; R 223; C 335]

The **transversospinal group of muscles** is located deep to the erector spinae muscle. The muscles in the transversospinal group attach to transverse processes and spinous processes (Fig. 1.11). The muscles of the transversospinal group cause rotational and lateral bending movements between adjacent vertebrae and act to stabilize the vertebral column. A number of muscles comprise this group: **semispinalis**, **multifidus**, and more deeply, **rotatores**.

SEMISPINALIS CAPITIS MUSCLE [G 325; L 19; N 175; R 222; C 333]

1. Identify the semispinalis capitis muscle (L. *semi*, half; L. *spinalis*, spine) (Fig. 1.11). The semi-

spinalis capitis muscle is the most superficial member of the transversospinal group of muscles. The semispinalis capitis muscle lies deep to the splenius muscles and its fibers course vertically, parallel to the long axis of the neck.

2. The inferior attachments of the semispinalis capitis muscle are the transverse processes of the upper thoracic vertebrae.

3. The superior attachment of the semispinalis capitis muscle is the occipital bone between the superior and inferior nuchal lines. Note that the greater occipital nerve passes through the semispinalis capitis muscle.

4. Do not dissect the semispinalis capitis muscle further at this time.

5. Do not dissect the other muscles of the transversospinal group.

Dissection Review

Use the dissected specimen to review the location, innervation, and action of each muscle or column of muscles in the deep group of back muscles.

SUBOCCIPITAL REGION

Dissection Overview

On a skull, identify (Fig. 1.2): [G 592; L 300, 301; N 8; R 32; C 536]

- **Superior nuchal line**
- **Inferior nuchal line**
- **External occipital protuberance**
- **Foramen magnum**

On the **atlas** (C1 vertebra), identify (Fig. 1.12): [G 295; L 7; N 17; R 198; C 342]

- **Posterior tubercle**
- **Posterior arch**
- **Groove for the vertebral artery**
- **Transverse process**
- **Foramen transversarium**

On the **axis** (C2 vertebra), identify (Fig. 1.12):

- **Spinous process**
- **Transverse process**
- **Foramen transversarium**

The order of dissection will be as follows: The greater occipital nerve will be identified and followed deeply. The semispinalis capitis muscle will be reflected. The muscles that bound the suboccipital triangle will be identified. The contents of the suboccipital region (vertebral artery and suboccipital nerve) will be studied.

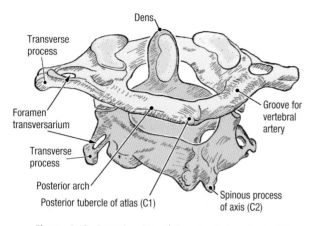

Figure 1.12. Posterior view of the atlas (C1) and axis (C2).

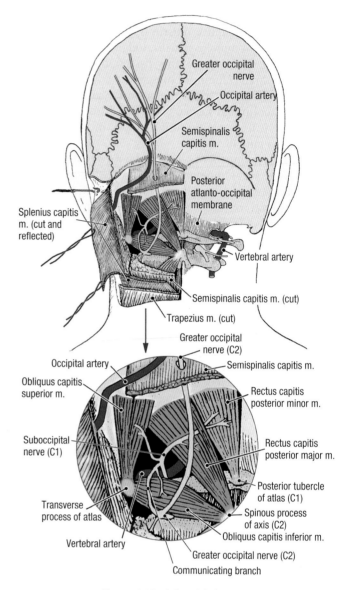

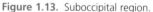

Figure 1.13. Suboccipital region.

Dissection Instructions

1. Identify the **semispinalis capitis muscle** (Fig. 1.13). [G 328; L 19, 20; N 176; R 238; C 333]
2. Once again, find the **greater occipital nerve**. Use blunt dissection to follow the greater occipital nerve deeply, through the semispinalis capitis muscle. Detach the semispinalis capitis muscle close to the occipital bone and reflect it inferiorly. Preserve the greater occipital nerve.
3. Deep to the semispinalis capitis muscle, follow the greater occipital nerve to the lower border of the **obliquus capitis inferior muscle**. Note that the greater occipital nerve (dorsal ramus of C2) emerges between vertebrae C1 and C2.
4. Identify and clean the three muscles that form the **boundaries of the suboccipital triangle** (Fig. 1.13): [G 331; L 20; N 178; R 238; C 341]
   - **Obliquus capitis inferior muscle** forms the inferior boundary of the suboccipital triangle. Verify that the proximal attachment of the obliquus capitis inferior muscle is the spinous process of the axis (C2). Its distal attachment is on the transverse process of the atlas (C1).
   - **Rectus capitis posterior major muscle** forms the medial boundary of the suboccipital triangle. Confirm that the proximal attachment of the rectus capitis posterior major muscle is the spinous process of the axis. Its distal attachment is the inferior nuchal line of the occipital bone.
   - **Obliquus capitis superior muscle** forms the lateral boundary of the suboccipital triangle. Confirm that the inferior attachment of the obliquus capitis superior muscle is the transverse process of the atlas. Its superior attachment is the occipital bone between the superior and inferior nuchal lines.
5. The muscles that bound the suboccipital triangle produce extension and lateral bending of the head

at the atlanto-occipital joints and rotation of the head at the atlantoaxial joints.

6. The **contents of the suboccipital triangle** are the **suboccipital nerve** and the **vertebral artery** (Fig. 1.13). Note that the suboccipital nerve (dorsal ramus of C1) emerges between the occipital bone and vertebra C1. The suboccipital nerve supplies motor innervation to the muscles of the suboccipital region. The suboccipital nerve is the only dorsal ramus that has no cutaneous distribution.

7. Identify the **vertebral artery**. Use an illustration to study the course of the vertebral artery through the neck and into the skull. [G 333; L 20; N 136; R 168; C 490]

Dissection Review

1. Review the actions of the suboccipital muscles.
2. Review the distribution of the branches of a thoracic dorsal ramus and compare the thoracic pattern to the distribution of the dorsal rami of spinal nerves C1 to C3.

VERTEBRAL CANAL, SPINAL CORD, AND MENINGES

Dissection Overview

The **vertebral canal** is a bony tube formed by the stacked **vertebral foramina** of the **cervical vertebrae**, **thoracic vertebrae**, **lumbar vertebrae**, and **sacral canal** (Fig. 1.14). The vertebral canal encloses and protects the **spinal cord**, its membranes (**spinal meninges**), and blood vessels. The spinal cord begins at the foramen magnum of the occipital bone and usually terminates in the adult at the level of the second lumbar vertebra. Because the spinal cord is shorter than the vertebral canal, *the spinal cord segments are found at higher vertebral levels than their names would suggest* (Fig. 1.14).

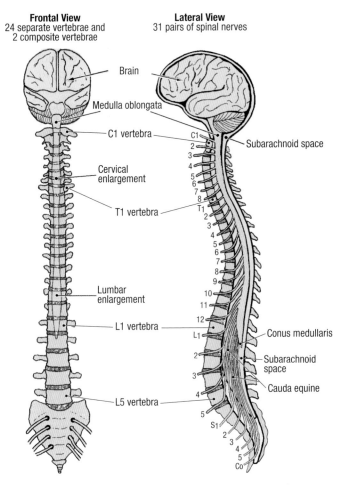

Frontal View
24 separate vertebrae and 2 composite vertebrae

Lateral View
31 pairs of spinal nerves

- Brain
- Medulla oblongata
- C1 vertebra
- Cervical enlargement
- T1 vertebra
- Lumbar enlargement
- L1 vertebra
- L5 vertebra
- Subarachnoid space
- Conus medullaris
- Subarachnoid space
- Cauda equine

Figure 1.14. The spinal cord within the vertebral canal.

The spinal cord is not uniform in diameter throughout its length. It has a **cervical enlargement** (Fig. 1.14) that corresponds to spinal cord segments C4 to T1 and a **lumbar enlargement** that corresponds to spinal cord segments L2 to S3. There are 31 pairs of **spinal nerves** (8 cervical, 12 thoracic, 5 lumbar, 5 sacral, and 1 coccygeal) (Fig. 1.14), which emerge between adjacent vertebrae. Most spinal nerves are numbered according to the vertebra above them as they pass through the intervertebral foramen (i.e., spinal nerve T1 exits the vertebral canal below vertebra T1). However, *in the cervical region, spinal nerves are numbered differently—they are numbered according to the vertebra below. For example, spinal nerve C1 exits the vertebral canal above vertebra C1 and the C8 spinal nerve does not have a correspondingly numbered vertebra.*

The order of dissection will be as follows: The erector spinae muscles will be removed from the lower back to expose the laminae of the vertebrae. The laminae will then be cut and removed (laminectomy) to expose the spinal meninges. The spinal meninges will be examined and will be opened to expose the spinal cord. The spinal cord will then be studied.

Dissection Instructions

1. *Wear eye protection for all steps that require the use of a chisel, bone saw, or bone cutters.*
2. Use a scalpel to remove the erector spinae muscles bilaterally from vertebral levels T4 to S3. The laminae must be cleanly exposed. Use scraping motions with a chisel to clean the muscle fragments off the laminae after the muscles have been removed.
3. Use a chisel or power saw to cut the laminae of vertebrae T6 to T12 on both sides of the spinous processes. Make this cut at the lateral end of the laminae to gain wide exposure to the vertebral canal. The cutting instrument should be angled at 45° to the vertical (Fig. 1.15).
4. Use a scalpel to cut the interspinous ligament between vertebrae T6 and T7 and between vertebrae T12 and L1. Preserve the interspinous ligaments between these levels to keep the intervening spines together.
5. Use a chisel to pry the six spinous processes and their laminae out as a unit. The dura mater will remain with the spinal cord and will be undamaged.
6. On the deep surface of the removed spinous specimen observe the **ligamenta flava**. The ligamenta flava connect the laminae of adjacent vertebrae.
7. Continue the laminectomy procedure inferiorly from the opening you have made in the vertebral canal. Exercise caution in lower lumbar and sacral regions, as the vertebral canal curves sharply posteriorly (superficially) (Fig. 1.16A). Do not drive the chisel or push the saw through the sacrum into the rectum.

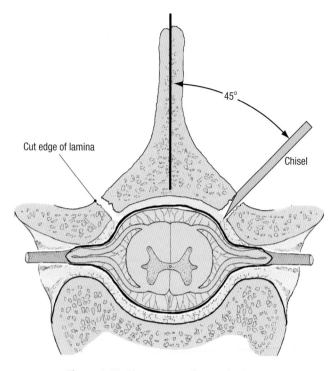

Figure 1.15. How to open the vertebral canal.

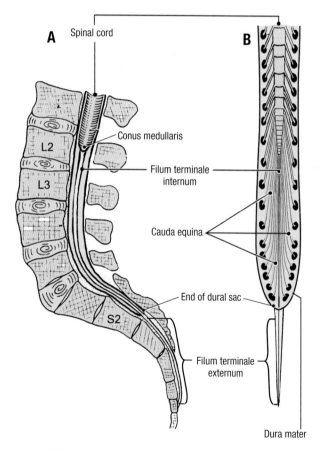

Figure 1.16. Lower portion of the vertebral canal and spinal cord. **A.** Lateral view. **B.** Posterior view.

8. When finished with the laminectomy, you should see the posterior surface of the dura mater from vertebral levels T6 to S2.

SPINAL MENINGES

1. Observe the **epidural (extradural) space**. Use blunt dissection to remove the **epidural fat** and the **posterior internal vertebral venous plexus** from the epidural space. [L 26; N 170; C 433]

CLINICAL CORRELATION

Vertebral Venous Plexuses

The veins of the vertebral venous plexuses are valveless, permitting blood to flow superiorly or inferiorly depending on blood pressure gradients. The vertebral venous plexuses can serve as routes for metastasis of cancer from the pelvis to the vertebrae, vertebral canal, and cranial cavity.

2. Identify the **dural sac**, which ends inferiorly at vertebral level S2 (Fig. 1.16A). [G 336; L 22, 24; R 230; C 357]

3. In the thoracic region, lift a fold of **dura mater** with forceps and use scissors to cut a small opening in its dorsal midline. Use scissors to extend the cut inferiorly to vertebral level S2. Attempt to do this without damaging the underlying arachnoid mater. Retract the dura mater and pin it open.

4. Identify the **arachnoid mater** (Fig. 1.17B). It is very delicate. Incise the arachnoid mater in the dorsal midline and observe the **subarachnoid space**. The subarachnoid space contains cerebrospinal fluid in the living person but not in the cadaver. [G 337; L 23; N 169; C 358]

5. Retract the arachnoid mater and observe the **spinal cord**. The spinal cord is completely invested by **pia mater**, which is on the surface of the spinal cord and cannot be dissected from it.

6. Identify the following features of the spinal cord: [G 334; L 22, 24; N 160; R 230; C 357]
   - **Lumbar enlargement** (spinal cord segments L2 to S3) provides nerves to the lower limb. The lumbar enlargement is located at lower thoracic vertebral levels.
   - **Conus medullaris (medullary cone)** is the end of the spinal cord located between vertebral levels L1 and L2.
   - **Cauda equina** (L., tail of horse) is a collection of ventral and dorsal roots in the lower vertebral canal (Fig. 1.16B).
   - **Filum terminale internum** (Fig. 1.16A, B) is a delicate filament continuous with the pia mater.

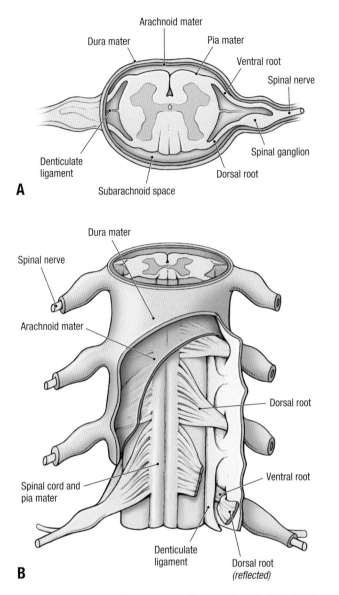

A

B

Figure 1.17. Relationships of the meninges to the spinal cord and nerve roots. **A.** Transverse section. **B.** Posterior view.

It arises from the inferior tip of the conus medullaris and ends at S2, where it is encircled by the lower end of the dural sac.

- Filum terminale externum (coccygeal ligament) (Fig. 1.16A, B) is the continuation of the filum terminale internum below vertebral level S2. The filum terminale externum passes through the sacral hiatus and ends by attaching to the coccyx.

7. The pia mater forms two **denticulate ligaments**, one on each side of the spinal cord (Fig. 1.17A, B). Each denticulate ligament has 21 teeth and each tooth is attached to the inner surface of the dura mater, anchoring the spinal cord. [G 335; L 23; N 169; R 231; C 358]

8. Use a probe to follow **dorsal roots** and **ventral roots** to the point where they pierce the dura

mater and enter the **intervertebral foramen** (Fig. 1.17B). The dorsal roots are on the dorsal side of the denticulate ligament and the ventral roots are on the ventral side of the denticulate ligament. The spinal nerve will be formed outside of the vertebral canal at the point where the dorsal and ventral roots join each other.

9. Observe small **blood vessels** that course along the ventral and dorsal roots. These are branches of posterior intercostal, lumbar, or vertebral arteries, depending upon vertebral level. They pass into the vertebral canal through the intervertebral foramen and supply the spinal cord. [G 341, 342; L 25; N 172; C 358]

10. In the thoracic region, expose one **spinal nerve**. Place a probe into an intervertebral foramen to protect the nerve within it. Use bone cutters to remove the posterior wall of the intervertebral foramen and expose the **spinal ganglion** (dorsal root ganglion) (Fig. 1.17A). Distal to the spinal ganglion, identify the spinal nerve and follow it distally to the point where it divides into a **dorsal ramus** and a **ventral ramus**.

CLINICAL CORRELATION

Lumbar Puncture

Cerebrospinal fluid (CSF) can be obtained from the subarachnoid space inferior to the conus medullaris (Fig. 1.18). At this level, there is no danger of penetrating the spinal cord with the puncture needle.

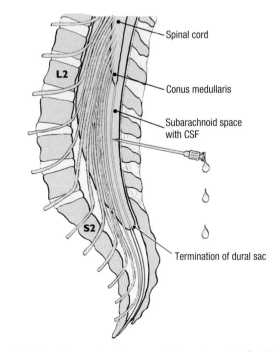

Figure 1.18. Lumbar puncture for removal of cerebrospinal fluid (CSF).

Dissection Review

1. Review the formation and branches of a typical spinal nerve.
2. Describe the way that the deep back muscles receive their innervation.
3. Review the coverings and parts of the spinal cord and study an illustration that shows the blood supply to the spinal cord.
4. Consult a dermatome chart and relate this pattern of cutaneous innervation to the spinal cord segments.
   [G 348; L 27; N 164; C 326]

CHAPTER 2

THE UPPER LIMB

The function of the upper limb is to place the hand in position to be effective as a grasping tool. As such, the upper limb has adapted into a body part with great freedom of motion. Muscles that control this motion extend across the back and thorax. If the back has previously been dissected, the superficial group of back muscles has been studied. If the upper limb is your first dissection unit, you will be instructed to dissect the superficial group of back muscles at the appropriate time.

SURFACE ANATOMY [G 476, 477; L 30; N 418; R 401, 402; C 28]

The upper limb is divided into four regions: **shoulder**, **arm (brachium)**, **forearm (antebrachium)**, and **hand (manus)**. The surface anatomy of the upper limb can be studied on a living subject or on the cadaver. Place the cadaver in the supine position (face up) and palpate the following superficial structures (Fig. 2.1):

- **Jugular notch**
- **Xiphisternal junction**
- **Costal margin**
- **Clavicle**
- **Acromion**
- **Anterior axillary fold**
- **Posterior axillary fold**
- **Deltoid muscle**
- **Biceps brachii muscle**
- **Triceps brachii muscle**
- **Cubital fossa**
- **Medial epicondyle**
- **Lateral epicondyle**
- **Olecranon**
- **Flexor muscle mass (in the forearm)**
- **Extensor muscle mass (in the forearm)**
- **Carpal bones (on the dorsum of the wrist)**
- **Styloid process of the radius**
- **Styloid process of the ulna**

ATLAS REFERENCES:
G = *Grant's Atlas*, 12th ed., page number
L = *LWW Atlas of Anatomy*, 1st ed., page number
N = *Netter's Atlas*, 4th ed., plate number
R = *Color Atlas of Anatomy*, 6th ed., page number

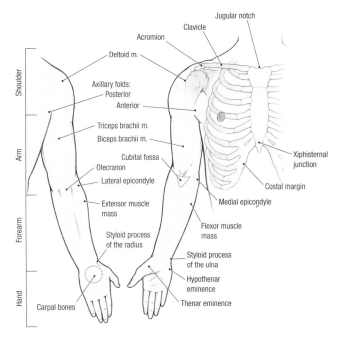

Figure 2.1. Surface anatomy of the upper limb.

- **Thenar eminence**
- **Hypothenar eminence**

SUPERFICIAL VEINS AND CUTANEOUS NERVES

Dissection Overview

The **superficial fascia** of the upper limb contains fat, **superficial veins,** and **cutaneous nerves**. In the living body, the superficial veins may be visible through the skin. They are frequently used for drawing blood and injecting medications. In the cadaver, the superficial veins are not conspicuous. The cutaneous nerves of the upper limb pierce the deep fascia to reach the superficial fascia and skin.

The order of dissection will be as follows: The anterior thoracic wall and the upper limb proximal to the wrist will be skinned. The objective is to remove only the skin, leaving the superficial fascia undisturbed. The superficial veins and selected cutaneous nerves will be dissected. The fat will then be removed so that the deep fascia may be observed. [G 484, 490; L 31; N 479, 480; R 400, 402; C 27]

Dissection Instructions

SKIN INCISIONS

1. Place the cadaver in the supine position.
2. Refer to Figure 2.2A. Before cutting, realize that the skin is thin on the anterior thoracic wall.
3. Make a midline skin incision from the jugular notch (A) to the xiphisternal junction (C).
4. Make a skin incision from the jugular notch (A) along the clavicle to the acromion (B). Continue this incision down the lateral side of the arm to a point that is approximately halfway down the arm (F).
5. At point F, make an incision around the anterior and posterior surfaces of the arm, meeting on the medial side (G).
6. Make an incision from the xiphisternal junction (C) along the costal margin to the midaxillary line (V).
7. Make an incision that begins at G on the medial surface of the arm and extends superiorly to the axilla. Extend this incision inferiorly along the lateral surface of the trunk to V.
8. Make a transverse skin incision from the middle of the manubrium to the midaxillary line, passing around the nipple.
9. Make a transverse skin incision from the xiphisternal junction (C) to the G–V incision.
10. Make a transverse skin incision halfway between the A–B incision and the incision made in step 8.
11. Remove the skin from medial to lateral. Leave the nipple attached to the superficial fascia. Detach the skin along the midaxillary line and place it in the tissue container.
12. If the back has not been dissected previously go to page 8, follow the skinning instructions that are provided there, and return to this page.
13. Refer to Figure 2.2B.
14. Make an incision that encircles the wrist (E). The skin is very thin (2 mm) on the anterior surface of the wrist.
15. Make a longitudinal incision on the anterior surface of the upper limb (E to G).
16. Remove the skin from the arm and forearm and place it in the tissue container. Do not damage the superficial veins and cutaneous nerves in the superficial fascia.

SUPERFICIAL VEINS [G 490; L 31; N 479, 480; R 398; C 27]

1. Use blunt dissection to demonstrate the superficial veins of the arm and forearm (Fig. 2.3).
2. Abduct the upper limb and have your dissection partner hold it in the abducted position.

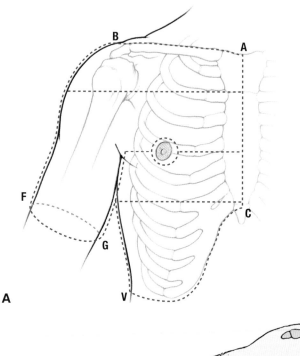

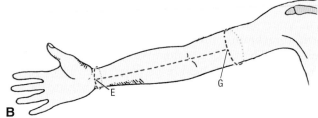

Figure 2.2. Skin incisions. **A.** Pectoral region. **B.** Upper limb.

3. In the posterior forearm, demonstrate the **basilic vein** and **cephalic vein**.
4. Use a probe to follow the cephalic and basilic veins proximally, freeing them from the surrounding fat and connective tissue.
5. Demonstrate that the cephalic and basilic veins are joined across the cubital fossa by the **median cubital vein**. This pattern can be quite variable and should be observed on other cadavers.
6. Follow the cephalic vein proximally into the pectoral region where it courses in the **deltopectoral groove** between the deltoid muscle and the pectoralis major muscle. Near the clavicle, the cephalic vein passes deeply through the **deltopectoral triangle** to join the axillary vein.
7. Follow the basilic vein proximally. Before reaching the axilla, it pierces the deep fascia to join the brachial vein.
8. Use a probe to elevate the superficial veins (Fig. 2.3). Note that **perforating veins** penetrate the deep fascia and connect the superficial veins to deep veins.

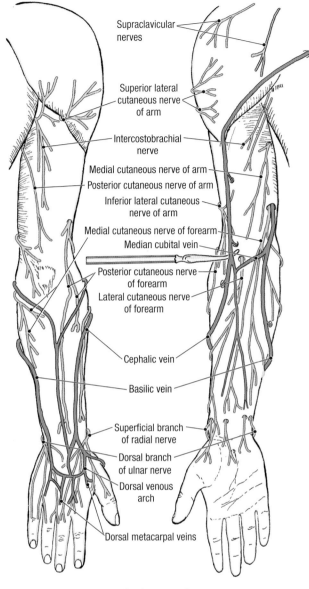

Figure 2.3. Superficial veins and cutaneous nerves.

- **Superficial branch of the radial nerve**
- **Dorsal branch of the ulnar nerve**

2. Dissect only four of the cutaneous nerves:
   - **Lateral cutaneous nerve of the forearm** – located at the level of the elbow in the superficial fascia lateral to the biceps brachii tendon. Note its close relationship to the cephalic vein and the median cubital vein.
   - **Medial cutaneous nerve of the forearm** – located on the medial side of the biceps brachii tendon. Note its close relationship to the basilic vein.
   - **Superficial branch of the radial nerve** – located in the superficial fascia near the styloid process of the radius. Expose only 2 or 3 cm of this nerve.
   - **Dorsal branch of the ulnar nerve** – located in the superficial fascia near the styloid process of the ulna. Expose only 2 or 3 cm of this nerve.

3. The cutaneous nerves to the digits will be studied with the hand.

4. Remove all remaining superficial fascia from the arm and forearm, preserving the superficial veins and nerves that you have dissected. Do not disturb the deep fascia. Place the superficial fascia in the tissue container.

5. Examine the **deep fascia** of the upper limb. Note that the deep fascia of the upper limb extends from the shoulder to the fingertips. It attaches to the bones of the upper limb and forms compartments that contain groups of muscles. The deep fascia of the upper limb is regionally named: **brachial fascia** in the arm and **antebrachial fascia** in the forearm. In the hand the deep fascia is called **palmar fascia** on the palmar surface and **dorsal fascia of the hand** on the dorsal surface.

CUTANEOUS NERVES [G 484; L 31; N 479, 480; R 400; C 27]

1. Before dissecting, use an illustration to familiarize yourself with the course and distribution of the **cutaneous nerves of the arm and forearm** (Fig. 2.3):
   - **Superior lateral cutaneous nerve of the arm**
   - **Inferior lateral cutaneous nerve of the arm**
   - **Posterior cutaneous nerve of the arm**
   - **Intercostobrachial nerve**
   - **Medial cutaneous nerve of the arm**
   - **Posterior cutaneous nerve of the forearm**
   - **Lateral cutaneous nerve of the forearm**
   - **Medial cutaneous nerve of the forearm**

Dissection Review

1. Review the superficial fascia of the upper limb.
2. Use the dissected specimen to trace the course of the superficial veins from distal to proximal.
3. Review the location of the cephalic vein, basilic vein, and median cubital vein in the cubital fossa and recall that these are important for venipuncture.
4. Use the dissected specimen to review the four cutaneous nerves that you have dissected. Use an illustration to review the pattern of distribution of the cutaneous nerves that you did not dissect.
5. Compare this pattern of cutaneous nerve distribution to a dermatome chart.
6. Review the deep fascia of the upper limb and name its parts. [G 483, 484; L 31; N 481, 482; C 26]

SUPERFICIAL GROUP OF BACK MUSCLES

Instructions for dissection of the superficial group of back muscles are found in Chapter 1, The Back. If you are dissecting the upper limb before the back, the superficial group of back muscles must be dissected now. Turn to pages 9 to 11, complete that dissection, and return to this page.

SCAPULAR REGION

Dissection Overview

There are six shoulder (scapulohumeral) muscles: **deltoid**, **supraspinatus**, **infraspinatus**, **teres minor**, **teres major**, and **subscapularis**. The order of dissection will be as follows: The deltoid muscle will be studied, and then it will be detached from its proximal attachment and the course of its nerve and artery will be studied. Subsequently, the four muscles arising from the dorsal surface of the scapula (supraspinatus, infraspinatus, teres major, teres minor) will be dissected and their nerves and blood vessels will be demonstrated. The subscapularis muscle will be dissected with the axilla.

SKELETON OF THE SCAPULAR REGION [G 518; L 31; N 421; R 371, 373; C 76, 77]

Refer to a skeleton. On the **scapula**, identify (Fig. 2.4):

- **Acromion**
- **Suprascapular notch**
- **Supraspinous fossa**
- **Spine**
- **Infraspinous fossa**
- **Supraglenoid tubercle**
- **Glenoid cavity**
- **Infraglenoid tubercle**
- **Coracoid process**

 On the **humerus**, identify (Fig. 2.4):

- **Head**
- **Anatomical neck**

- **Greater tubercle**
- **Lesser tubercle**
- **Intertubercular sulcus (bicipital groove)**
- **Surgical neck**
- **Deltoid tuberosity**
- **Radial groove**

Dissection Instructions

1. Place the cadaver in the prone position (face down). Abduct the upper limb to 45°. If a block is available, place it under the chest.
2. Use blunt dissection to define the borders of the **deltoid muscle**. The proximal attachments of the deltoid muscle are the spine of the scapula, the acromion of the scapula, and the lateral one-third of the clavicle. The distal attachment of the deltoid muscle is the deltoid tuberosity of the humerus. The deltoid muscle abducts the humerus. [G 513; L 36; N 424; R 382; C 328]
3. Use a scalpel to detach the deltoid muscle from its proximal attachments. Make your cuts close to the bone. Leave the muscle attached to its distal attachment on the humerus. Reflect the deltoid muscle laterally, taking care not to tear the vessels and nerve that course along its deep surface.
4. Observe the **axillary nerve** and the **posterior circumflex humeral artery and vein** on the deep surface of the deltoid muscle near its attachment to the humerus. Use a probe to clean the nerve and vessels and trace them around the surgical neck of the humerus (Fig. 2.5). [G 528; L 37; N 426; R 383; C 43]
5. Note that the axillary nerve innervates the deltoid muscle and the **teres minor muscle**.
6. Follow the axillary nerve and the posterior circumflex humeral artery and vein deeply. Push your finger parallel to the nerve and vessels to open the **quadrangular space** (Fig. 2.5). Define the **borders of the quadrangular space**:
   - **Superior border** – inferior border of the teres minor muscle
   - **Lateral border** – surgical neck of the humerus
   - **Medial border** – long head of the triceps brachii muscle
   - **Inferior border** – superior border of the teres major muscle
7. Identify the **long head of the triceps brachii muscle**. Observe that the long head of the triceps brachii muscle passes anterior to the teres minor muscle and posterior to the teres major muscle.
8. Use a probe to clean and define the borders of the **teres minor muscle**. The proximal attachment of

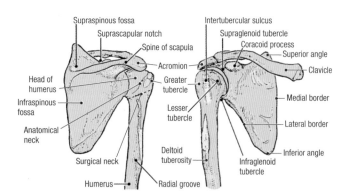

Supraspinous fossa
Suprascapular notch
Spine of scapula
Acromion
Head of humerus
Infraspinous fossa
Anatomical neck
Surgical neck
Humerus
Radial groove
Greater tubercle
Lesser tubercle
Deltoid tuberosity
Intertubercular sulcus
Supraglenoid tubercle
Coracoid process
Superior angle
Clavicle
Medial border
Lateral border
Inferior angle
Infraglenoid tubercle

Figure 2.4. Skeleton of the scapular region.

Posterior view

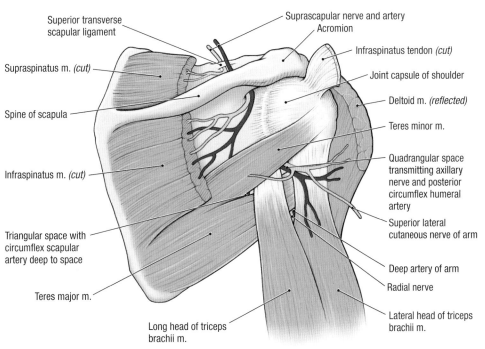

Figure 2.5. Blood and nerve supply to the posterior aspect of the shoulder.

the teres minor muscle is the lateral border of the scapula. The distal attachment of the teres minor muscle is the inferior facet of the greater tubercle of the humerus. The teres minor muscle laterally rotates the humerus.

9. Clean and define the borders of the **teres major muscle**. The proximal attachment of the teres major muscle is the inferior angle of the scapula. The distal attachment of the teres major muscle is the medial lip of the intertubercular sulcus of the humerus. The teres major muscle adducts and medially rotates the humerus.

10. Define the **borders of the triangular space**:
    • **Superior border** – inferior border of the teres minor muscle
    • **Lateral border** – tendon of the long head of the triceps brachii muscle
    • **Inferior border** – superior border of the teres major muscle

11. Note that the circumflex scapular artery may be found deep within the triangular space.

12. Reflect the trapezius muscle superiorly, leaving it attached along the "hinge" of cervical fascia that was created during the back dissection.

13. Clean and define the borders of the **supraspinatus muscle**. The proximal attachment of the supraspinatus muscle is the supraspinous fossa of the scapula. The distal attachment of the supraspinatus muscle is the highest facet of the greater tubercle of the humerus. The supraspinatus muscle initiates abduction of the humerus.

14. Use a probe to define the borders of the **infraspinatus muscle**. The proximal attachment of the infraspinatus muscle is the infraspinous fossa of the scapula. The distal attachment of the infraspinatus muscle is the middle facet of the greater tubercle of the humerus. The infraspinatus muscle laterally rotates the humerus.

15. The **suprascapular artery** and the **suprascapular nerve** are found deep to the supraspinatus muscle (Fig. 2.5). To see them, the supraspinatus muscle must be reflected. [G 528; L 37; N 426; R 406; C 25]

16. Use a scalpel to transect the supraspinatus muscle about 5 cm lateral to the superior angle of the scapula but medial to the suprascapular notch. Hold a disarticulated scapula over the scapula of the cadaver to help you locate the proper level of the cut.

17. Use blunt dissection to loosen, from the supraspinous fossa, the portion of the supraspinatus muscle that is distal to the transection. Reflect it laterally. Leave it attached to the humerus.

18. Identify the **suprascapular artery and nerve**. Follow the artery and nerve superiorly. Observe that the suprascapular artery passes superior to the **superior transverse scapular ligament** and the suprascapular nerve passes inferior to it (Fig. 2.5). This relationship can be remembered by use of a

mnemonic device: "*A*rmy (*a*rtery) goes over the bridge; *N*avy (*n*erve) goes under the bridge."

19. Transect the **infraspinatus muscle** about 5 cm lateral to the vertebral border of the scapula (Fig. 2.5).
20. Use blunt dissection to loosen, from the infraspinous fossa, the portion of the infraspinatus muscle that is distal to the transection. Reflect it laterally.
21. Follow the **suprascapular artery** and the **suprascapular nerve** inferiorly. Note that they reach the infraspinatus muscle by coursing deep (anterior) to the spine of the scapula (Fig. 2.5).
22. The suprascapular artery contributes to the collateral circulation of the scapular region. Use an illustration to study the **scapular anastomosis**. [G 504; L 38; N 427; R 406]
23. The four muscles of the **rotator cuff** are the **supraspinatus, infraspinatus, teres minor,** and **subscapularis.** The subscapularis muscle will be dissected with the axilla. Use an illustration to study the distal attachments of the rotator cuff muscles. [G 516, 517, 534; L 45; N 420, 421; R 383; C 33]

Dissection Review

1. Replace the muscles of the scapular region in their correct anatomical positions.
2. Use an illustration and the dissected specimen to review the proximal attachment and distal attachment of each muscle of the scapular region. List the action of each muscle and the combined action of the rotator cuff group of muscles.
3. Review the origin, course, and distribution of the transverse cervical artery, dorsal scapular artery, and suprascapular artery.
4. Review the scapular anastomosis.
5. Review the relationship of the suprascapular artery and the suprascapular nerve to the superior transverse scapular ligament.
6. Review the innervation of each muscle dissected today.

PECTORAL REGION

Dissection Overview

The **pectoral region** (L., *pectus*, chest) covers the anterior thoracic wall and part of the lateral thoracic wall. The order of dissection will be as follows: The breast will be dissected in female cadavers. The superficial fascia will be removed in cadavers of both sexes.

Dissection Instructions

BREAST [G 4, 5; L 39; N 182; R 290; C 4–6]

The breast is dissected in female cadavers only. Students with male cadavers must observe at another dissection table. Because of the advanced age of some cadavers, it may be difficult to dissect and identify all of the structures listed. Expect the lobes of the gland to be replaced by fat with advanced age.

The **breast** extends from the lateral border of the sternum to the midaxillary line, and from rib 2 to rib 6. The mammary gland is a modified sweat gland that is contained within the superficial fascia of the breast (Fig. 2.6). The breast is positioned anterior to the **pectoral fascia** (the deep fascia of the pectoralis major muscle). The pectoral fascia is attached to the overlying skin by the **suspensory ligaments of the breast** that pass between the lobes of the mammary gland.

1. Identify the **areola** and the **nipple** (Fig. 2.6).
2. Use the handle of a forceps to scoop the fat out of several compartments between **suspensory ligaments.** These areas between suspensory ligaments once contained lobes of functional glandular tissue.
3. Make a parasagittal (superior to inferior) cut through the nipple that divides the breast into a medial half and a lateral half (Fig. 2.6).
4. On the cut edge of the breast, use a probe to dissect through the fat deep to the nipple. Confine

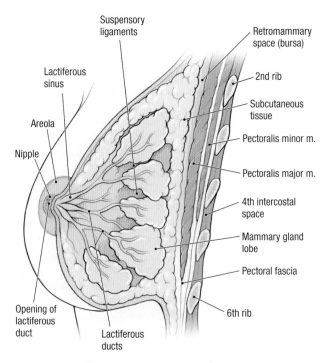

Figure 2.6. Breast in sagittal section.

your search area to within 3 cm deep to the areola. Find and clean one of the 15 to 20 **lactiferous ducts** that converge on the nipple. Identify the **lactiferous sinus**, which is an expanded part of the lactiferous duct located deep to the nipple.

5. Trace one lactiferous duct to the nipple and attempt to identify its opening.
6. Use an illustration to study the **lymphatic drainage of the mammary gland**. [G 9; L 40; N 184; R 290; C 7]
7. Insert your fingers behind the breast and open the **retromammary space**. Note that the normal breast can be easily separated from the underlying deep fascia of the pectoralis major muscle.
8. Remove the breast from the anterior surface of the pectoralis major muscle with the aid of a scalpel.
9. Store the breast in a plastic bag.

CLINICAL CORRELATION

Breast

For descriptive purposes, clinicians divide the breast into four quadrants. The superolateral (upper outer) quadrant contains a large amount of glandular tissue and is a common site for breast cancers to develop. From this quadrant, an "axillary tail" of breast tissue often extends into the axilla.

In advanced stages of breast cancer, the tumor may invade the underlying pectoralis major muscle and its fascia. When this happens, the tumor and breast become fused to the chest wall, a condition that can be detected by palpation during a physical examination. As the breast tumor enlarges, it places traction on the suspensory ligaments, resulting in dimpling of the skin overlying the tumor.

SUPERFICIAL FASCIA

1. Dissection of the superficial fascia must be performed on both male and female cadavers.
2. The **platysma muscle** is a muscle of facial expression that may extend inferior to the clavicle into the superficial fascia of the superior thorax. It is very thin, but broad. If the platysma muscle is present in the thorax, dissect it from the superficial fascia that lies deep to it and reflect it superiorly. Do not extend the dissection field superior to the clavicles.
3. Make a vertical cut through the superficial fascia in the midline of the sternum. Make additional cuts through the superficial fascia corresponding

to skin incisions A–B–F, C–V, and G–V (Fig. 2.2A).
4. Use blunt dissection to remove the superficial fascia, proceeding from medial to lateral.
5. Study an illustration of the **cutaneous branches of a typical spinal nerve** (Fig 2.7). The **anterior cutaneous branches** are small and emerge from the intercostal space lateral to the border of the sternum. Do not attempt to find them. [G 20; L 161; N 192; R 214; C 8]
6. As you peel back the superficial fascia, identify an intercostal space by palpation. Palpate the **lateral cutaneous branches** of the intercostal nerves where they leave the intercostal space and enter the superficial fascia. Identify one lateral cutaneous branch (from intercostal space 4, 5, or 6) while the superficial fascia is being removed. Trace its **anterior and posterior branches** for a short distance and preserve them.
7. Detach the superficial fascia along the midaxillary line and place it in the tissue container.

Dissection Review

1. Review the location and parts of the breast.
2. Use an illustration to review the vascular supply to the breast.
3. Discuss the pattern of lymphatic drainage of the breast and identify by name the lymph node groups that are involved.
4. Use an illustration of the branching pattern of a typical spinal nerve to review the innervation of the anterior thoracic wall and breast (Fig. 2.7).

MUSCLES OF THE PECTORAL REGION

Dissection Overview

The muscles of the pectoral region are the pectoralis major, pectoralis minor, and subclavius muscles. The muscles of the pectoral region attach the upper limb to the thoracic skeleton. The pectoral muscles are positioned immediately deep to the superficial fascia (deep to the breast).

The dissection will proceed as follows: The pectoralis major muscle will be studied and reflected. The pectoralis minor muscle and clavipectoral fascia will be studied. The subclavius muscle will be identified. The pectoralis minor muscle will be reflected, and the branches of the thoracoacromial artery will be dissected.

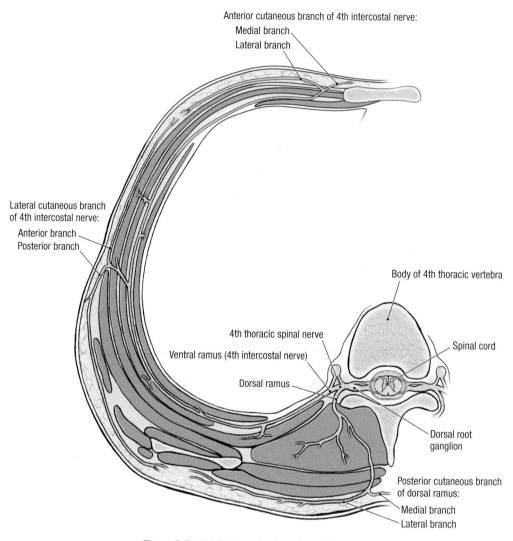

Anterior cutaneous branch of 4th intercostal nerve:
Medial branch
Lateral branch

Lateral cutaneous branch
of 4th intercostal nerve:
Anterior branch
Posterior branch

Body of 4th thoracic vertebra

4th thoracic spinal nerve

Ventral ramus (4th intercostal nerve)

Dorsal ramus

Spinal cord

Dorsal root
ganglion

Posterior cutaneous branch
of dorsal ramus:
Medial branch
Lateral branch

Figure 2.7. Distribution of a thoracic spinal nerve.

Dissection Instructions

1. Clean the superficial surface of the **pectoralis major muscle**, using your fingers to define its borders (Fig. 2.8). Study an illustration and note that the deep fascia on the surface of the pectoralis major muscle is called **pectoral fascia** and that it is continuous with the **axillary fascia** that forms the floor of the axilla. [G 498; L 41; N 424; R 408; C 13]

2. Identify the two heads of the pectoralis major muscle: **clavicular head** and **sternocostal head** (Fig. 2.8). Observe that the juncture of these two heads is at the sternoclavicular joint.

3. Use your fingers to trace the tendon of the pectoralis major muscle to its distal attachment on the humerus. The pectoralis major muscle flexes, adducts, and medially rotates the humerus.

4. Between the clavicular head of the pectoralis major muscle and the adjacent deltoid muscle, use

blunt dissection to define the borders of the **deltopectoral triangle** and find the **cephalic vein**. Preserve the cephalic vein in subsequent steps of this dissection.

5. Relax the sternal head of the pectoralis major muscle by flexing and adducting the arm. Gently insert your fingers posterior to the inferior border of the pectoralis major muscle. Create a space between the posterior surface of the pectoralis major and the **clavipectoral fascia**. Push your fingers superiorly to open this space.

6. Use scissors to detach the sternoscostal head of the pectoralis major muscle from its attachment to the sternum (Fig. 2.8, dashed line).

7. Palpate the deep surface of the pectoralis major muscle to locate the **medial and lateral pectoral nerves and vessels**. Preserve these nerves and vessels.

8. Use scissors to cut the clavicular head of the pectoralis major muscle close to the clavicle (Fig. 2.8).

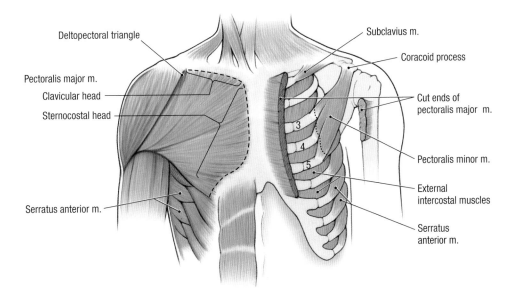

Figure 2.8. Cuts for reflection of the pectoralis major and pectoralis minor muscles.

Preserve the cephalic vein. Note that the **lateral pectoral nerve** and the **pectoral branch of the thoracoacromial artery** enter the deep surface of the clavicular head.

9. Reflect the pectoralis major muscle laterally. Attempt to preserve the nerves and vessels that enter its deep surface.

10. Deep to the pectoralis major muscle are the **clavipectoral fascia, pectoralis minor muscle,** and **subclavius muscle**. [G 498; L 41; N 428; R 409]

11. Identify the pectoralis minor muscle. The proximal attachment of the pectoralis minor muscle is ribs 3 to 5 near their costal cartilages. Its distal attachment is onto the coracoid process of the scapula. The pectoralis minor muscle draws the glenoid cavity of the scapula anteriorly and inferiorly.

12. Note that the **medial pectoral nerve** pierces the pectoralis minor muscle and then enters the pectoralis major muscle, innervating both.

13. Identify the **subclavius muscle**, which is located inferior to the clavicle (Fig. 2.8). The subclavius muscle, which is attached to the clavicle and the first rib, depresses the clavicle.

14. Read a description of the **clavipectoral fascia** and understand that it is immediately deep to the pectoralis major muscle. The clavipectoral fascia is attached to the clavicle. It passes both superficial and deep to the subclavius muscle and the pectoralis minor muscle. The clavipectoral fascia is attached to the axillary fascia inferiorly.

15. Clean the **cephalic vein** where it crosses the anterior surface of the pectoralis minor tendon. The cephalic vein passes through the **costocoracoid**

membrane (part of the clavipectoral fascia) medial to the pectoralis minor tendon. The **thoracoacromial artery** and the **lateral pectoral nerve** also pass through the costocoracoid membrane.

16. Use scissors to detach the pectoralis minor muscle from its proximal attachments on ribs 3 to 5 (Fig. 2.8, dashed line).

17. Reflect the pectoralis minor muscle superiorly. Leave the muscle attached to the coracoid process of the scapula. [G 500; L 42; N 427; R 412; C 15]

18. Clean and define the branches of the thoracoacromial artery (Fig. 2.9):
    • **Acromial branch** passes laterally across the coracoid process toward the acromion.
    • **Deltoid branch** courses laterally in the **deltopectoral groove** between the deltoid muscle

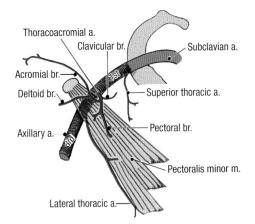

Figure 2.9. Blood supply to the pectoral region.

and pectoralis major muscle. The deltoid branch accompanies the cephalic vein.

- **Pectoral branch** passes between the pectoralis major muscle and the pectoralis minor muscle and supplies both.
  - **Clavicular branch** courses superiorly and medially to supply the subclavius muscle.
19. Along the lateral border of the pectoralis minor muscle, identify the **lateral thoracic artery** (Fig. 2.9). Do not follow the lateral thoracic artery at this time.
20. Identify the **serratus anterior muscle** (Fig. 2.8). Note its extensive proximal attachment on the upper eight ribs. The distal attachment of the serratus anterior muscle is the deep surface of the scapula along the entire length of its medial border. You cannot see the distal attachment at this time.

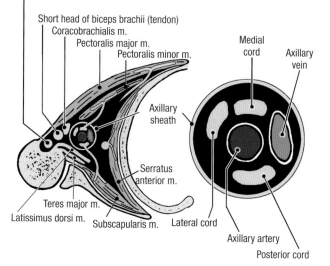

Figure 2.10. Walls and contents of the axilla (transverse section).

Dissection Review

1. Replace the pectoral muscles into their correct anatomical positions.
2. Review the attachments of the pectoralis major, pectoralis minor, and subclavius muscles. Review their actions, innervations, and blood supply.
3. Review the relationship of the clavipectoral fascia to the muscles, vessels, and nerves of this region.
4. Be sure that you understand the role played by the clavipectoral fascia in supporting the floor of the axilla.
5. Name all branches of the thoracoacromial artery and the structures supplied by each branch.

AXILLA

Dissection Overview

The **axilla** is the region between the pectoral muscles, the scapula, the arm, and the thoracic wall (Fig. 2.10). It is a region of passage for vessels and nerves that course from the root of the neck into the upper limb. The **contents of the axilla** are the **axillary sheath, brachial plexus, axillary vessels and their branches, lymph nodes and lymphatic vessels, portions of three muscles,** and a considerable amount of fat and connective tissue.

Study a diagram and note the following **boundaries of the axilla**: [G 502; N 428]

- **Apex of the axilla** – bounded by the clavicle anteriorly, the upper border of the scapula posteriorly, and the first rib medially
- **Base of the axilla** – skin and fascia of the armpit
- **Anterior wall** – pectoralis major muscle, pectoralis minor muscle, and clavipectoral fascia

- **Posterior wall** – posterior axillary fold (teres major and latissimus dorsi muscles) and the subscapularis muscle that covers the anterior surface of the scapula
- **Medial wall** – upper portion of the thoracic wall and the serratus anterior muscle, which overlies this wall
- **Lateral wall** – intertubercular sulcus of the humerus

The order of dissection will be as follows: The pectoralis major and pectoralis minor muscles will be reflected to expose the contents of the axilla. The axillary vein and its tributaries will be removed. The branches of the axillary artery will be dissected. The brachial plexus will be studied.

Dissection Instructions

1. Review the pectoralis major muscle, the pectoralis minor muscle, and the clavipectoral fascia.
2. Reflect the pectoralis major muscle laterally.
3. Reflect the pectoralis minor muscle superiorly.
4. Abduct the arm to about 45°.
5. Identify the **axillary sheath** (Fig. 2.10). The axillary sheath is a connective tissue structure that surrounds the axillary vessels and brachial plexus. The axillary sheath extends from the lateral border of the first rib to the inferior border of the teres major muscle.
6. Use scissors to open the anterior surface of the axillary sheath.
7. Identify the **axillary vein** within the axillary sheath. Note that the axillary vein is formed at the lateral border of the teres major muscle by the joining of the two brachial veins. The axillary vein

ends at the lateral border of the first rib where it is continuous with the subclavian vein.

8. To enhance dissection of the arteries and nerves in the axilla, the axillary vein must be removed. Cut the cephalic vein where it joins the axillary vein and preserve the cephalic vein. Cut the axillary vein at the lateral border of the first rib and bluntly dissect it distally as far as possible. Use a probe to dissect the axillary vein from the structures that lie posterior to it (axillary artery and brachial plexus). Cut the axillary vein at the lateral border of the teres major muscle and remove it. [G 501; N 429; R 411; C 14]

9. As the dissection proceeds, remove veins that are tributary to the axillary vein. Preserve the accompanying arteries. Note the presence of lymph nodes that are associated with the veins.

AXILLARY ARTERY [G 508, 509; L 44; N 427; R 412; C 16]

The **axillary artery** begins at the lateral border of the first rib where it is the continuation of the **subclavian artery** (Fig. 2.11). The axillary artery ends at the inferior border of the teres major muscle where its name changes to **brachial artery**. The axillary artery is surrounded by the brachial plexus (Fig. 2.10, inset). *The brachial plexus must be retracted and preserved during dissection of the axillary artery and its branches.*

1. Identify the **three parts of the axillary artery** (Fig. 2.11):

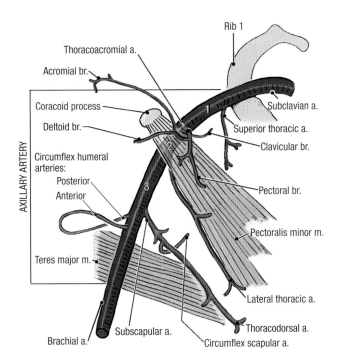

Figure 2.11. Branches arising from the axillary artery.

- **First part** extends from the lateral border of the first rib to the medial border of the pectoralis minor muscle.
- **Second part** lies posterior to the pectoralis minor muscle.
- **Third part** extends from the lateral border of the pectoralis minor muscle to the inferior border of the teres major muscle.

Dissection note: The branching pattern of the axillary artery may vary from that which is commonly illustrated. If the pattern is different in your specimen, note that the branches are named according to their distribution rather than by their origin.

2. The first part of the axillary artery has one branch, the **superior thoracic artery**. Follow the superior thoracic artery to its area of distribution in the first and second intercostal spaces.

3. The second part of the axillary artery has two branches (Fig. 2.11):
   - **Thoracoacromial artery** arises at the medial border of the pectoralis minor muscle and penetrates the costocoracoid membrane.
   - **Lateral thoracic artery** arises at the lateral border of the pectoralis minor muscle (65%) and descends along the lateral border of the pectoralis minor muscle. The lateral thoracic artery may arise from the subscapular artery or from the thoracoacromial artery.

4. Use blunt dissection to open the clavipectoral fascia and identify the thoracoacromial artery on the medial side of the pectoralis minor muscle.

5. Review the branches of the thoracoacromial artery that have been dissected previously:
   - **Acromial branch** passes laterally across the coracoid process to the acromion.
   - **Deltoid branch** courses laterally in the deltopectoral groove. It accompanies the cephalic vein.
   - **Pectoral branch** passes between the pectoralis major and pectoralis minor muscles and supplies both.
   - **Clavicular branch** courses superiorly and medially to supply the subclavius muscle.

6. Identify the **lateral thoracic artery** and follow it along the lateral border of the pectoralis minor muscle (Fig. 2.11). The lateral thoracic artery supplies the pectoral muscles, the serratus anterior muscle, the axillary lymph nodes, and the lateral thoracic wall. In females, the lateral thoracic artery also supplies the lateral portion of the mammary gland.

7. The third part of the axillary artery has three branches: **subscapular artery, posterior circumflex humeral artery**, and **anterior circumflex humeral artery**.

8. Identify the **subscapular artery**. It is the largest branch of the axillary artery. The subscapular artery courses inferiorly for a short distance before dividing into the **circumflex scapular artery** (to muscles on the posterior surface of the scapula) and the **thoracodorsal artery** (to the latissimus dorsi muscle). The subscapular artery gives off several unnamed muscular branches.

9. Find the **anterior and posterior circumflex humeral arteries**, which arise from the axillary artery distal to the origin of the subscapular artery. Occasionally, these two arteries may arise from a short common trunk. They supply the deltoid muscle.

10. Observe that the **posterior circumflex humeral artery** is the larger of the two circumflex humeral arteries. Follow it as it passes posterior to the surgical neck of the humerus with the axillary nerve. Demonstrate that the posterior circumflex humeral artery and the axillary nerve pass through the quadrangular space.

11. The **anterior circumflex humeral artery** courses around the anterior surface of the humerus at the surgical neck. It passes deep to the tendon of the long head of the biceps brachii muscle.

BRACHIAL PLEXUS [G 508; L 43; N 429; R 413; C 14]

The brachial plexus begins in the root of the neck superior to the clavicle. It passes distally toward the base of the axilla where its **terminal branches** arise. Only the **infraclavicular part of the brachial plexus** will be dissected at this time. The **supraclavicular part** will be dissected with the neck.

The **three cords of the brachial plexus** (lateral, medial, and posterior) are named according to their relationship to the second part of the axillary artery (posterior to the pectoralis minor muscle) (Fig. 2.12).

1. Identify the **musculocutaneous nerve**. It is the most lateral terminal branch of the brachial plexus and enters the coracobrachialis muscle.

2. To find the **lateral cord**, use your fingers to follow the musculocutaneous nerve proximally.

3. Observe that the lateral cord gives rise to one other large branch, the **lateral root of the median nerve**. Follow the lateral root distally and identify the **median nerve.**

4. To find the **medial cord**, trace the **medial root of the median nerve** proximally.

5. A portion of the medial cord continues distally as the **ulnar nerve**.

6. Note that the three **terminal branches** (musculocutaneous nerve, median nerve, and ulnar nerve) that you have just identified form the letter M anterior to the third part of the axillary artery (Fig. 2.12).

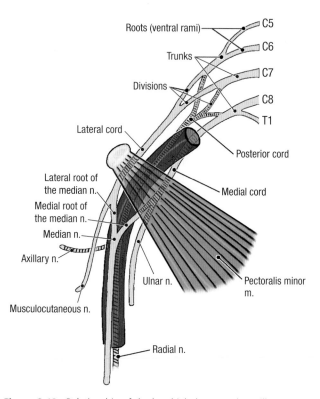

Figure 2.12. Relationship of the brachial plexus to the axillary artery.

7. Trace the **medial** and **lateral pectoral nerves** from the reflected pectoral muscles to their origins from the medial and lateral cords, respectively.

8. Identify two branches that arise from the inferior edge of the medial cord. They are the **medial cutaneous nerve of the forearm** and the **medial cutaneous nerve of the arm**. Use your fingers to trace these nerves a short distance (7.5 cm) into the arm.

9. Retract the axillary artery, the lateral cord, and the medial cord in the superior direction. This procedure exposes the **posterior cord** of the brachial plexus. The branches of the posterior cord are the **axillary nerve, radial nerve**, and three **subscapular nerves (upper, middle, and lower)**.

10. Use blunt dissection to clean the **axillary nerve**. Observe that the axillary nerve passes posterior to the humerus and courses through the quadrangular space with the posterior circumflex humeral artery (Fig. 2.13).

11. Use blunt dissection to clean the **radial nerve** and confirm that it leaves the axilla by passing posterior to the humerus. The radial nerve is the motor and sensory nerve to the posterior portion of the upper limb.

12. Identify the subscapular nerves that arise from the posterior cord (Fig. 2.13) and verify that they run

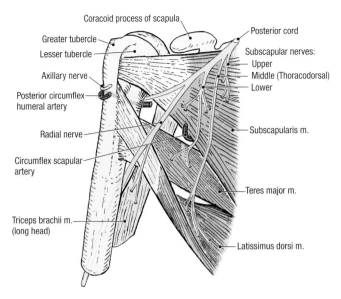

Figure 2.13. Posterior wall of the axilla and posterior cord of the brachial plexus.

in the loose connective tissue on the anterior surface of the subscapularis muscle:

- **Upper subscapular nerve** innervates the subscapularis muscle.
- **Middle subscapular nerve (thoracodorsal nerve)** innervates the latissimus dorsi muscle.
- **Lower subscapular nerve** innervates the subscapularis muscle and the teres major muscle.

13. Identify the three muscles that form the posterior wall of the axilla: **latissimus dorsi**, **teres major**, and **subscapularis** (Fig. 2.13).

14. Examine the **subscapularis muscle**. The proximal attachment of the subscapularis muscle is the subscapular fossa of the scapula. The distal attachment of the subscapularis muscle is the lesser tubercle of the humerus. The subscapularis muscle medially rotates the humerus. The subscapularis muscle is a member of the **rotator cuff group of muscles**.

15. Verify that the medial wall of the axilla is formed by the **serratus anterior muscle** (Fig. 2.10). Use an illustration to study the attachments of the serratus anterior muscle. The proximal attachments of the serratus anterior muscle are the external surfaces of ribs 1 to 8. Its distal attachment is the anterior surface of the medial border of the scapula. The serratus anterior muscle protracts the scapula. The serratus anterior muscle also rotates the scapula, especially when the arm is abducted above the horizontal plane. [G 511; L 41; N 429; R 412; C 14]

16. Use your fingers to follow the serratus anterior muscle posteriorly toward the medial margin of the scapula. On the superficial surface of this mus-

cle, use a probe to free the **long thoracic nerve**. Note the vertical course of this nerve. Observe its branches to the serratus anterior muscle. Follow the nerve superiorly as far as possible toward the apex of the axilla.

Nerve Injuries

The **long thoracic nerve** is vulnerable to stab wounds and to surgical injury during radical mastectomy. Injury of the long thoracic nerve affects the serratus anterior muscle. When a patient with paralysis of the serratus anterior muscle is asked to push with both hands against a wall, the medial border of the scapula protrudes on the affected side, a condition known as "winged scapula."

The **thoracodorsal nerve** is vulnerable to compression injuries and surgical trauma during mastectomy. Injury of the thoracodorsal nerve affects the latissimus dorsi muscle resulting in a weakened ability to extend, adduct, and medially rotate the arm.

The **axillary nerve** courses around the surgical neck of the humerus and may be injured during a fracture or during an inferior dislocation of the shoulder joint. Injury of the axillary nerve affects the deltoid muscle and teres minor muscle, resulting in a weakened ability to abduct and laterally rotate the arm.

Dissection Review

1. Replace the pectoralis major muscle and the pectoralis minor muscle into their correct anatomical positions and review their attachments.
2. Review the boundaries of the axilla.
3. Use the dissected specimen to observe the relationship of the three parts of the axillary artery to the pectoralis minor muscle.
4. Recite the names of all of the branches of the axillary artery and identify each branch on your dissected specimen.
5. Test your understanding of the brachial plexus by drawing a picture that shows its structure and branches. Extend this exercise to the cadaver by demonstrating the divisions, cords, and terminal branches of the infraclavicular portion of the brachial plexus.
6. Review the motor nerve supply to the muscles of the scapular region. Name each muscle and the nerve that supplies it. Realize that some of these nerves arise from the supraclavicular portion of the brachial plexus and that they have not yet been dissected completely.

7. Review the movements of the scapula.
8. Examine other cadavers to gain an appreciation of variations in the branching patterns of arteries and nerves.
9. Use an illustration to review the lymphatic drainage of the axilla.

ARM AND CUBITAL FOSSA

Dissection Overview

The **brachial fascia (deep fascia of the arm)** is a sleeve of tough connective tissue that is continuous at its proximal end with the pectoral fascia, the axillary fascia, and the deep fascia that covers the deltoid and latissimus dorsi muscles. Distally, the brachial fascia is continuous with the **antebrachial fascia (deep fascia of the forearm)**. The brachial fascia is connected to the medial and lateral sides of the humerus by intermuscular septa (Fig. 2.14), creating an **anterior (flexor) compartment** and a **posterior (extensor) compartment** for the muscles of the arm. The anterior compartment contains three muscles (biceps brachii, brachialis, and coracobrachialis) and the musculocutaneous nerve. The posterior compartment contains two muscles (triceps brachii and anconeus), the radial nerve, and the deep artery and vein of the arm.

The order of dissection will be as follows: The anterior compartment of the arm will be opened and its contents will be studied. Nerves and blood vessels will then be traced distally through the arm to the elbow region. The cadaver will be turned to the prone position to complete the dissection of the posterior compartment of the arm.

SKELETON OF THE ARM AND CUBITAL REGION [G 544; L 32, 33; N 436; R 373, 374; C 77, 84]

Refer to a skeleton. On the **humerus,** identify (Fig. 2.15):

*   **Medial epicondyle**
*   **Lateral epicondyle**
*   **Olecranon fossa**

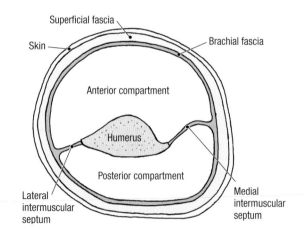

Figure 2.14. Compartments of the right arm.

On the **radius,** identify:

*   **Head**
*   **Neck**
*   **Tuberosity**

On the **ulna,** identify:

*   **Olecranon**
*   **Coronoid process**

Dissection Instructions

ANTERIOR COMPARTMENT OF THE ARM [G 522, 523; L 46; N 431; R 415; C 34, 35]

1. Place the cadaver in the supine position.
2. Use scissors to make a longitudinal incision in the anterior surface of the brachial fascia from the level of the pectoralis major tendon to the elbow.
3. Use your fingers to separate the brachial fascia from the underlying muscles. Work laterally and medially from the incision and note the presence of the **lateral intermuscular septum** and the **medial intermuscular septum**.
4. Use your fingers to separate the three muscles in the anterior compartment of the arm: **coracobrachialis, brachialis,** and **biceps brachii** (Fig. 2.16).
5. The **biceps brachii muscle** has two proximal attachments on the scapula:
    *   **Short head of the biceps brachii muscle** attaches to the coracoid process of the scapula.
    *   **Long head of the biceps brachii muscle** attaches to the supraglenoid tubercle of the scapula.
6. The tendon of the **long head of the biceps brachii muscle** courses through the intertubercular sulcus of the humerus posterior to the **transverse humeral ligament,** then enters the shoulder joint. Do not follow the tendon of the long head to its attachment on the scapula.
7. Identify the **biceps brachii tendon** at the level of the elbow (Fig. 2.16). The distal attachment of the biceps brachii muscle is on the tuberosity of the radius. The biceps brachii muscle supinates and flexes the forearm.
8. Identify the **bicipital aponeurosis** (Fig. 2.16). The bicipital aponeurosis is a broad extension of the biceps tendon that attaches to the antebrachial fascia. The bicipital aponeurosis is located on the medial side of the biceps brachii tendon.
9. Find the **musculocutaneous nerve** in the axilla (Fig. 2.16). Follow the musculocutaneous nerve distally until it enters the **coracobrachialis muscle.** Note that the musculocutaneous nerve inner-

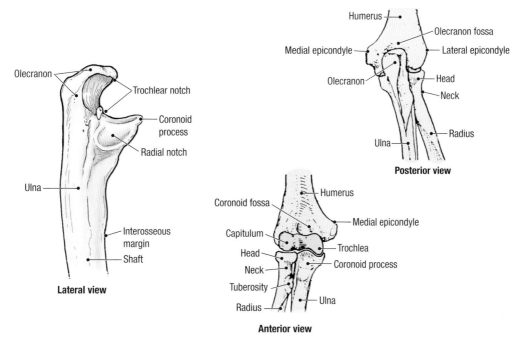

Figure 2.15. Skeleton of the elbow region.

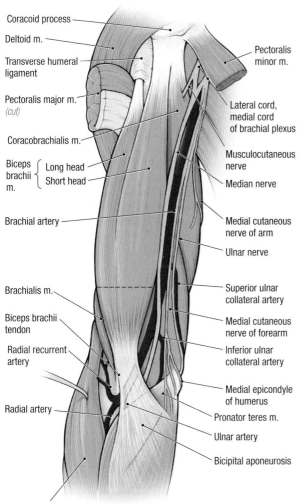

Figure 2.16. Contents of the anterior compartment of the arm.

vates the three muscles of the anterior compartment of the arm.

10. Use your fingers to confirm that the proximal attachment of the coracobrachialis muscle is the coracoid process and that its distal attachment is on the medial side of the shaft of the humerus. The coracobrachialis muscle adducts and flexes the humerus.

11. Use scissors to transect the biceps brachii muscle about 5 cm proximal to the elbow (Fig. 2.16, dashed line). Preserve the musculocutaneous nerve. Reflect the two portions of the biceps brachii muscle proximally and distally, respectively.

12. Observe the **brachialis muscle**, which is deep to the biceps brachii muscle. The proximal attachment of the brachialis muscle is the anterior surface of the distal one-half of the humerus and its distal attachment is on the coronoid process of the ulna. The brachialis muscle flexes the forearm.

13. Find the **musculocutaneous nerve** where it emerges from the coracobrachialis muscle. Follow the musculocutaneous nerve through the plane of loose connective tissue between the biceps brachii muscle and brachialis muscle.

14. After the musculocutaneous nerve gives off its muscular branches, it continues distally as the **lateral cutaneous nerve of the forearm**. Follow the lateral cutaneous nerve of the forearm to the cubital fossa where it emerges near the lateral side of the biceps brachii tendon. Review the relationship

of the lateral cutaneous nerve of the forearm to the cephalic vein.

15. Follow the **medial cutaneous nerve of the forearm** from the brachial plexus to the level of the elbow (Fig. 2.16). Note its relationship to the basilic vein at the level of the elbow.

16. Find the **median nerve** where it arises from the brachial plexus (Fig. 2.16). Use blunt dissection to follow the median nerve from the axilla to the cubital fossa. The median nerve courses distally within the **medial intermuscular septum**.

17. Use blunt dissection to follow the **ulnar nerve** from the medial cord of the brachial plexus to the medial epicondyle of the humerus (Fig. 2.16). Note that the ulnar nerve is in contact with the posterior surface of the medial epicondyle of the humerus. Palpate the ulnar nerve on yourself where it passes posterior to the medial epicondyle.

18. Identify the **brachial artery**. The brachial artery is the continuation of the axillary artery. The brachial artery begins at the inferior border of the teres major muscle and ends at the level of the elbow by branching into the **ulnar artery** and **radial artery** (Fig. 2.16). Verify that the brachial artery courses with the median nerve within the medial intermuscular septum, and that the median nerve is the only large structure to cross the anterior surface of the brachial artery. [G 525; L 46; N 433; R 415; C 35, 36]

19. The brachial artery has three named branches in the arm: **deep artery of the arm**, **superior ulnar collateral artery**, and **inferior ulnar collateral artery**. Several unnamed muscular branches also arise along the length of the brachial artery.

20. Remove the brachial veins and their tributaries to clear the dissection field. Preserve the branches of the brachial artery.

21. In the proximal arm, find the **deep artery of the arm (deep brachial artery, profunda brachii artery)** where it arises from the brachial artery (Fig. 2.17). The deep artery of the arm courses around the posterior surface of the humerus, where it accompanies the radial nerve in the radial groove. The course of the deep artery of the arm will be seen when the posterior compartment of the arm is dissected.

22. Identify the **superior ulnar collateral artery** (Fig. 2.16). It arises from the brachial artery near the middle of the arm. It courses distally with the ulnar nerve and passes posterior to the medial epicondyle of the humerus.

23. Find the **inferior ulnar collateral artery** (Fig. 2.16). It arises from the brachial artery about 3 cm above the medial epicondyle of the humerus and passes anterior to the medial epicondyle between the **brachialis muscle** and the **pronator teres muscle**.

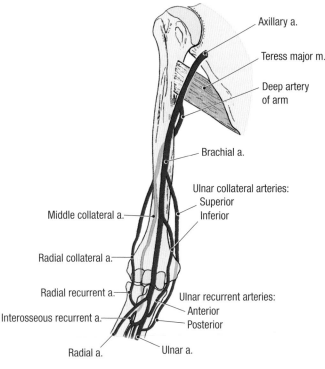

Figure 2.17. Brachial artery and its branches.

Brachial Artery [G 550; L 48, 75; N 434; R 397; C 17]

Use an illustration to study the collateral circulation around the elbow joint (Fig. 2.17). The brachial artery may become blocked at any level distal to the deep artery of the arm without completely blocking blood flow to the forearm and hand.

In the arm, the brachial artery lies medial to the biceps brachii muscle and close to the shaft of the humerus. The brachial artery is compressed at this location when taking a blood pressure reading.

CUBITAL FOSSA [G 538–540; L 46; N 433; R 419–421; C 46, 50]

The **cubital fossa** (L., *cubitus*, elbow) is the depression on the anterior aspect of the elbow. The cubital fossa is clinically important because it contains superficial veins that are used for venipuncture. Large nerves and vessels pass through this region to enter the forearm.

1. Note the **boundaries of the cubital fossa**:
   • **Lateral boundary** – brachioradialis muscle
   • **Medial boundary** – pronator teres muscle
   • **Superior boundary** – an imaginary line connecting the medial and lateral epicondyles of the humerus

- **Superficial boundary (roof of the cubital fossa)** – antebrachial fascia reinforced by the bicipital aponeurosis
- **Deep boundary (floor of the cubital fossa)** – brachialis and supinator muscles

2. Review the positions of the cephalic vein, basilic vein, and median cubital vein in the cubital fossa. To gain access to deeper structures it may be necessary to cut the median cubital vein and retract its cut ends medially and laterally, respectively.
3. Find the **tendon of the biceps brachii muscle** in the cubital fossa.
4. Cut the **bicipital aponeurosis** near the biceps brachii tendon and reflect the aponeurosis medially. Do not cut the brachial artery, which lies deep to the bicipital aponeurosis.
5. Follow the **median nerve** and the **brachial artery** from the arm into the cubital fossa. Remove any fat that may be obstructing your view of these structures.
6. Observe the relative positions of the structures in the cubital fossa (Fig. 2.16): The biceps brachii tendon is lateral, the brachial artery is intermediate, and the median nerve is medial. Note that the bicipital aponeurosis passes superficial to the brachial artery and median nerve, but it lies deep to the superficial veins. The bicipital aponeurosis protects the brachial artery and median nerve from injury during venipuncture.

POSTERIOR COMPARTMENT OF THE ARM [G 527, 528; L 47; N 432; R 403, 404; C 38]

1. Place the cadaver in the prone position.
2. To gain better access to the posterior compartment, rotate the arm medially.
3. Use scissors to open the posterior compartment of the arm by making a longitudinal incision through the brachial fascia from the level of the olecranon of the ulna to the teres minor muscle.
4. Use your fingers to clean and define the borders of the **triceps brachii muscle**. The triceps brachii muscle has three proximal attachments:
   - **Long head of the triceps brachii muscle** attaches to the infraglenoid tubercle of the scapula.
   - **Lateral head of the triceps brachii muscle** attaches to the posterior surface of the humerus superior to the radial groove.
   - **Medial head of the triceps brachii muscle** attaches to the posterior surface of the humerus inferior to the radial groove.
5. Observe the distal attachment of the triceps brachii tendon on the olecranon of the ulna. The triceps brachii muscle extends the forearm.

6. Use your fingers to separate the **long head of the triceps brachii** from the **lateral head**. Observe that the teres major muscle crosses the anterior surface of the long head.
7. Inferior to the teres major muscle is an opening between the long head of the triceps brachii muscle and lateral head of the triceps brachii muscle (Fig. 2.18). Use a probe to widen this opening and identify the **radial nerve** and the **deep artery of the arm**.

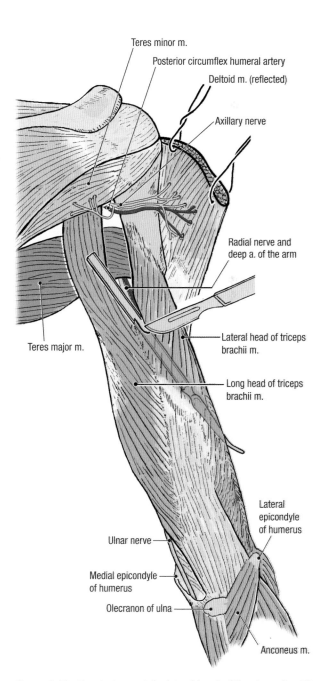

Figure 2.18. How to transect the lateral head of the triceps brachii muscle.

8. Push a probe distally along the course of the radial nerve. The probe should be positioned between the lateral head of the triceps brachii muscle and the humerus (Fig. 2.18).

9. Use a scalpel to transect the lateral head of the triceps brachii muscle over the probe. This cut will separate the lateral head of the triceps brachii muscle from the medial head.

10. Use a probe to clean the radial nerve and the deep artery of the arm. Observe that the radial nerve and deep artery of the arm lie directly on the posterior surface of the humerus in the **radial groove**.

11. Confirm the course of the radial nerve through the posterior compartment to the elbow. To do this, return to the cubital fossa. On the lateral aspect of the forearm, identify the **brachioradialis muscle**. Use your fingers to open the connective tissue plane between the brachioradialis muscle and the brachialis muscle. Deep in this plane of connective tissue, find the radial nerve and follow it proximally.

12. Note that the radial nerve passes on the flexor side of the elbow joint and that it is accompanied by the radial recurrent artery at that location (Fig. 2.16).

13. Identify the **anconeus muscle** (Fig. 2.18). The proximal attachment of the anconeus muscle is the lateral epicondyle of the humerus. The distal attachment is the lateral surface of the olecranon and superior part of the posterior surface of the ulna. The anconeus muscle assists the triceps brachii muscle in extension of the forearm.

Dissection Review

1. Replace the muscles of the anterior and posterior compartments of the arm in their correct anatomical positions.

2. Review the proximal attachment, distal attachment, nerve, and action of each muscle.

3. Use the dissected specimen to review the origin, course, termination, and branches of the brachial artery.

4. Trace each nerve that you have dissected from the brachial plexus to the elbow, reviewing relationships.

5. Review a drawing of a cross section of the arm and notice the position of the brachial fascia and the intermuscular septa relative to the structures that you have dissected.

6. Review the nerve territories of the brachial region (Fig. 2.19).

7. Recall the rules of innervation of the muscles of the arm:

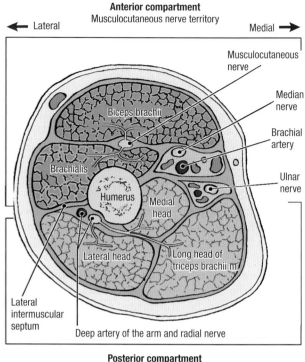

Anterior compartment
Musculocutaneous nerve territory

← Lateral   Medial →

Posterior compartment
Radial nerve territory

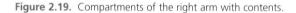

Figure 2.19. Compartments of the right arm with contents.

- **All muscles in the anterior compartment of the arm are innervated by the musculocutaneous nerve.** [L 76]
- **All muscles in the posterior compartment of the arm are innervated by the radial nerve.** [L 79]
- *The median nerve and the ulnar nerve do not innervate muscles in the arm.*

FLEXOR REGION OF THE FOREARM

Dissection Overview

The antebrachial fascia is a sleeve of connective tissue that invests the forearm. Intermuscular septa project inward from it and attach the antebrachial fascia to the radius and ulna (Fig. 2.20). The intermuscular septa, the interosseous membrane, the radius, and the ulna combine to divide the forearm into an **anterior (flexor) compartment** and a **posterior (extensor) compartment**.

The muscles in the anterior compartment of the forearm can be divided into a **superficial group of flexor muscles** and a **deep group of flexor muscles**. Muscles of the superficial flexor group arise primarily from the medial epicondyle of the humerus and its supracondylar ridge. Muscles of the deep flexor group arise from the anterior surfaces of the radius, ulna, and interosseous membrane. Study a transverse section through the midlevel of the forearm (Fig. 2.20). Note that the ulnar artery, ulnar nerve,

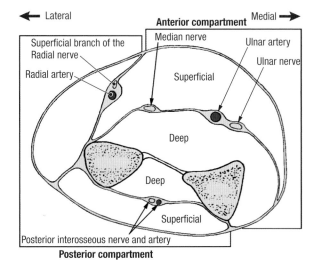

Figure 2.20. Compartments of the right forearm.

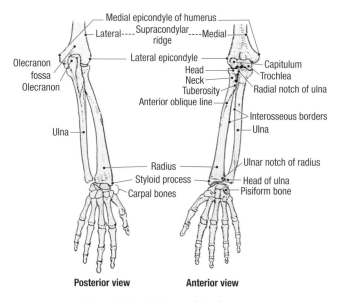

Figure 2.21. Skeleton of the forearm.

and median nerve are in a connective tissue plane that separates the superficial flexor group from the deep flexor group.

SKELETON OF THE FOREARM [G 552, 574; L 33; N 436, 439; R 373, 374; C 77, 84]

Refer to a skeleton. On the **humerus**, identify (Fig. 2.21):

- **Medial epicondyle**
- **Medial supracondylar ridge**
- **Lateral epicondyle**
- **Lateral supracondylar ridge**
- **Capitulum**
- **Trochlea**
- **Olecranon fossa**

On the **radius**, identify (Fig. 2.21):

- **Head**
- **Neck**
- **Tuberosity**
- **Anterior oblique line**
- **Ulnar notch**
- **Styloid process**
- **Interosseous border** for attachment of the **interosseous membrane**

On the **ulna**, identify (Fig. 2.21):

- **Olecranon**
- **Trochlear notch**
- **Radial notch**
- **Head**
- **Interosseous border** for attachment of the interosseous membrane

On the palmar surface of the articulated hand, identify the **pisiform bone** (Fig. 2.21).

On the skeleton, examine the **elbow joint**. The elbow joint is the articulation between the trochlear notch of the

ulna and the trochlea of the humerus, and the articulation between the head of the radius and the capitulum of the humerus. These two articulations account for the hinge action of the elbow joint.

Observe the **proximal radioulnar joint** between the head of the radius and the radial notch of the ulna. Observe the **distal radioulnar joint** between the head of the ulna and the ulnar notch of the radius. Pronate and supinate the hand of the skeleton and notice the rotational movements that occur in the proximal and distal radioulnar joints. In the position of supination (anatomical position), the radius and the ulna are parallel. In the position of pronation, the radius crosses the ulna.

The order of dissection will be as follows: The structures in the superficial fascia will be reviewed and the antebrachial fascia will be removed. At the level of the wrist, the relative positions of tendons, vessels, and nerves will be studied. The superficial group of flexor muscles will be studied and then reflected. Vessels and nerves that lie between the superficial and deep groups of flexor muscles will be studied. The deep group of flexor muscles will be dissected.

Dissection Instructions

SUPERFICIAL GROUP OF FLEXOR MUSCLES [G 554, 555; L 52; N 446; R 422; C 46]

1. Place the cadaver in the supine position and abduct the upper limb. Forcefully supinate the hand and have your dissection partner hold it in this position.
2. Use blunt dissection to remove the remnants of the superficial fascia, taking care to preserve the cephalic and basilic veins.

3. Use scissors to incise the anterior surface of the antebrachial fascia from the cubital fossa to the wrist. Use your fingers or a probe to separate the antebrachial fascia from the muscles that lie deep to it. Detach the antebrachial fascia from its attachments to the radius and ulna and place it in the tissue container.

4. Use blunt dissection to clean the **superficial group of flexor muscles**. There are five muscles in this group: **pronator teres, flexor carpi radialis, palmaris longus, flexor carpi ulnaris**, and **flexor digitorum superficialis**. The flexor digitorum superficialis muscle is located deep to the other four muscles in this group.

5. Note that part of the proximal attachment of the superficial group of flexor muscles is from a **common flexor tendon**. The common flexor tendon is attached to the medial epicondyle of the humerus.

6. Note the distal attachment and action of each muscle of the superficial group of flexors:
    -   **Pronator teres muscle** attaches to the middle of the lateral surface of the radius. The pronator teres muscle pronates the hand and flexes the forearm.
    -   **Flexor carpi radialis tendon** attaches to the base of the second metacarpal bone. The flexor carpi radialis muscle flexes and abducts the hand.
    -   **Palmaris longus tendon** attaches to the palmar aponeurosis. The palmaris longus muscle flexes the hand.
    -   **Flexor carpi ulnaris tendon** attaches to the pisiform bone, the hamate bone, and the base of the fifth metacarpal bone. The flexor carpi ulnaris muscle flexes and adducts the hand.
    -   **Flexor digitorum superficialis tendon** attaches to the middle phalanx of digits 2 to 5. The flexor digitorum superficialis muscle flexes the middle phalanx of digits 2 to 5.

7. Use your fingers to separate the tendons of the superficial group of flexor muscles. Note that the muscle bellies cannot be easily separated from each other. From lateral to medial, identify the superficial structures at the wrist (Fig. 2.22): [G 558, 559; L 52; N 446; R 422; C 46]
    -   Tendon of the **abductor pollicis longus muscle**
    -   **Radial artery**
    -   Tendon of the **flexor carpi radialis muscle**
    -   **Median nerve**
    -   Tendon of the **palmaris longus muscle** (absent in 13% of limbs)
    -   Four tendons of the **flexor digitorum superficialis muscle**

-   **Ulnar artery** and **ulnar nerve**
-   Tendon of the **flexor carpi ulnaris muscle**

8. Palpate the tendons listed above in your own wrist. Feel the pulse of the radial artery between the abductor pollicis longus and flexor carpi radialis tendons. The median nerve is superficial at the wrist and can be easily injured. Palpate the distal attachment of the flexor carpi ulnaris tendon on the pisiform bone. Palpate the ulnar nerve and artery, which lie immediately lateral to the pisiform bone.

VESSELS AND NERVES [G 556; L 53, 54; N 447; R 422; C 50]

1. On the lateral side of the proximal forearm, identify the **brachioradialis muscle**. At the point where the pronator teres muscle passes deep to the brachioradialis muscle, use your fingers to open the connective tissue plane that is medial to the brachioradialis muscle. In this intermuscular plane, identify the **superficial branch of the ra-**

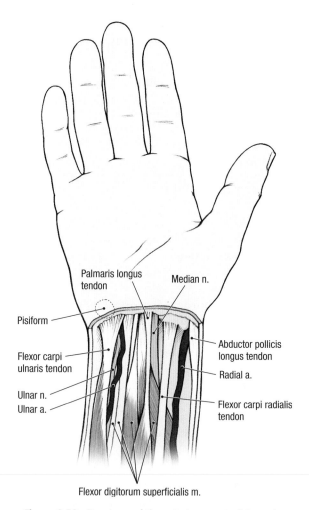

Figure 2.22. Structures of the anterior aspect of the wrist.

dial nerve, which courses distally on the deep surface of the brachioradialis muscle. Trace the superficial branch of the radial nerve to the distal one-third of the forearm and confirm that it emerges on the dorsal side of the brachioradialis tendon to become a cutaneous nerve.

2. Once again, identify the **brachial artery** in the cubital fossa. Use blunt dissection to trace the brachial artery distally until it bifurcates into the **radial artery** and the **ulnar artery**.

CLINICAL CORRELATION

High Bifurcation of the Brachial Artery

In about 3% of upper limbs, the brachial artery bifurcates in the arm. When it does, the ulnar artery may course superficial to the superficial group of flexor muscles. When this happens, the ulnar artery may be mistaken for a vein. When certain drugs are injected into an artery, the capillary bed is damaged, followed by gangrene. In the example of an injection into a superficial ulnar artery, the hand could be severely injured.

---

3. Use a probe to clean the radial artery and follow it distally to the level of the wrist. The radial vein and its tributaries may be removed to clear the dissection field. The radial artery gives rise to several unnamed muscular branches in the forearm.

4. Find the **radial recurrent artery,** which arises from the radial artery near its origin from the brachial artery. The radial recurrent artery courses proximally in the connective tissue plane between the brachioradialis muscle and the brachialis muscle. The radial recurrent artery anastomoses with the radial collateral branch of the deep artery of the arm. The radial recurrent artery is part of the anastomotic network around the elbow (Fig. 2.17).

5. Identify the **median nerve** in the cubital fossa. It is medial to the brachial artery. The median nerve innervates most of the muscles of the flexor compartment of the forearm.

6. Follow the median nerve distally. The median nerve courses deep to the superficial group of flexor muscles. To expose the median nerve, use scissors to cut the tendon of the palmaris longus muscle about 3 cm proximal to the wrist and reflect the muscle belly proximally. Cut the tendon of the flexor carpi radialis muscle about 5 cm proximal to the wrist and reflect it proximally.

7. Insert a probe through the pronator teres muscle along the anterior surface of the median nerve. Use scissors to cut the portion of the pronator teres muscle that lies anterior to the median nerve. Use a probe to release the median nerve and follow it distally.

8. Observe that the median nerve passes deep to the flexor digitorum superficialis muscle. Use scissors to detach the flexor digitorum superficialis muscle from its proximal attachment on the radius. Retract the muscle medially, leaving its ulnar and humeral attachments undisturbed.

9. Use a probe to free the median nerve from the loose connective tissue that lies between the superficial and deep groups of forearm flexor muscles (Fig. 2.20). Observe that the median nerve innervates the palmaris longus, flexor carpi radialis, flexor digitorum superficialis, and pronator teres muscles.

10. Find the **ulnar artery** in the cubital fossa. The ulnar artery passes posterior to the deep part of the pronator teres muscle. To follow the ulnar artery distally, release it from the pronator teres muscle by inserting a probe through the pronator teres muscle along the anterior surface of the ulnar artery (posterior to the deep part of the pronator teres muscle). Use scissors to cut the deep part of the pronator teres muscle. The pronator teres muscle is now completely transected and it may be reflected to broaden the dissection field.

11. Use a probe to clean the ulnar artery and follow it from the cubital fossa to the wrist. The ulnar vein and its tributaries may be removed to clear the dissection field. Observe that the median nerve crosses anterior to the ulnar artery in the cubital fossa. Note that the ulnar artery passes between the flexor digitorum superficialis and the flexor digitorum profundus muscles to reach the ulnar (medial) side of the forearm.

12. Find the **common interosseous artery**. It arises about 3 cm distal to the origin of the ulnar artery from the brachial artery. The common interosseous artery is usually quite short. It passes posterolaterally toward the interosseous membrane before dividing into the **anterior interosseous artery** and the **posterior interosseous artery**.

13. Identify the **anterior interosseous artery** on the anterior surface of the interosseous membrane. The anterior interosseous artery supplies the deep group of flexor muscles.

14. The **posterior interosseous artery** passes posteriorly over the proximal end of the interosseous membrane to reach the posterior compartment of the forearm. The posterior interosseous artery

supplies the extensor group of forearm muscles. Identify it, but do not attempt to follow it into the posterior compartment at this time.

15. Two other named vessels arise from the ulnar artery in the proximal forearm: **anterior ulnar recurrent artery** and **posterior ulnar recurrent artery**. They anastomose with the inferior and superior ulnar collateral branches of the brachial artery, respectively (Fig. 2.17). Do not attempt to find these vessels. Note that unnamed muscular branches arise from the ulnar artery in the forearm.

16. Observe that the ulnar artery joins the **ulnar nerve** about one-third of the way down the forearm.

17. Follow the ulnar nerve proximally and observe that it passes between the two heads of the flexor carpi ulnaris muscle. The ulnar nerve innervates the flexor carpi ulnaris muscle and the medial one-half of the flexor digitorum profundus muscle.

DEEP GROUP OF FLEXOR MUSCLES [G 557; L 54; N 448; R 423; C 51]

1. Three muscles comprise the **deep group of flexor muscles**: **flexor digitorum profundus**, **flexor pollicis longus**, and **pronator quadratus**.

2. The proximal attachment of the **flexor digitorum profundus muscle** is the anterior surface of the ulna and interosseous membrane. Its four tendons lie deep to the four tendons of the flexor digitorum superficialis muscle. Distally, the flexor digitorum profundus tendons attach to the distal phalanx of digits 2 to 5. The flexor digitorum profundus muscle flexes the distal phalanx of digits 2 to 5. The lateral one-half of the flexor digitorum profundus muscle is innervated by the median nerve. The medial one-half of the flexor digitorum profundus muscle is innervated by the ulnar nerve.

3. The proximal attachment of the **flexor pollicis longus muscle** is the anterior surface of the radius and interosseous membrane. The distal attachment of the flexor pollicis longus tendon is the distal phalanx of digit 1 (thumb). The flexor pollicis longus muscle flexes digit 1.

4. The **pronator quadratus muscle** lies deep to the tendons of the superficial and deep flexor muscles. The fibers of the pronator quadratus muscle run transversely from the ulna to the radius in the distal one-fourth of the forearm. Retract the tendons of the superficial and deep groups of flexor muscles and find the pronator quadratus muscle. The pronator quadratus muscle pronates the hand.

5. Observe that the **anterior interosseous artery and nerve** pass deep to the pronator quadratus muscle.

Dissection Review

1. Replace the flexor muscles in their correct anatomical positions.

2. Use the dissected specimen to review the proximal attachment, distal attachment, and action of each muscle dissected.

3. Organize the flexor muscles into a superficial group and a deep group and recall that the nerves and vessels that course through the forearm are found between the two groups.

4. Follow the brachial artery from its origin in the proximal arm to its bifurcation in the cubital fossa.

5. Review all of the branches of the radial and ulnar arteries. Trace the course of these two arteries from the elbow to the wrist.

6. Review the course of the median nerve from the brachial plexus to the wrist.

7. Review the course of the ulnar nerve from the brachial plexus to the wrist.

8. Recall the rule for innervation of the muscles in the anterior compartment of the forearm:

   • **All muscles of the anterior compartment of the forearm are innervated by the median nerve** *except the flexor carpi ulnaris muscle and the medial one-half of the flexor digitorum profundus muscle, which are innervated by the ulnar nerve.*[L 77, 78]

PALM OF THE HAND

Dissection Overview

By definition, **intrinsic hand muscles** are muscles that have their proximal and distal attachments within the hand. There are two superficial groups of intrinsic hand muscles: The **thenar group of muscles** forms the **thenar eminence**, and the **hypothenar group of muscles** forms the **hypothenar eminence**. Deep in the hand is a third group of intrinsic hand muscles: the interosseous muscles and the adductor pollicis muscle.

In the middle of the palm, the palmar fascia is thickened to form the palmar aponeurosis. The palmar fascia over the thenar and hypothenar eminences is much thinner. Deep to the palmar aponeurosis are the tendons of the flexor digitorum superficialis and flexor digitorum profundus muscles. These tendons reach the palm through the carpal tunnel and are responsible for flexing the digits. In the deepest part of the palm are muscles that abduct and adduct the digits.

The palm is supplied with blood by two arterial arches. The superficial palmar arch is mainly derived from the ulnar artery and the deep palmar arch from the radial artery. The nerve supply of the palmar aspect of the hand is derived from the median and ulnar nerves.

The order of dissection will be as follows: The palmar aponeurosis will be studied and removed. The superficial palmar arch will be dissected, followed by the tendons of the muscles of the anterior compartment of the forearm. The flexor retinaculum will be cut and the flexor tendons will be released from the palm. The muscles of the thenar group will be dissected, followed by the muscles of the hypothenar group. The deep palmar arch will be dissected along with the deep branch of the ulnar nerve. The interosseous muscles will be studied.

SKELETON OF THE HAND [G 552, 554; L 60, 61; N 456; R 376, 377; C 90, 91]

Refer to an articulated skeleton of the hand and identify (Fig. 2.23):

- **Eight carpal bones** (Gr. *karpos*, wrist)
- **Five metacarpal bones**
- **14 phalanges**

Be able to identify the eight carpal bones in an articulated skeleton. Digit 1 (thumb) has two phalanges: proximal and distal. Digits 2 to 5 (fingers) have three phalanges: proximal, middle, and distal.

Identify the **pisiform bone** and the **hook of the hamate** on the medial side of the wrist. On the lateral side of the wrist, identify the **tubercle of the scaphoid** and the **tubercle of the trapezium**. The **flexor retinaculum** bridges these four bones (Fig. 2.24). The space between the carpal bones and the flexor retinaculum is the **carpal tunnel**, which allows passage of the flexor tendons and the median nerve into the hand.

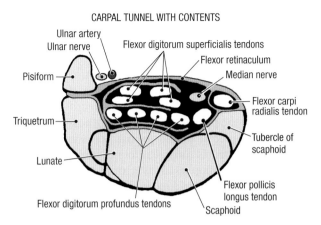

Figure 2.24. Transverse section through the left carpal tunnel.

Dissection Instructions

SKIN INCISIONS

1. Refer to Figure 2.25.
2. Force open the clenched hand and let your dissection partner hold it open.
3. Make a longitudinal incision across the palm (E to M).
4. Make a transverse incision at the level of the webs of the fingers (N to O).
5. Make a longitudinal incision on the anterior surface of digits 2 to 5 (from incision N/O to P).
6. Make a longitudinal incision along the palmar surface of the thumb (E to Q).
7. Remove the skin from the palmar and dorsal surfaces of the hand and digits 1 to 5. *When skinning the digits, proceed with caution.* Note that the subcutaneous tissue on the palmar surface of the digits is very thin, especially at the skin creases. There are digital nerves, vessels, and fibrous digital sheaths immediately deep to the skin.

SUPERFICIAL PALM [G 561; L 62; N 459, 460; R 426; C 64, 65]

1. Use scraping motions with a dull scalpel blade to clean the fat from the **palmar aponeurosis**. Observe that the palmar aponeurosis has four

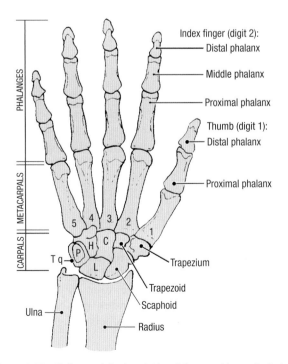

Figure 2.23. Skeleton of the hand. The eight carpal bones include a proximal row of four bones (scaphoid; lunate, *L*; triquetrum, *Tq*; pisiform, *P*) and a distal row of four bones (trapezium; trapezoid; capitate, *C*; hamate, *H*).

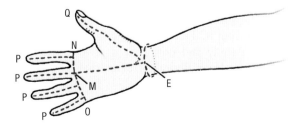

Figure 2.25. Skin incisions.

bands of **longitudinal fibers**, one band to each of digits 2 to 5. These longitudinal fibers end by attaching to the fibrous digital sheath near the base of the proximal phalanx of each digit.

2. Identify the palmar fascia covering the **thenar muscles** lateral to the palmar aponeurosis.

3. Identify the palmar fascia covering the hypothenar muscles medial to the palmar aponeurosis. The **palmaris brevis muscle** is found superficial to the hypothenar muscles. It is a thin, fragile muscle. The proximal attachment of the palmaris brevis muscle is the medial aspect of the palmar aponeurosis. Its distal attachment is the skin over the hypothenar eminence.

4. Detach the palmaris brevis muscle from the palmar aponeurosis and reflect it medially.

5. Find the tendon of the **palmaris longus muscle** where you transected it in the forearm. Follow the palmaris longus tendon distally into the palm where it is attached to the palmar aponeurosis. Although the palmaris longus muscle may be absent, the palmar aponeurosis is always present.

6. To remove the palmar aponeurosis, use a scalpel and skinning motions to detach the palmar aponeurosis from the underlying deep structures. Begin at its proximal end and proceed distally. Use the palmaris longus tendon to apply traction to the palmar aponeurosis during its removal. Do not cut too deeply, as the superficial palmar arch is in contact with the deep surface of the palmar aponeurosis.

7. Near the proximal end of digits 2 to 5, remove each band of longitudinal fibers of the palmar aponeurosis. Use blunt dissection to clean the **fibrous digital sheath** on the flexor surface of digit 3 (Fig. 2.26).

8. Find the **ulnar artery** in the forearm. Use a probe to dissect the ulnar artery and follow it into the palm. The ulnar artery passes lateral to the pisiform bone with the ulnar nerve, then divides into a **superficial branch** and a **deep palmar branch.** The superficial branch of the ulnar artery crosses the palm to form the **superficial palmar arch.** The superficial palmar arch is completed by a smaller contribution from the **superficial palmar branch of the radial artery** (Fig. 2.27). [G 566; L 63; N 460; R 426; C 70]

9. Use a probe to clean the superficial palmar arch and the three **common palmar digital arteries** arising from it. Trace one common palmar digital artery distally and note that it divides into two **proper palmar digital arteries** that supply the adjacent sides of two digits.

10. Find the **ulnar nerve** lateral to the pisiform bone. Use a probe to dissect the **superficial branch of**

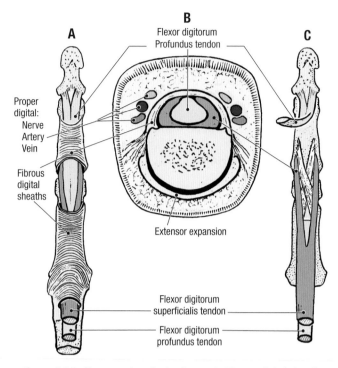

Figure 2.26. Flexor tendons in the finger. **A.** Fibrous digital sheath showing the two osseofibrous tunnels. **B.** Transverse section of a finger showing the fibrous digital sheath surrounding the flexor tendons. **C.** Distal attachment of the flexor tendons.

the ulnar nerve, which supplies cutaneous innervation to digit 5 and the medial side of digit 4. The **deep branch of the ulnar nerve** disappears into the hypothenar muscles. Identify the initial portion of the deep branch of the ulnar nerve but do not follow it at this time.

CARPAL TUNNEL [G 567; L 63, 65; N 461; R 429; C 67]

1. Identify the **flexor retinaculum** between the thenar and hypothenar eminences (Fig. 2.27). Use an illustration to review the flexor retinaculum and its role in the formation of the **carpal tunnel** (Fig. 2.24).

2. Insert a probe from proximal to distal, deep to the flexor retinaculum (Fig. 2.28). Use a scalpel to cut through the flexor retinaculum to the probe. Open the carpal tunnel.

3. Examine the **contents of the carpal tunnel**: **median nerve, four tendons of the flexor digitorum superficialis muscle, four tendons of the flexor digitorum profundus muscle,** and the **tendon of the flexor pollicis longus muscle** (Fig. 2.24).

4. Find the median nerve at the level of the wrist and follow it through the carpal tunnel. Identify the **recurrent branch of the median nerve,** which

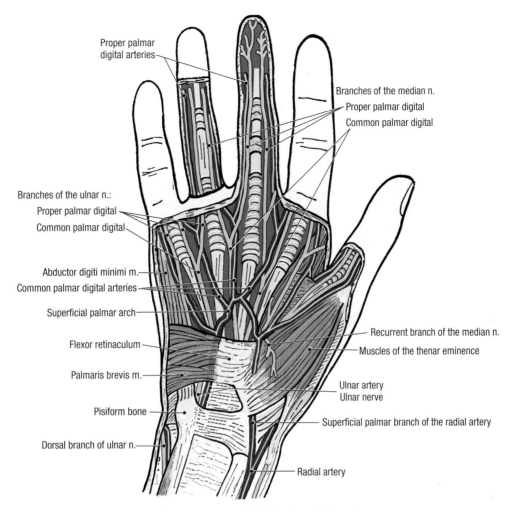

Proper palmar digital arteries

Branches of the median n.
Proper palmar digital
Common palmar digital

Branches of the ulnar n.:
Proper palmar digital
Common palmar digital

Abductor digiti minimi m.
Common palmar digital arteries
Superficial palmar arch
Flexor retinaculum
Palmaris brevis m.
Pisiform bone
Dorsal branch of ulnar n.

Recurrent branch of the median n.
Muscles of the thenar eminence
Ulnar artery
Ulnar nerve
Superficial palmar branch of the radial artery
Radial artery

Figure 2.27. Superficial dissection of the palm.

innervates the three thenar muscles (Fig. 2.28). The median nerve also innervates **lumbrical muscles 1 and 2**.

5. Follow the **common palmar digital branches** of the median nerve into the lateral 3½ digits (Fig. 2.27). Note that the common palmar digital nerves typically divide to give rise to two **proper palmar digital nerves**, which accompany the proper palmar digital arteries. Use an illustration to study the cutaneous distribution of the median nerve in the hand. [G 579; L 62; N 472; R 423; C 26]

6. Identify the flexor tendons that pass through the carpal tunnel. Observe that these tendons pass through the palm of the hand posterior to the superficial palmar arch and digital nerves. The flexor tendons enter the **fibrous digital sheaths** on the anterior surfaces of the digits (Fig. 2.26).

7. Use an illustration to study the extent of the synovial tendon sheaths deep to the flexor retinaculum and extending into the palm. There are two sets of synovial sheaths: one **common flexor syn-** ovial sheath (ulnar bursa) and three **digital synovial sheaths**. The tendon of the flexor pollicis longus muscle has it own synovial sheath (**radial bursa**). [G 568; L 65; N 462, 463; R 392, 393; C 65]

CLINICAL CORRELATION

Carpal Tunnel Syndrome

A swelling of the common flexor synovial sheath may encroach on the available space in the carpal tunnel. As a result, the median nerve may be compressed, resulting in pain and paresthesia of the thumb and index and middle fingers, and weakness of the thenar muscles.

8. In the distal forearm, use your fingers to separate the tendons of the **flexor digitorum superficialis muscle** from the tendons of the **flexor digitorum**

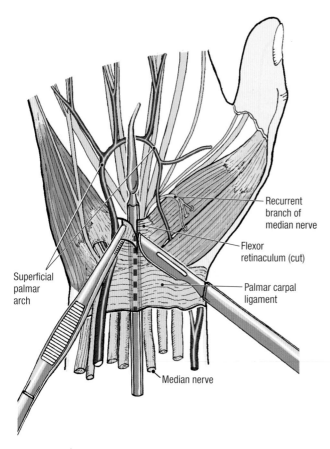

Figure 2.28. How to open the carpal tunnel.

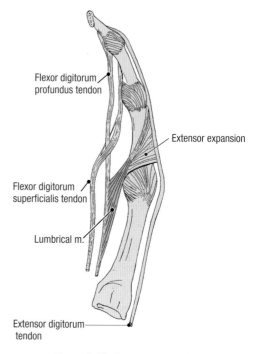

Figure 2.29. Extensor expansion.

profundus muscle. About 5 cm proximal to the wrist, use scissors to transect the tendons of the flexor digitorum superficialis muscle. Reflect the tendons distally, pulling them through the carpal tunnel. During this procedure, the common flexor synovial sheath will be destroyed. To reflect the tendons even further, cut the superficial palmar arch in the midline of the palm, retract the common digital branches of the median and ulnar nerves, and make a longitudinal slit in the fibrous digital sheaths of digits 2 to 5.

9. In the palm, observe the tendons of the **flexor digitorum profundus muscle**. Identify four **lumbrical muscles** that are attached to the four tendons of the flexor digitorum profundus muscle. The distal attachment of the lumbrical muscles is the radial side of the **extensor expansions** of digits 2 to 5 (Fig. 2.29). The lumbrical muscles flex the metacarpophalangeal joints and extend the interphalangeal joints.

10. In digit 3, study the **relationship of the tendons of the flexor digitorum superficialis** and **flexor digitorum profundus muscles** (Fig. 2.29). Note that the flexor digitorum profundus tendon passes through the flexor digitorum superficialis tendon. Verify that the flexor digitorum superficialis ten-

don attaches to the middle phalanx, whereas the flexor digitorum profundus tendon attaches to the distal phalanx. This pattern is true of digits 2 to 5.

11. Identify the **flexor pollicis longus muscle** in the forearm. Follow its tendon distally through the carpal tunnel into the palm. Pull on the tendon to confirm that the flexor pollicis longus muscle attaches to the distal phalanx of the thumb.

THENAR MUSCLES [G 568, 570; L 63; N 465; R 426; C 66, 67]

1. Use blunt dissection to clean the palmar fascia off the thenar muscles. Preserve the recurrent branch of the median nerve.

2. The thenar group contains three muscles: **abductor pollicis brevis**, **flexor pollicis brevis**, and **opponens pollicis** (L. *pollex*, thumb; genitive, *pollicis*). The proximal attachments of the thenar muscles are the scaphoid, trapezium, and flexor retinaculum.
   - **Abductor pollicis brevis muscle** attaches to the lateral side of the proximal phalanx of the thumb and abducts the thumb.
   - **Flexor pollicis brevis muscle** attaches to the lateral side of the proximal phalanx of the thumb and flexes the thumb.
   - **Opponens pollicis muscle** attaches to the lateral side of the shaft of the first metacarpal bone and opposes the thumb.

3. Observe the **recurrent branch of the median nerve**. The recurrent branch of the median nerve

crosses the superficial surface of the flexor pollicis brevis muscle, then disappears deep to the abductor pollicis brevis muscle.

4. Use a probe to separate the abductor pollicis brevis muscle from the flexor pollicis brevis muscle. Use the recurrent branch of the median nerve to help you locate the correct plane of separation.

5. Use a probe to elevate the abductor pollicis brevis muscle and transect it with scissors.

6. Observe the **opponens pollicis muscle** deep to the abductor pollicis brevis muscle. Note that the opponens pollicis muscle attaches to the lateral side of the entire length of the shaft of the first metacarpal bone.

CLINICAL CORRELATION

Recurrent Branch of the Median Nerve

The recurrent branch of the median nerve is superficial and it can easily be severed by "minor" cuts over the thenar eminence. If the recurrent branch of the median nerve is injured, the thenar muscles are paralyzed and the thumb cannot be opposed.

HYPOTHENAR MUSCLES [G 568, 570; L 63, 64; N 465; R 426; C 66, 67]

1. Use blunt dissection to clean the palmar fascia off the hypothenar muscles. The hypothenar group contains three muscles: **abductor digiti minimi, flexor digiti minimi brevis**, and **opponens digiti minimi**. The proximal attachments of the hypothenar muscles are the pisiform, hamate, and flexor retinaculum.
   - **Abductor digiti minimi muscle** attaches to the medial side of the base of the proximal phalanx of digit 5 and abducts digit 5.
   - **Flexor digiti minimi brevis muscle** attaches to the medial side of the base of the proximal phalanx of digit 5 and flexes digit 5.
   - **Opponens digiti minimi muscle** attaches to the medial border of the fifth metacarpal bone and opposes digit 5.

2. Find the tendons of the abductor digiti minimi and flexor digiti minimi brevis muscles near their distal attachments on the base of the proximal phalanx. Use a probe to separate and define the borders of the muscles using their tendons to aid in this separation.

3. Use a probe to elevate the abductor digiti minimi brevis muscle and detach it from its proximal at-

tachment on the flexor retinaculum. Preserve the deep branches of the ulnar artery and ulnar nerve. Reflect the muscle distally.

4. Observe the **opponens digiti minimi muscle**. Note that the opponens digiti minimi muscle attaches to the entire length of the shaft of the fifth metacarpal bone.

DEEP PALM [G 570, 571; L 64; N 465, 466; R 426; C 71]

1. Transect the flexor digitorum profundus muscle in the distal one-third of the forearm. Reflect its tendons and the associated lumbrical muscles distally as far as possible. The deep palm is now exposed.

2. Find the ulnar nerve and the ulnar artery on the lateral side of the pisiform bone.

3. The **deep branch of the ulnar nerve** and the **deep palmar branch of the ulnar artery** pass between the proximal attachments of the flexor digiti minimi brevis and abductor digiti minimi muscles.

4. Push a probe parallel to the deep branch of the ulnar nerve where it pierces the opponens digiti minimi muscle. Use a scalpel to cut down to the probe. Use blunt dissection to follow the deep branch of the ulnar nerve into the palm.

5. Observe that the deep branch of the ulnar nerve lies on the anterior surface of the interosseous muscles (Fig. 2.30A).

6. Observe the **deep palmar arch.** The deep palmar arch courses with the deep branch of the ulnar nerve. The deep palmar arch arises from the **radial artery**. The deep palmar arch is completed by the deep branch of the ulnar artery. Use an illustration to study the branches of the deep palmar arch.

7. Identify the **adductor pollicis muscle** (Fig 2.30A). Use blunt dissection to define its borders. The adductor pollicis muscle has two heads: **oblique** and **transverse**. The proximal attachments of the oblique head are the bases of metacarpal bones 2 and 3 and the adjacent carpal bones. The proximal attachment of the transverse head is the anterior surface of the shaft of metacarpal bone 3. Both heads attach to the medial side of the base of the proximal phalanx of the thumb. The adductor pollicis muscle draws the thumb toward digit 3 (adduction).

8. Use an illustration to study the three **palmar interosseous muscles** (Fig. 2.30A). The palmar interosseous muscles are unipennate muscles that attach to the metacarpal bones of digits 2, 4, and 5. Distally, each palmar interosseous muscle attaches to the base of the proximal phalanx and the extensor expansion of the same digit on which it origi-

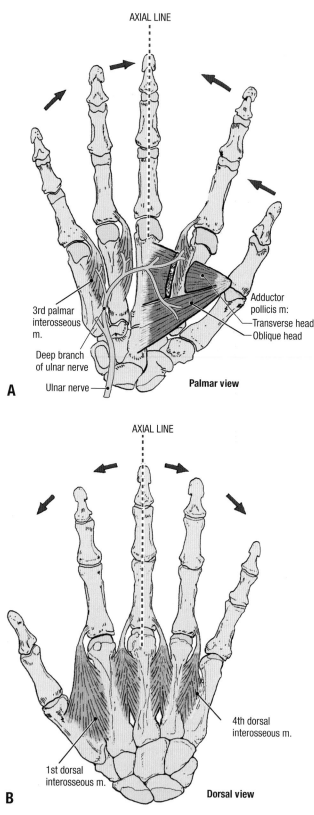

AXIAL LINE

3rd palmar interosseous m.

Deep branch of ulnar nerve

Ulnar nerve

Adductor pollicis m:
- Transverse head
- Oblique head

A **Palmar view**

AXIAL LINE

4th dorsal interosseous m.

1st dorsal interosseous m.

B **Dorsal view**

Figure 2.30. A. The three unipennate **P**almar interosseous muscles **AD**duct (**PAD**) the fingers (arrows) in relation to the axial line. **B.** The four bipennate **D**orsal interosseous muscles **AB**duct (**DAB**) the fingers (arrows).

nates. Do not attempt to dissect these muscles. [G 565; L 64; N 465; R 430; C 68]

9. Use an illustration to study the four **dorsal interosseous muscles** (Fig. 2.30B). The dorsal interosseous muscles are bipennate muscles that attach to metacarpal bones 1 to 5. Distally, the dorsal interosseous muscles attach to the bases of the proximal phalanges and the extensor expansions of digits 2 to 4. Look at the dorsum of the dissected hand and note that the dorsal interosseous muscles occupy the intervals between the metacarpal bones. Do not dissect these muscles.

10. Study the actions of the interosseous muscles (Fig. 2.30A, B). The three **P**almar interosseous muscles are **AD**ductors (**PAD**). They adduct digits 2, 4, and 5 toward an imaginary axial line drawn through the long axis of digit 3. The four **D**orsal interosseous muscles are **AB**ductors (**DAB**). They move digits 2 to 4 away from the imaginary axial line. The two dorsal interosseous muscles that attach to digit 3 move it to either side of the imaginary axial line. The interosseous muscles are innervated by the deep branch of the ulnar nerve.

Dissection Review

1. Place the muscles, tendons, and nerves that you have dissected back into their correct anatomical positions.
2. Review the movements of the fingers and thumb. Define flexion, extension, abduction, and adduction. Review the muscles that are responsible for each action.
3. Use the dissected specimen to follow the median nerve from the forearm into the hand. Review its recurrent branch and list the five muscles that the recurrent branch innervates.
4. Follow the ulnar artery from the elbow to the hand. In the hand, trace the superficial branch and deep palmar branch of the ulnar artery.
5. Follow the ulnar nerve from the medial epicondyle of the humerus to the hand. In the hand, trace the superficial and deep branches of the ulnar nerve.
6. Review an illustration that demonstrates the cutaneous distribution of the ulnar and median nerves in the hand.
7. Recall the rule for innervation of the muscles in the hand:

- **All intrinsic muscles of the hand are innervated by the ulnar nerve** *except the muscles of the thenar group and the first two lumbrical muscles, which are innervated by the median nerve.* [L 77, 78; N 472; R 400; C 27]

EXTENSOR REGION OF THE FOREARM AND DORSUM OF THE HAND

Dissection Overview

The posterior compartment of the forearm contains the extensor muscles of the hand and digits. They can be divided into a superficial group and a deep group (Fig. 2.20). The muscles of the superficial group extend the wrist and the proximal phalanges. The muscles of the deep group of extensors cause supination of the hand, extension of digit 2, and abduction and extension of the thumb. The deep branch of the radial nerve innervates the extensor muscles of the forearm. Nerves and vessels of the posterior compartment run in the connective tissue plane that divides the superficial group of extensor muscles from the deep group of extensor muscles (Fig. 2.20).

In the dorsum of the hand, the bones are superficial. There are no intrinsic muscles in the dorsum of the hand, so no motor innervation is required. The radial, ulnar, and median nerves share the cutaneous innervation of the dorsum of the hand.

The order of dissection will be as follows: The antebrachial fascia will be removed from the elbow to the wrist. The muscles of the superficial extensor group will be identified and followed to their distal attachments in the hand. The tendons of the superficial extensor muscles will be released from the extensor retinaculum and retracted to permit the muscles of the deep extensor group to be studied. The contents of the anatomical snuffbox will be identified.

Dissection Instructions

SUPERFICIAL GROUP OF EXTENSOR MUSCLES [G 576; L 58; N 444; R 417; C 54]

1. Place the cadaver in the supine position.
2. Use blunt dissection to remove the remnants of the superficial fascia from the posterior forearm and dorsum of the hand, taking care to preserve the dorsal venous arch.
3. Identify the **extensor retinaculum**, which is a specialization of the antebrachial fascia located on the posterior surface of the distal forearm.
4. Use scissors to incise the posterior surface of the antebrachial fascia from the olecranon to the extensor retinaculum. Preserve the extensor retinaculum. Use your fingers or a probe to separate the antebrachial fascia from the muscles that lie deep to it. Detach the antebrachial fascia from its attachments to the radius and ulna and place it in the tissue container.

5. Six muscles comprise the **superficial extensor group**: **brachioradialis**, **extensor carpi radialis longus**, **extensor carpi radialis brevis**, **extensor digitorum**, **extensor digiti minimi**, and **extensor carpi ulnaris**. Note that four of the muscles in the superficial extensor group (extensor carpi radialis brevis, extensor digitorum, extensor digiti minimi, and extensor carpi ulnaris) attach to the lateral epicondyle of the humerus by way of a **common extensor tendon**.

6. Use tendon patterns at the wrist and distal attachments to positively identify the muscles of the superficial extensor group:
   - **Brachioradialis tendon** attaches to the lateral surface of the distal radius.
   - **Extensor carpi radialis longus tendon** attaches to the base of metacarpal bone 2.
   - **Extensor carpi radialis brevis tendon** attaches to the base of metacarpal bone 3.
   - **Extensor digitorum tendons** attach to the extensor expansions of digits 2 to 5.
   - **Extensor digiti minimi tendon** attaches to the extensor expansion of digit 5.
   - **Extensor carpi ulnaris tendon** attaches to the base of metacarpal bone 5.

7. Note that the tendons of the extensor digitorum muscle are tied together by **intertendinous connections** on the posterior surface of the hand. [G 582; L 58; N 470; R 418; C 62]

8. Observe the **extensor expansion** of digit 3 (Fig. 2.29). The extensor expansion is wrapped around the dorsum and the sides of the proximal phalanx and the distal end of the metacarpal bone. The hood-like expansion retains the extensor tendon in the midline of the digit. The tendons of the lumbrical and interosseous muscles attach to the extensor expansion. [G 583; L 59; N 464; R 417; C 67]

9. Cut through the **extensor retinaculum** to release the tendons of the extensor digitorum muscle. Retract the tendons medially. Note that the other extensor tendons are also contained within individual osseofibrous tunnels. Synovial sheaths line these tunnels.

DEEP GROUP OF EXTENSOR MUSCLES [G 577; L 59; N 445; R 417; C 56]

1. Five muscles comprise the **deep extensor group**: **abductor pollicis longus**, **extensor pollicis brevis**, **extensor pollicis longus**, **extensor indicis**, and **supinator**.
2. The proximal attachments of four muscles of the deep extensor group (abductor pollicis longus, extensor pollicis brevis, extensor pollicis longus, and extensor indicis) are the posterior surfaces of the radius, ulna, and interosseous membrane. These

four muscles emerge from the interval between the extensor digitorum muscle and the extensor carpi radialis brevis muscle.

3. Observe the tendon of each of the following muscles and follow it to its distal attachment:
   - **Abductor pollicis longus tendon** attaches to the base of metacarpal bone 1.
   - **Extensor pollicis brevis tendon** attaches to the base of the proximal phalanx of digit 1.
   - **Extensor pollicis longus tendon** attaches to the base of the distal phalanx of digit 1.
   - **Extensor indicis tendon** attaches to the extensor expansion of digit 2.

4. Identify the **anatomical snuffbox** (Fig. 2.31). The anatomical snuffbox is a depression on the posterior surface of the wrist that is bounded anteriorly by the **abductor pollicis longus tendon** and the **extensor pollicis brevis tendon**. The posterior boundary of the anatomical snuffbox is the **extensor pollicis longus tendon**. [G 584, 585; L 58; N 469; R 418; C 75]

5. Within the anatomical snuffbox, find the **radial artery**. Use a probe to clean the radial artery and follow it distally until it disappears between the two heads of the **first dorsal interosseous muscle**. Note that the **dorsal carpal arch** is a branch of the radial artery that arises in the anatomical snuff box. The dorsal carpal arch supplies arterial blood to the dorsum of the hand (Fig. 2.31). Do not dissect its branches.

6. Near the elbow, use your fingers to retract the brachioradialis muscle and observe the **supinator muscle**. The proximal attachments of the supinator muscle are the lateral epicondyle of the humerus, the radial collateral and anular ligaments of the elbow, and the lateral surface of the ulna. The distal attachment of the supinator muscle is the proximal one-third of the radius. The supinator muscle supinates the hand.

7. On the lateral aspect of the elbow, once again find the radial nerve in the connective tissue plane between the brachioradialis muscle and the brachialis muscle. Observe that the radial nerve divides into a superficial branch and a deep branch. The **deep branch of the radial nerve** enters the supinator muscle.

8. Turn the upper limb and look for the deep branch of the radial nerve where it emerges from the distal border of the supinator muscle.

9. When the deep branch of the radial nerve emerges from the supinator muscle, its name changes to **posterior interosseous nerve**. The posterior interosseous nerve provides motor branches to the extensor muscles.

10. Observe that the posterior interosseous nerve is accompanied by the **posterior interosseous artery**, which is a branch of the common interosseous artery.

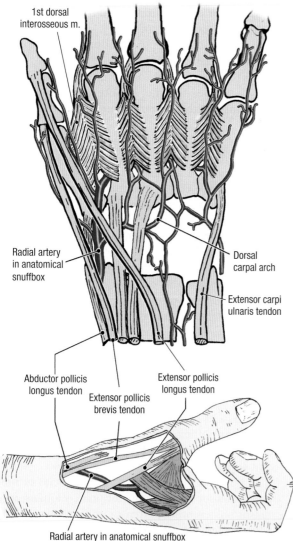

Figure 2.31. Radial artery in the anatomical snuffbox.

Dissection Review

1. Replace the muscles of the posterior compartment of the forearm into their correct anatomical positions.
2. Use the dissected specimen to review the attachments of the extensor tendons.
3. Note that the tendons of three strong extensor muscles (extensor carpi radialis longus, extensor carpi radialis brevis, and extensor carpi ulnaris) attach to the proximal ends of metacarpal bones. These three extensors of the wrist work synergistically with the flexors of the digits: A firm grasp requires an extended wrist.

4. Review the extensor expansion of digit 3. Recall the muscles that insert there and the action of each muscle.
5. Review the course of the common interosseous branch of the ulnar artery and observe how the posterior interosseous artery enters the posterior compartment of the forearm.
6. Review the course of the radial artery from the cubital fossa to the deep palmar arch.
7. Palpate the anatomical snuffbox on yourself. Feel the pulsations of the radial artery within its boundaries.
8. Recall the rule for innervation of the posterior compartment of the forearm:
   - **The radial nerve innervates all of the muscles in the posterior compartment of the forearm.** [L 79]
   - *Note that there are no intrinsic muscles in the dorsum of the hand. Therefore, there are no muscles in the hand that are innervated by the radial nerve.*

JOINTS OF THE UPPER LIMB

Dissection Overview

Dissect joints in one upper limb. Keep the soft tissue structures of the other limb intact for review purposes.

The order of dissection will be as follows: The sternoclavicular and acromioclavicular joints will be dissected. The glenohumeral joint will be dissected. The elbow joint and radioulnar joints will be studied. The wrist joint will be dissected. Finally, the joints of the digits will be studied. During this dissection, the muscles of one limb will be removed. Take advantage of this opportunity to review the proximal attachment, distal attachment, innervation, and action of each muscle as it is removed.

Dissection Instructions

STERNOCLAVICULAR JOINT [G 506; L 71; N 419; R 378; C 104]

1. Use an articulated skeleton to observe the relationships between the sternum and clavicle. Identify the **clavicular notch of the manubrium**. The medial end of the clavicle articulates with the clavicular notch and the adjacent part of the first costal cartilage (Fig. 2.32).
2. Place the cadaver in the supine position. The tendon of the sternocleidomastoid muscle is attached to the anterior surface of the sternoclavicular joint. Detach the tendon and reflect the sternocleidomastoid muscle superiorly.
3. Identify the **anterior sternoclavicular ligament**, which spans from the sternum to the clavicle.
4. Use blunt dissection to clean the **costoclavicular ligament**, which runs obliquely from the first costal cartilage to the inferior surface of the clavicle near its medial end.
5. Use a scalpel to remove the anterior sternoclavicular ligament. Within the joint cavity, observe the **articular disc**. Inferiorly, the articular disc is attached to the first costal cartilage. Superiorly, the articular disc is attached to the clavicle. Observe that the articular disc is attached in such a manner that it resists medial displacement of the clavicle.
6. Palpate the movements of the sternoclavicular joint on yourself. Place your left hand on your right sternoclavicular joint and circumduct your right upper limb through a large circle. Observe that the sternoclavicular joint allows a limited amount of movement in every direction.

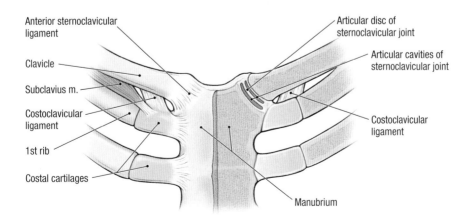

Figure 2.32. Sternoclavicular joint.

ACROMIOCLAVICULAR JOINT [G 532, 535; L 71; N 423; R 378; C 78]

1. Review the bony features that are relevant to the **acromioclavicular joint** (Fig. 2.33):
    • **Acromion**
    • **Coracoid process of the scapula**
    • **Lateral end of the clavicle**
2. Detach the trapezius muscle from the lateral end of the clavicle. Detach the coracobrachialis and pectoralis minor muscles from the coracoid process. The acromioclavicular joint is now exposed. The acromioclavicular joint is a plane synovial joint between the acromion and the distal end of the clavicle.
3. Identify the **coracoclavicular ligament**, which supports the acromioclavicular joint. Use a probe to clean the ligament. Identify its two parts:
    • **Conoid ligament**
    • **Trapezoid ligament**
4. Open the acromioclavicular joint by completely removing the joint capsule. Separate the acromion from the lateral end of the clavicle.
5. Note the shape of the articulating surfaces. The angle of the articulating surfaces causes the acromion to move inferior to the distal end of the clavicle when the acromion is forced medially. The conoid and trapezoid ligaments prevent the acromion from moving inferiorly relative to the clavicle, strengthening the joint.

GLENOHUMERAL JOINT [G 532, 533; L 71; N 423; R 378; C 80-82]

The **glenohumeral joint (shoulder joint)** is a ball-and-socket synovial joint with a wide range of motion. The shoulder joint has a greater degree of movement than any other joint in the body. This is due to the small area of contact between the head of the humerus and the glenoid fossa of the scapula and the loose joint capsule. Stability of the shoulder joint depends on the function of the muscles of the rotator cuff.

1. Place the cadaver in the supine position.
2. Review the bony features pertinent to dissection of the **glenohumeral joint** (Fig. 2.34):
    • **Glenoid fossa of the scapula**
    • **Head of the humerus**
    • **Anatomical neck of the humerus**
3. To expose the **capsule of the glenohumeral joint**, the muscles and tendons that span the joint must be removed. Review the proximal attachment and distal attachment of each muscle as you remove it.
4. Remove the coracobrachialis muscle and the short head of the biceps brachii muscle. Leave the subscapularis muscle intact.
5. Place the cadaver in the prone position. Observe that the tendons of the supraspinatus, infraspinatus, and teres minor muscles blend with the joint capsule. Remove these tendons.

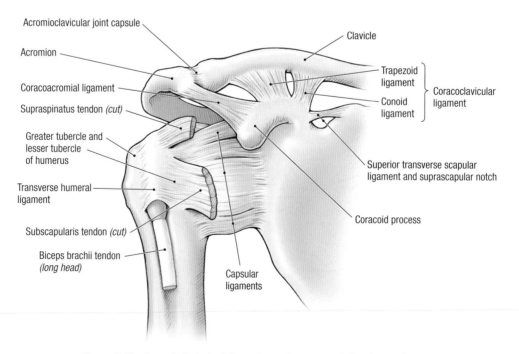

Figure 2.33. Acromioclavicular joint and anterior aspect of glenohumeral joint.

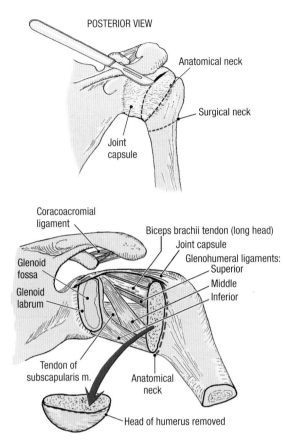

POSTERIOR VIEW

Anatomical neck

Surgical neck

Joint capsule

Coracoacromial ligament

Biceps brachii tendon (long head)

Joint capsule

Glenohumeral ligaments:
Superior
Middle
Inferior

Glenoid fossa

Glenoid labrum

Tendon of subscapularis m.

Anatomical neck

Head of humerus removed

Figure 2.34. How to open the glenohumeral joint capsule and remove the head of the humerus.

6. Remove the long head of the triceps brachii muscle.
7. The posterior surface of the **joint capsule** is now exposed. Verify that the joint capsule is attached to the anatomical neck of the humerus.
8. Use a scalpel to open the posterior surface of the joint capsule (Fig. 2.34).
9. Use a saw or a chisel to remove the head of the humerus at the anatomical neck.
10. Use a probe to explore the **glenoid cavity**. Identify the **glenoid labrum** and attempt to demonstrate the three **glenohumeral ligaments**, which strengthen the anterior wall of the fibrous capsule (Fig. 2.34).
11. Observe that the **tendon of the long head of the biceps brachii muscle** passes through the glenoid cavity and is attached to the supraglenoid tubercle.
12. Place the cadaver in the supine position. Define and clean the **coracoacromial ligament**, which spans from the coracoid process to the acromion. The coracoacromial ligament, the acromion, and the coracoid process prevent superior displacement of the head of the humerus.
13. Use the dissected specimen to perform the movements of the glenohumeral joint: flexion, extension, abduction, adduction, and circumduction.

Note that this freedom of motion is obtained at the loss of joint stability.

ELBOW JOINT AND PROXIMAL RADIOULNAR JOINT
[G 546, 547; L 72; N 436, 438; R 379; C 85–88]

1. Review the bony features of the elbow region (Fig. 2.35).
2. Use an articulated skeleton to verify that the elbow joint consists of two parts:
   - A **hinge joint** between the trochlea of the humerus and the trochlear notch of the ulna
   - A **gliding joint** between the capitulum of the humerus and the head of the radius
3. Remove the brachialis muscle from the anterior surface of the joint capsule.
4. Detach the triceps brachii tendon from the olecranon and the posterior surface of the joint capsule.
5. Remove the superficial flexor muscles of the forearm from their attachment to the medial epicondyle. Review the common flexor tendon and the five muscles that attach to it.
6. Identify the **ulnar collateral ligament** on the medial side of the elbow joint (Fig. 2.35). Observe that it consists of a strong anterior cord and a fan-like posterior portion.
7. Remove the superficial extensor muscles of the forearm from their attachment to the lateral epicondyle of the humerus. Review the common extensor tendon and the muscles that attach to it.
8. Remove the supinator muscle.
9. Identify the **radial collateral ligament**. It fans out from the lateral epicondyle of the humerus to the radius and anular ligament.
10. The **proximal radioulnar joint** is a pivot joint that occurs between the head of the radius and the radial notch of the ulna. The **anular ligament** and the radial notch of the ulna completely encircle the head of the radius (Fig. 2.35). Note that the radius can freely rotate in the anular ligament. Place the hand of the cadaver specimen into the pronated position. Now pull on the biceps brachii tendon. Note the strong supinating action of the biceps brachii muscle.
11. Open the elbow joint by making a transverse cut through the anterior surface of the joint capsule between the ulnar collateral ligament and the radial collateral ligament.
12. Use a probe to explore the extent of the **synovial cavity**. Observe the smooth articular surfaces of the humerus, ulna, and radius.
13. Use the dissected specimen to perform the movements of the elbow joint: flexion and extension. Observe the joint surfaces and the collateral ligaments during these movements.

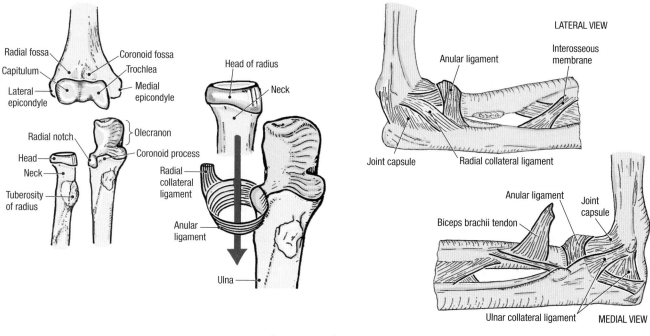

Figure 2.35. Elbow joint.

INTERMEDIATE RADIOULNAR JOINT [G 551; L 72, 73; N 439; R 380; C 88]

1. The radius and ulna are joined throughout their length by the **interosseous membrane**. This is a fibrous joint. Use an illustration to study this joint.

DISTAL RADIOULNAR JOINT [G 590, 591; L 73; N 455; R 381; C 88]

1. The distal radioulnar joint is the pivot joint that occurs between the head of the ulna and the ulnar notch of the radius (Fig. 2.36).
2. Remove all tendons and soft tissue structures that cross the wrist. Review the distal attachment of each tendon and the action of each muscle.
3. Note that the anterior and posterior surfaces of the wrist joint are reinforced by **radiocarpal ligaments**.
4. To open the distal radioulnar joint, extend the hand. On the anterior surface of the joint capsule, cut transversely through the radiocarpal ligaments. This cut should be made proximal to the flexor retinaculum and carpal tunnel. Leave the hand attached to the forearm by the posterior part of the joint capsule.
5. Use a probe to explore the articulation between the radius and the ulna. Note that the distal radioulnar joint contains an **articular disc**. Verify that the articular disc holds the distal ends of the radius and the ulna together.

WRIST JOINT [G 590, 592; L 73, 74; N 454, 455; R 380, 381; C 92, 93]

1. The **wrist joint (radiocarpal joint)** is the articulation between the distal end of the **radius** and the proximal **carpal bones** (Fig. 2.36). Note that the distal end of the radius articulates with only two carpal bones: **scaphoid** and **lunate**.

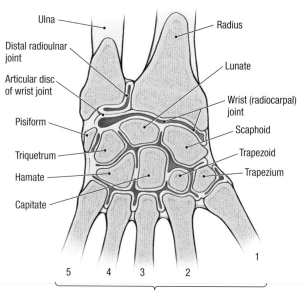

Figure 2.36. Distal radioulnar and wrist joints.

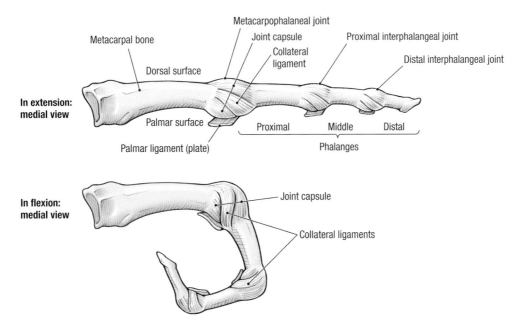

Figure 2.37. Metacarpophalangeal and interphalangeal joints.

2. Identify the smooth proximal surfaces of the **scaphoid**, **lunate**, and **triquetrum**. Study the corresponding **articular surface of the radius**. Notice that the **scaphoid** and **lunate** bones must transmit forces from the hand to the forearm. Therefore, these carpal bones are the ones most commonly fractured in a fall on the outstretched hand.

3. Once again, identify the articular disc. The articular disc articulates with the triquetrum when the hand is adducted.

4. Use the dissected specimen to perform the movements of the wrist joint: flexion, extension, adduction, abduction, and circumduction. Observe the articular surfaces during these movements.

METACARPOPHALANGEAL JOINTS [G 595; L 74; N 458; R 381; C 92, 93]

1. Dissect digit 3 as a representative example.

2. Remove the tendons of the flexor digitorum superficialis and flexor digitorum profundus muscles. Note their attachments on the phalanges.

3. Remove the interosseous muscles and the extensor expansion to expose the metacarpophalangeal joint capsule.

4. Clean the collateral ligaments (Fig. 2.37). Move the digit to confirm that the ligaments are slack during extension and taut during flexion. Therefore, the digits cannot be spread (abducted) unless they are extended.

5. Use the dissected specimen to perform the movements of the digit at the metacarpophalangeal joint: flexion, extension, abduction, and adduction. Confirm that the metacarpophalangeal joints are condyloid joints.

INTERPHALANGEAL JOINTS [G 595; L 74; N 458; R 381; C 93]

1. Clean the collateral ligaments of the interphalangeal joints of digit 3 (Fig. 2.37).

2. Use a probe to explore the synovial cavity of one interphalangeal joint. Inspect the articular surfaces that are covered with smooth cartilage.

3. Use the dissected specimen to perform flexion and extension of the interphalangeal joint and confirm that the collateral ligaments limit the range of motion. Confirm that the interphalangeal joints are hinge joints.

CHAPTER 3

THE THORAX

The main function of the thorax is to house and protect the heart and lungs. The protective function of the thoracic wall is combined with mobility to accommodate volume changes during respiration. These two dissimilar functions, protection and flexibility, are accomplished by the alternating arrangement of the ribs and intercostal muscles.

The superficial fascia of the thorax contains the usual elements that are common to superficial fascia in all body regions: blood vessels, lymph vessels, cutaneous nerves, and sweat glands. In addition, the superficial fascia of the anterior thoracic wall in the female contains the mammary glands, which are highly specialized organs unique to the superficial fascia of the thorax.

SURFACE ANATOMY [G 2; L 160; N 181; C 101]

The surface anatomy of the thorax can be studied on a living subject or on the cadaver. Turn the cadaver to the supine position and palpate the following structures (Fig. 3.1):

- **Clavicle**
- **Acromion of the scapula**
- **Jugular notch (suprasternal notch)**
- **Manubrium**
- **Sternal angle**
- **Body of the sternum**
- **Xiphisternal junction**
- **Xiphoid process**
- **Seventh costal cartilage**
- **Costal margin**
- **Anterior axillary fold (lateral border of the pectoralis major muscle)**

SKELETON OF THE THORAX

If you have previously dissected the back, review the parts of a **thoracic vertebra**. If you have not dissected the back, you must study the vertebrae now. Turn to pages 6 to 7, complete that exercise, and return to this page.

Refer to a skeleton. Examine a **rib** from the midthorax level and identify (Fig. 3.2): [G 13 L 164; N 186; R 197; C 106]

- **Head**
- **Neck**

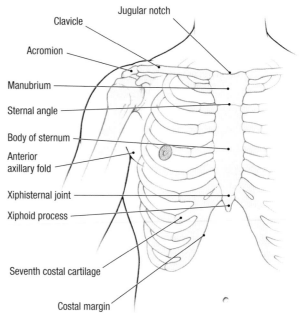

Figure 3.1. Surface anatomy of the anterior thoracic wall.

- **Tubercle**
- **Costal angle**
- **Shaft (body)**
- **Costal groove**

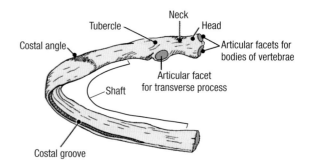

Figure 3.2. Typical left rib, posterior view.

ATLAS REFERENCES
G = *Grant's Atlas*, 12th ed., page number
L = *LWW Atlas of Anatomy*, 1st ed., page number
N = *Netter's Atlas*, 4th ed., plate number
R = *Color Atlas of Anatomy*, 6th ed., page number
C = *Clemente's Atlas*, 5th ed., plate number

On an articulated skeleton, note the following features:

- The **first rib** is the highest, shortest, broadest, and most sharply curved rib.
- The **head** of a rib usually articulates with two vertebral bodies and their intervertebral disc. For example, the head of rib 5 articulates with vertebral bodies T4 and T5 (Fig. 3.3). The 1st, 10th, 11th, and 12th ribs are exceptions to this rule—their heads articulate with only one vertebral body.
- The **tubercle** of a rib articulates with the transverse costal facet on the transverse process of the thoracic vertebra of the same number (Fig. 3.3).
- A **costal cartilage** is attached to the anterior end of each rib.

Ribs are classified by the way their costal cartilage articulates (Fig. 3.4):

- **True ribs (ribs 1 to 7)** – costal cartilage is attached directly to the sternum.
- **False ribs (ribs 8 to 10)** – costal cartilage is attached to the costal cartilage of the rib above.
- **Floating ribs (ribs 11 and 12)** − costal cartilage is not attached to a skeletal element, but ends in the abdominal musculature.

Examine the **sternum** and identify (Fig. 3.4): [G 12; L 163; N 186; R 193; C 105]

- **Jugular notch** (suprasternal notch)
- **Manubrium** (L. *manubrium*, handle)
- **Sternal angle** (at the attachment of the second costal cartilage; also at the level of the T4/T5 intervertebral disc)
- **Body**
- **Xiphoid process** (Gr. *xiphos*, sword)

Examine a **scapula** and identify (Fig. 3.4): [G 479; L 32; N 185; R 189; C 76]

- **Acromion**
- **Coracoid process**

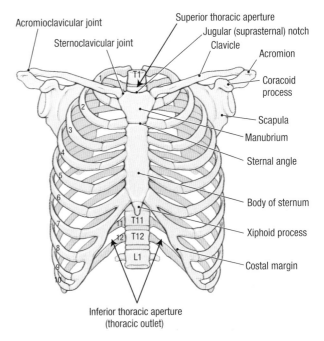

Figure 3.4. Skeleton of the thoracic region.

Observe that the medial end of the **clavicle** articulates with the manubrium of the sternum (**sternoclavicular joint**) and the lateral end of the clavicle articulates with the acromion of the scapula (**acromioclavicular joint**) (Fig. 3.4).

PECTORAL REGION

Instructions for dissection of the pectoral region are found in Chapter 2, The Upper Limb. If you are dissecting the thorax before the upper limb, the pectoral region must be dissected now. Turn to pages 24 to 28, complete that dissection, and return to this page.

INTERCOSTAL SPACE AND INTERCOSTAL MUSCLES

Dissection Overview

The interval between adjacent ribs is called the **intercostal space**. The intercostal space is truly a space only in a skeleton, as three layers of muscle fill the intercostal space in the living body and the cadaver. From superficial to deep, the three layers of muscle are **external intercostal muscle**, **internal intercostal muscle**, and **innermost intercostal muscle**.

There are 11 intercostal spaces on each side of the thorax. Each is numbered according to the rib that forms its superior boundary. For example, the fourth intercostal space is located between ribs 4 and 5.

The order of dissection will be as follows: The external intercostal muscle will be studied in the fourth intercostal

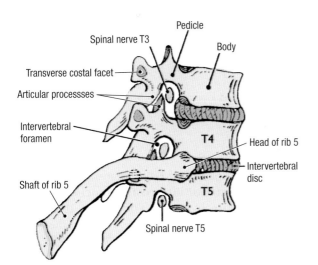

Figure 3.3. Part of the thoracic vertebral column.

space and will be reflected. The internal intercostal muscle will then be studied in the fourth intercostal space and will be reflected. Branches of intercostal nerves and blood vessels will be identified. The innermost intercostal muscle will be identified.

Dissection Instructions

1. Detach the **serratus anterior muscle** from its proximal attachments on ribs 1 to 8 and reflect it laterally.
2. Palpate the ribs and the intercostal spaces. Begin at the level of the sternal angle (attachment of the second costal cartilage) and identify each intercostal space by number.
3. Dissect intercostal space 4 (the space between ribs 4 and 5).
4. Identify the **external intercostal muscle** (Fig. 3.5). The external intercostal muscle attaches to the inferior border of the rib above and the superior border of the rib below. The external intercostal muscle elevates the rib below. Note that the fibers of the external intercostal muscles pass diagonally toward the anterior midline as they descend. [G 19; L 166; N 426; R 198; C 102]
5. Identify the **external intercostal membrane**, which is located at the anterior end of the intercostal space between the **costal cartilages**. Note that the fibers of the external intercostal muscle end at the lateral edge of the external intercostal membrane.
6. Insert a probe deep to the external intercostal membrane just lateral to the border of the sternum in the fourth intercostal space. Push the probe laterally and note that it passes deep to the external intercostal muscle.

7. With the probe as a guide, use scissors to cut the external intercostal muscle from the rib above and reflect it inferiorly (Fig. 3.5). Continue the cut laterally to the midaxillary line.
8. Identify the **internal intercostal muscle**. The internal intercostal muscle attaches to the superior border of the rib below and the inferior border of the rib above. The internal intercostal muscle depresses the rib above. Note that the fiber direction of the internal intercostal muscle is perpendicular to the fiber direction of the external intercostal muscle (Fig. 3.5).
9. Begin at the lateral border of the sternum and detach the internal intercostal muscle from its attachment on rib 5. Continue to detach the internal intercostal muscle as far laterally as the midaxillary line. Reflect the muscle superiorly (Fig. 3.5).
10. Identify the fourth **intercostal nerve** and the fourth **posterior intercostal artery and vein** inferior to rib 4. The intercostal nerve and vessels run in the plane between the **internal intercostal muscle** and **innermost intercostal muscle** (Fig. 3.6). The **innermost intercostal muscle** has the same fiber direction, attachments, and action as the internal intercostal muscle, but it does not extend as far anteriorly in the intercostal space. [G 20; L 170; N 192; R 214; C 8]
11. The intercostal nerve and vessels supply the intercostal muscles, the skin of the thoracic wall, and the parietal pleura. Use Figure 3.6 to study the course and distribution of a typical intercostal nerve.

Pleural Tap (Thoracocentesis)

The aspiration of pathologic material from the pleural cavity (serous fluid, fluid mixed with tumor cells, blood, pus, etc.) may be done through the intercostal space. The pleural tap is performed in the midaxillary line or slightly posterior to it. Usually, intercostal space 6, 7, or 8 is selected for the puncture to avoid penetrating abdominal viscera. A large-bore needle is inserted low in the intercostal space to avoid injury to the intercostal nerve and vessels (Fig. 3.7).

12. The anterior end of the intercostal space is supplied by **anterior intercostal branches** of the **internal thoracic artery**. The internal thoracic artery runs a vertical course just lateral to the border of the sternum and crosses the deep surfaces of the costal cartilages. [G 22; L 167, 168; N 189; R 209; C 102]

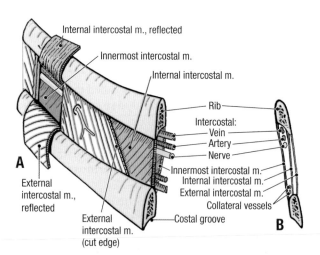

Figure 3.5. Structures in the intercostal space. **A.** Anterior view. **B.** Coronal section at the midaxillary line.

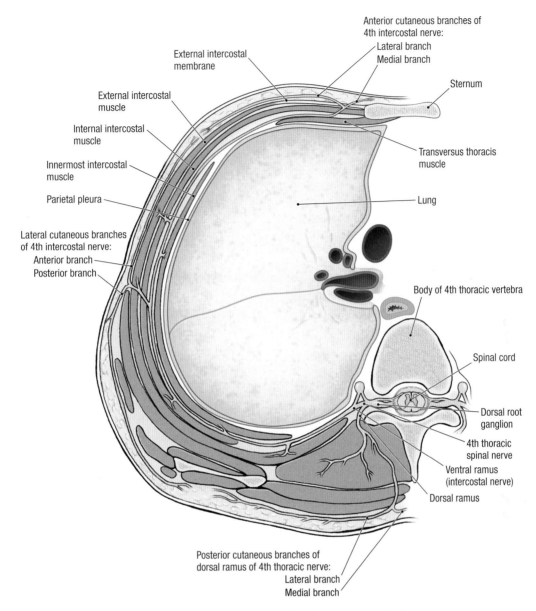

Figure 3.6. Course and distribution of the fourth thoracic spinal nerve.

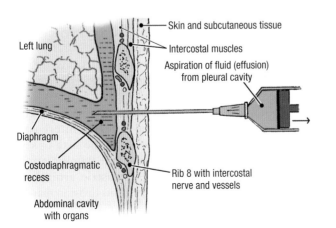

Figure 3.7. Anatomical relationships associated with a pleural tap.

Dissection Review

1. Replace the internal and external intercostal muscles in their correct anatomical positions.
2. Review the muscles that lie in the intercostal space. Review their actions. Understand how they assist respiration by elevating and depressing the ribs.
3. Use an illustration and your dissected specimen to review the origin, course, and branches of the posterior intercostal artery and intercostal nerve.
4. Consult a dermatome chart and compare the dermatome pattern to the distribution of the intercostal nerves. [G 348; L 162; N 164; C 8]

REMOVAL OF THE ANTERIOR THORACIC WALL

Dissection Overview

To view the contents of the thoracic cavity, the anterior thoracic wall must be removed. The goal of this dissection is to remove the thoracic wall with the **costal parietal pleura** attached to its inner surface. The structures to be removed include the proximal ends of both clavicles, the manubrium and body of the sternum, the anterior and lateral portions of ribs 1 through 5, and the contents of intercostal spaces 1 to 4.

The order of dissection will be as follows: The sternocleidomastoid muscle and infrahyoid neck muscles will be detached from their sternal and clavicular attachments. The clavicles will be cut at their midlength. The costal cartilages and sternum will be cut at the level of the xiphisternal joint. The ribs and contents of the intercostal spaces will be cut at the midaxillary line. The thoracic wall will be removed and the inner surface of the thoracic wall will be studied.

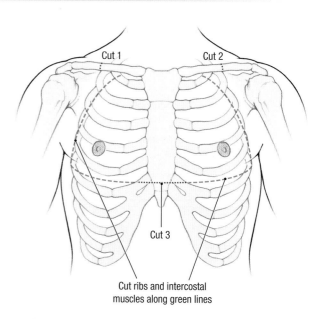

Figure 3.8. Cuts used to remove the anterior thoracic wall.

Dissection Instructions [G 761; L 308; N 28, 29; R 174, 175; C 470]

1. Reflect the pectoralis major muscle laterally. Reflect the pectoralis minor muscle superiorly. Reflect the serratus anterior muscle laterally.

2. Use scissors to cut the sternocleidomastoid muscle where it is attached to the superior margin of the sternum and the superior surface of the clavicle. Use blunt dissection to loosen the distal 5 cm of the sternocleidomastoid muscle and reflect it superiorly.

3. Use your fingers to push the infrahyoid muscles posteriorly with enough force to tear their attachments to the deep surface of the sternum.

4. Cut both clavicles at their midlength using a saw (Fig. 3.8, cuts 1 and 2).

5. At the level of the xiphisternal joint (approximately at the level of intercostal space 5), use a saw to make a transverse cut across the sternum and costal cartilages (Fig. 3.8, cut 3). Allow the saw to pass through the bone and cartilage, but not into the deeper tissues.

6. Use a saw or bone cutters to cut ribs 1 to 5 in the midaxillary line on both sides of the thorax.

7. With a scalpel, make a series of vertical cuts through the muscles in intercostal spaces 1 to 5 in the midaxillary line. The cuts should be aligned with the cut ribs. Make the cut deep enough to cut the parietal pleura.

8. Use scissors to cut the intercostal muscles and underlying costal parietal pleura from the upper border of rib 6 on both sides of the thorax.

9. Gently, elevate the inferior end of the sternum along with the attached portions of the severed costal cartilages and ribs. Near the lower end of the sternum, identify the **right and left internal thoracic vessels** (Fig. 3.8). Cut the internal thoracic vessels at the level of the fifth sternocostal joint.

10. Continue to elevate the inferior end of the thoracic wall and cut the parietal pleura with scissors where it reflects from the inner surface of the thoracic wall onto the mediastinum.

11. Cut the internal thoracic vessels at the level of the first rib. Remove the anterior thoracic wall with the internal thoracic vessels attached.

12. Observe the internal surface of the anterior thoracic wall and identify the **costal parietal pleura**. Use blunt dissection to remove the parietal pleura from the inner surface of the anterior thoracic wall.

13. Identify the **transversus thoracis muscle** [G 23; L 168; N 191; R 206; C 111]. Observe that the inferior attachment of the transversus thoracis muscle is on the sternum and its superior attachments are on costal cartilages 2 to 6. The transversus thoracis muscle depresses the ribs.

14. The **internal thoracic artery and veins** are located between the transversus thoracis muscle and the costal cartilages.

15. Follow the internal thoracic artery inferiorly and identify at least one of the **anterior intercostal branches**. Note that posterior to the sixth or seventh costal cartilage, the internal thoracic artery divides into the **superior epigastric artery** and the **musculophrenic artery**. This division may be seen on the cadaver rather than on the thoracic wall specimen.

Dissection Review

1. Replace the anterior thoracic wall in its correct anatomical position.
2. Replace the serratus anterior muscle in its correct anatomical position.
3. Replace the pectoralis minor muscle, making sure that its proximal attachments touch ribs 3, 4, and 5.
4. Replace the pectoralis major muscle in its correct anatomical position.
5. Review the attachments and the action of the pectoral muscles, the serratus anterior muscle, and the transversus thoracis muscle.
6. Study the course of the internal thoracic artery from its origin to its bifurcation and name its branches.

CLINICAL CORRELATION

Anterior Thoracic Wall

The anterior and lateral approaches to the contents of the thorax are the two most common surgical approaches. In the anterior approach, the sternum is split vertically in the midline. This approach does not cross major vessels and allows good access to the heart. The incision through the sternum is closed with stainless steel wires. In the lateral approach, an intercostal space is incised to provide access to the lungs or to structures posterior to the heart.

PLEURAL CAVITIES

Dissection Overview

The thorax has two apertures (Fig. 3.4). The **superior thoracic aperture (thoracic inlet)** is relatively small and bounded by the manubrium of the sternum, the right and left first ribs, and the body of the first thoracic vertebra. Structures pass between the thorax, the neck, and the upper limb through the superior thoracic aperture (e.g., **trachea, esophagus, vagus nerves, thoracic duct, major blood vessels**).

The **inferior thoracic aperture (thoracic outlet)** is larger and bounded by the xiphisternal joint, the costal margin, ribs 11 and 12, and the body of vertebra T12. The **diaphragm** attaches to the structures that form the boundaries of the inferior thoracic aperture and it separates the thoracic cavity from the abdominal cavity. Several large structures (e.g., **aorta, inferior vena cava, esophagus, vagus nerves**) pass between the thorax and abdomen through openings in the diaphragm.

The thorax contains two **pleural cavities** (right and left) and the **mediastinum**. The two pleural cavities occupy the lateral parts of the thoracic cavity and each contains one **lung**. The mediastinum (L. *quod per medium stat*, that which stands in the middle) is the region between the two pleural cavities. It contains the **heart, aorta, trachea, esophagus**, and other structures that pass to or from the head and neck. [G 28; L 173; N 196; R 243; C 109]

Each pleural cavity is lined by a serous membrane called the **parietal pleura** (Fig. 3.9). The parietal pleura has subdivisions that are regionally named:

- **Costal pleura** – lines the inner surface of the thoracic wall
- **Mediastinal pleura** – lines the mediastinum
- **Diaphragmatic pleura** – lines the superior surface of the diaphragm
- **Cervical pleura (cupula)** – extends superior to the first rib

The parietal pleura is sharply folded where the costal pleura meets the diaphragmatic pleura, and where the costal pleura meets the mediastinal pleura. The folds are called **lines of pleural reflection**. The lines of pleural reflection are acute, and the inner surfaces of the parietal pleurae are in contact with one another (Fig. 3.9). The areas where parietal pleura contacts parietal pleura are called **pleural recesses**. The two **costomediastinal recesses** (left and right) occur posterior to the sternum where costal pleura meets mediastinal pleura. The two **costodiaphragmatic recesses** (left and right) are located at the most inferior limits of the parietal pleura (Fig. 3.9). During quiet inspiration, the inferior border of the lung does not extend into the costodiaphragmatic recess. [G 28; L 172; N 196; R 265; C 113]

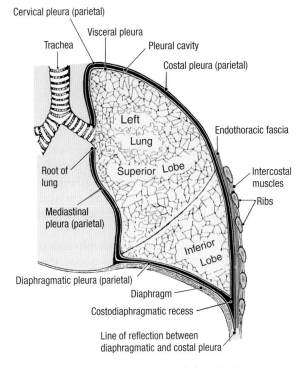

Figure 3.9. The pleurae and pleural cavity

The **endothoracic fascia** is a small amount of connective tissue between the thoracic wall and the costal parietal pleura. Endothoracic fascia provides a cleavage plane for surgical separation of the pleura from the thoracic wall.

Each lung is completely covered with **visceral pleura (pulmonary pleura)**. At the root of the lung the visceral pleura becomes continuous with the mediastinal parietal pleura.

The **pleural cavity** is the space between the visceral pleura and the parietal pleura (Fig. 3.9). In the living body, the pleural cavity is a potential space and visceral pleura touches parietal pleura.

Dissection Instructions

1. Explore the right and left pleural cavities. *Caution: The cut ends of the ribs are sharp and can cut you.* To reduce the risk of injury, use a mallet or the side of the bone cutters to hit and blunt the ends of ribs 1 to 5. As an additional precaution, place paper towels over the cut ends of the ribs before you begin to palpate the pleural cavities.

CLINICAL CORRELATION

Pleural Cavity

Under pathological conditions, the potential space of the pleural cavity may become a real space. For example, if air enters the pleural cavity (pneumothorax), the lung collapses due to the elasticity of its tissue.

Excess fluid may accumulate in the pleural cavity, compress the lung, and produce breathing difficulties. The fluid could be serous fluid (plural effusion) or blood resulting from trauma (hemothorax).

2. Use paper towels or a large syringe to remove fluid that may have collected in the pleural cavity.
3. Identify the parts of the **parietal pleura**: **costal**, **diaphragmatic**, **mediastinal**, and **cervical**. Part of the costal pleura was removed with the anterior thoracic wall.
4. Place your fingers in the **costodiaphragmatic recess**. Follow it posteriorly and notice the acute angle that the diaphragm makes with the inner surface of the thoracic wall.
5. Place your hand between the lung and the mediastinum and palpate the root of the lung. At the root of the lung the mediastinal parietal pleura is continuous with the visceral pleura. Palpate the

pulmonary ligament, which extends inferior to the root of the lung.
6. The root of the lung is attached to the mediastinum. All other parts of the lung should slide freely against the parietal pleura. Pleural adhesions may occur between visceral and parietal pleurae. Pleural adhesions are the result of disease processes, and you should use your fingers to break them.

Dissection Review

1. Replace the anterior thoracic wall in its correct anatomical position.
2. Use an illustration and the dissected specimen to project the lines of pleural reflection to the anterior thoracic wall.
3. Review the course of the intercostal nerves and understand that they are the source of somatic innervation (including pain fibers) to the costal parietal pleura.

LUNGS

Dissection Overview

The order of dissection will be as follows: The surface features and relationships of the lungs that can be seen from an anterior view will be studied with the lungs in the thorax. Then the lungs will be removed and the study of surface features and relationships of the lungs will be completed. The hilum of the lung will be studied.

Dissection Instructions

LUNGS IN THE THORAX

1. Observe the lungs in situ (Fig. 3.10). [G 25; L 174, 175; N 198; R 268; C 113]
2. Each lung has three surfaces: **costal**, **mediastinal**, and **diaphragmatic**. You can see only the costal surface with the lung in situ.
3. Observe the **oblique fissure** on both lungs. Replace the anterior thoracic wall and observe that the oblique fissure lies deep to the fifth rib laterally and that it is deep to the sixth costal cartilage anteriorly. Clinicians may refer to the oblique fissure as the **major fissure**.
4. Remove the anterior thoracic wall and identify the **horizontal fissure** on the right lung. Replace the anterior thoracic wall and observe that the horizontal fissure lies deep to the fourth rib and fourth

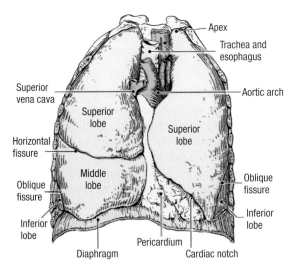

Figure 3.10. The lungs in situ.

costal cartilage. Clinicians may refer to the horizontal fissure as the **minor fissure** or **transverse fissure**.

5. Note that the right lung has three lobes (**superior**, **middle**, and **inferior**). The left lung has two lobes (**superior** and **inferior**).

6. Observe that the **apex** of the lung occupies the cupula of the pleura and that both rise as high as the neck of the first rib (superior to the body of the first rib). Therefore, the apex of the lung and the cupula of the pleura lie superior to the plane of the superior thoracic aperture and are actually located in the neck.

7. Identify the **pericardium** that occupies the midline between the lungs. The pericardium contains the heart.

8. Palpate the **root of the lung**. Feel the hard structures within the root of the lung. These are the

pulmonary vessels filled with clotted blood, and the main (primary) bronchus.

9. Observe that the **phrenic nerve** and **pericardiacophrenic vessels** pass anterior to the root of the lung and medial (deep) to the mediastinal pleura. Use an illustration to observe that the **vagus nerve** passes posterior to the root of the lung. [G 80, 81; L 194, 195; N 230, 231; R 280, 281; C 126, 127]

REMOVAL OF THE LUNGS

1. Preserve the phrenic nerve, pericardiacophrenic vessels, and vagus nerve during lung removal.

2. Place your hand into the pleural cavity between the lung and mediastinum. Retract the lung laterally, to stretch the root of the lung.

3. While retracting the lung, use scissors to transect the root of the lung halfway between the lung and the mediastinum. Take care not to cut into the mediastinum or the lung. Remove both lungs.

4. Compare the two lungs (Fig. 3.11). Note that the right lung is shorter, but has greater volume than the left lung. [G 32; L 189; R 249; C 118]

5. Identify the **surfaces of the lung**: **costal**, **mediastinal**, and **diaphragmatic**.

6. Identify the **borders of the lung**: **anterior**, **posterior**, and **inferior**.

7. Recall that each lung has a **superior** lobe and an **inferior lobe** separated by the **oblique fissure**. Observe the lung from the lateral view, and note that most of the inferior lobe lies posteriorly and that most of the superior lobe lies anteriorly (Fig. 3.11).

8. Recall that the right lung has a **horizontal fissure**, which defines a small **middle lobe** (Fig. 3.11). Identify the middle lobe.

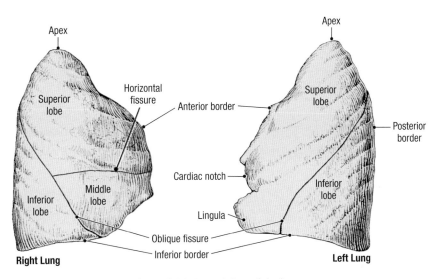

Figure 3.11. Lateral view of the lungs.

9. Identify the **cardiac notch** on the superior lobe of the left lung (Fig. 3.11). The cardiac notch is located on the anterior border of the left lung, and in the anatomical position it is anterior to the heart.

10. Identify the **lingula** of the left lung. The lingula is the inferior, medial portion of the superior lobe of the left lung. It is the homolog of the middle lobe of the right lung.

11. Identify several **contact impressions** on the mediastinal surface of each lung (Figs. 3.12 A,B). These impressions are artifacts of embalming and illustrate the close proximity of the mediastinal structures to the lung.

    On the mediastinal surface of the **right lung**, identify: [G 34, 35; L 190; N 199; R 249; C 120]

- **Cardiac impression**
- **Esophagus impression**
- **Arch of the azygos vein impression**
- **Superior vena cava impression**

    On the mediastinal surface of the **left lung**, identify:

- **Cardiac impression**
- **Aortic arch impression**
- **Thoracic aorta impression**

12. Examine the **hilum of the lung** (Figa. 3.12 A,B). Identify the **main bronchus, pulmonary artery,** and **pulmonary veins**. At the hilum, the main bronchus usually lies posterior to the pulmonary vessels, and the pulmonary artery is superior to the pulmonary veins. To help distinguish the arteries from the veins, compare the relative thickness of the walls of the vessels (the arteries have thicker walls). To distinguish the main bronchus from the pulmonary vessels, look for cartilage in its wall.

13. At the hilum of each lung, use blunt dissection to follow the **main bronchus** into the lung.

14. In the left lung, identify the **superior** and **inferior lobar (secondary) bronchi**. [G 41; L 192; N 203; R 247; C 122]

15. In the right lung, identify the **superior, middle,** and **inferior lobar bronchi**. Note that the **right superior lobar bronchus** passes superior to the

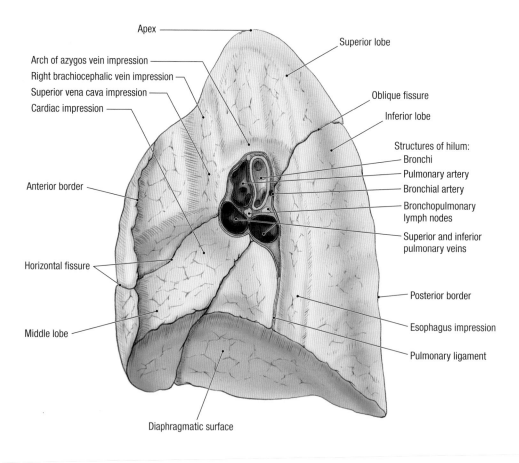

Figure 3.12A. Mediastinal surface of the right lung.

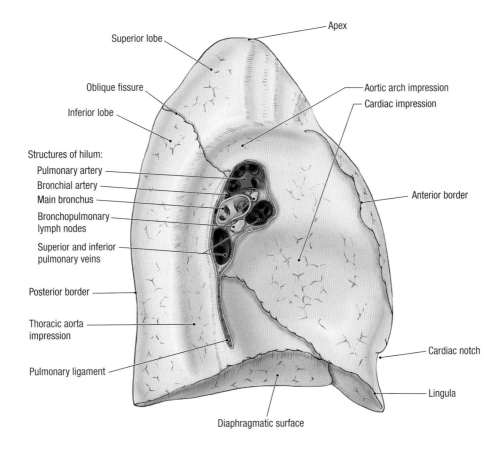

Superior lobe

Apex

Oblique fissure

Inferior lobe

Aortic arch impression

Cardiac impression

Structures of hilum:
Pulmonary artery
Bronchial artery
Main bronchus
Bronchopulmonary
lymph nodes
Superior and inferior
pulmonary veins

Anterior border

Posterior border

Thoracic aorta
impression

Pulmonary ligament

Cardiac notch

Lingula

Diaphragmatic surface

Figure 3.12B. *continued* Mediastinal surface of the left lung.

right pulmonary artery and, therefore, it is also called the "**eparterial bronchus**."

16. Use blunt dissection to follow one lobar bronchus approximately 3 to 4 cm deeper into the lung tissue until it branches into several **segmental bronchi**. The right lung contains 10 segmental bronchi and the left lung contains 9. Each segmental bronchus supplies one **bronchopulmonary segment** of the lung. In your textbook, read a description of the bronchopulmonary segments and the internal organization of the lung.

17. Identify the **bronchial artery**. The bronchial artery courses along the surface of the main bronchus. The lumen of the bronchial artery may be seen where the main bronchus was cut during lung removal.

18. The hilum of the lung contains lymph nodes, lymph vessels, and autonomic nerve fibers. Use an illustration to confirm this. [G 42, 43; L 190; N 208, 209; R 275; C 126, 127]

19. Note that the lungs have a rich nerve supply via the anterior and posterior pulmonary plexuses. Sympathetic contributions are received from the right and left sympathetic trunks, while parasympathetic contributions are received from the right and left vagus nerves.

Dissection Review

1. Review the parts of the lungs.
2. Replace the lungs in their correct anatomical positions within the pleural cavities.
3. Replace the anterior thoracic wall. Project the borders, surfaces, and fissures of the lungs to the surface of the thoracic wall.
4. Review the relationship of the pleural reflections to the thoracic wall.
5. Review the costomediastinal and costodiaphragmatic recesses.

MEDIASTINUM

Dissection Overview

The region between the two pleural cavities is the mediastinum. The **boundaries of the mediastinum** are:

- **Superior boundary** – superior thoracic aperture
- **Inferior boundary** – diaphragm
- **Anterior boundary** – sternum
- **Posterior boundary** – bodies of vertebrae T1 to T12
- **Lateral boundaries** – mediastinal parietal pleurae (left and right)

For descriptive purposes, the mediastinum is divided into four parts (Fig. 3.13). An imaginary transverse plane at the level of the **sternal angle** intersects the intervertebral disk between vertebrae T4 and T5. The **plane of the sternal angle** separates the **superior mediastinum** from the **inferior mediastinum**. The pericardium divides the inferior mediastinum into three parts: [G 29; L 194, 195; R 243; C 130]

- **Anterior mediastinum** – the part that lies between the sternum and the pericardium. In children and adolescents, part of the thymus may be found in the anterior mediastinum.
- **Middle mediastinum** – the part that contains the pericardium, the heart, and the roots of the great vessels.
- **Posterior mediastinum** – the part that lies posterior to the pericardium and anterior to the bodies of vertebrae T5 to T12. The posterior mediastinum contains structures that pass between the neck, thorax, and abdomen (esophagus, vagus nerves, azygos system of veins, thoracic duct, thoracic aorta).

The plane of the sternal angle is an important thoracic landmark that marks the level of the:

- **Superior border of the pericardium**
- **Bifurcation of the trachea**

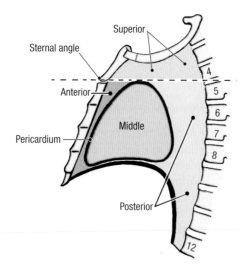

Figure 3.13. Subdivisions of the mediastinum.

- **End of the ascending aorta**
- **Beginning *and* end of the arch of the aorta**
- **Beginning of the thoracic aorta**

It is worth noting that some structures that course through the mediastinum (esophagus, vagus nerve, phrenic nerve, and thoracic duct) pass through more than one mediastinal subdivision.

The order of dissection will be as follows: The mediastinal pleura will be examined and mediastinal structures will be palpated. The costal and mediastinal pleurae will then be removed.

Dissection Instructions

1. Observe the **mediastinal pleura**. You may be able to see structures through the mediastinal pleura. [G 80, 81; L 194, 195; N 230, 231; R 280, 281]
2. Palpate the mediastinal structures through the mediastinal pleura. Observe that, as you move from anterior to posterior, the mediastinal pleura is in contact with the **pericardium** and **root of the lung**, and either the **esophagus (right side)** or the **thoracic aorta (left side)**.
3. Follow the mediastinal pleura further posteriorly until it contacts the sides of the vertebral bodies. At this location the **mediastinal pleura** becomes the **costal pleura**.
4. To examine the mediastinum more closely, the pleura must be removed bilaterally.
5. Use your fingers to pick up the costal pleura in the midaxillary line at the cut ends of ribs 1 to 5. Note that the **endothoracic fascia** provides a natural cleavage plane for separation of costal pleura from the thoracic wall. Peel the costal pleura off the inner surface of the posterior thoracic wall, moving from lateral to medial.
6. Continue to remove the parietal pleura where it covers the vertebral column, esophagus or aorta, and pericardium.
7. Identify the left and right **phrenic nerves** and the left and right **pericardiacophrenic vessels**. The phrenic nerve and pericardiacophrenic vessels are located between the mediastinal pleura and the pericardium about 1.5 cm anterior to the root of the lung. Follow the phrenic nerve and pericardiacophrenic vessels to the diaphragm. Each phrenic nerve (right or left) is the only motor innervation to that half of the diaphragm.

Dissection Review

1. Review the parts of the parietal pleura.
2. Note that the transition from parietal to visceral pleura occurs at the root of the lung.

3. Compare and contrast the structures that can be seen on the right side of the mediastinum to those that can be seen on the left side of the mediastinum.
4. Review the relationship of the phrenic nerve to the root of the lung and pericardium.

MIDDLE MEDIASTINUM

Dissection Overview

The **middle mediastinum** contains the **pericardium**, the **heart**, and the **roots of the great vessels**. The **pericardium** is a sac that encloses the heart and it is pierced by the great vessels (aorta, pulmonary trunk, superior vena cava, inferior vena cava, and four pulmonary veins). The outer surface of the pericardium is fibrous, whereas the inner surface of the pericardium is serous and smooth. The pericardium is attached to the central tendon of the diaphragm. Thus, the heart moves with the diaphragm during inspiration and expiration.

The order of dissection will be as follows: The pericardium will be opened and its relationship to the heart and great vessels will be explored. The characteristics of the parietal serous pericardium will then be studied. The heart will be removed by cutting the great vessels.

Dissection Instructions

HEART IN THE THORAX [G 49; L 177, 178; N 212; R 268; C 134]

1. Open the pericardium in the following manner (Fig. 3.14). Use forceps to elevate the anterior surface of the pericardium. Use scissors to make a longitudinal incision from the diaphragm to the aorta. Make the transverse incisions illustrated in Figure 3.14 and open the flaps widely.
2. Identify the following structures (Fig. 3.15): **superior vena cava**, **ascending aorta**, **arch of the aorta**, and **pulmonary trunk**.
3. Use your fingers to gently open the interval between the concavity of the aortic arch and pulmonary trunk, and identify the **ligamentum arteriosum** (Fig. 3.15). The ligamentum arteriosum connects the left pulmonary artery to the arch of the aorta.
4. Use a probe to dissect the **left vagus nerve** where it crosses the left side of the aortic arch (Fig. 3.15). Identify the initial portion of the **left recurrent laryngeal nerve**. The left recurrent laryngeal nerve is located inferior to the aortic arch and posterior to the ligamentum arteriosum.
5. Examine the heart and identify the chambers that can be seen from the anterior view: **right atrium**,

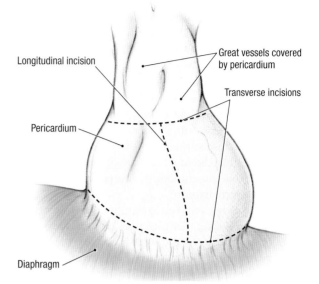

Figure 3.14. How to open the pericardium.

right ventricle, and **left ventricle** (Fig. 3.15). Note that the right ventricle forms most of the anterior surface of the heart.

6. Identify the **borders of the heart**:
   - **Right border** – formed by the right atrium
   - **Inferior border** – formed by the right ventricle and a small part of the left ventricle
   - **Left border** – formed by the left ventricle
   - **Superior border** – formed by the right and left atria and auricles

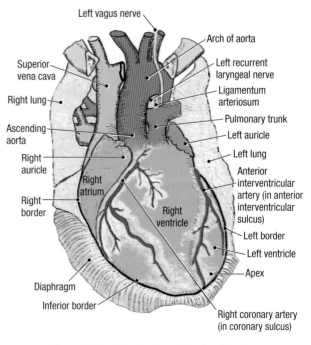

Figure 3.15. Anterior view of the heart in situ.

7. Identify the **apex of the heart**. Note that the apex of the heart is part of the left ventricle. The apex of the heart is normally located deep to the left fifth intercostal space, approximately 9 cm from the midline.

8. Identify the **base of the heart**. The left atrium and part of the right atrium form the base of the heart. Clinicians often refer to the emergence of the great vessels from the heart as its base.

9. Observe that the inner surface of the pericardium is lined by the smooth, shiny **parietal layer of serous pericardium**.

10. Use the cadaver and an illustration to observe that the parietal layer of serous pericardium is reflected onto the heart as the **visceral layer of serous pericardium (epicardium).** The line of reflection of parietal serous pericardium to visceral serous pericardium occurs at the roots of the great vessels. [G 49; L 178; N 212; R 269; C 134]

11. The **pericardial cavity** is a potential space between the parietal and visceral layers of serous pericardium. Normally it contains only a thin film of serous fluid that lubricates the serous surfaces and allows free movement of the heart within the pericardium.

12. Place your right hand in the pericardial cavity with your fingers posterior to the heart. Lift the heart gently and push your fingers superiorly until they are stopped by the reflection of serous pericardium. Your fingertips are located in the **oblique pericardial sinus** (Fig. 3.16). Remove your hand from the oblique pericardial sinus. [G 51; L 179; N 215; R 272; C 135]

13. In the transverse plane, push your right index finger posterior to the pulmonary trunk and ascending aorta. Proceed from left to right until your fingertip emerges between the superior vena cava and the aortic arch. Your finger is in the **transverse pericardial sinus** (Fig. 3.16).

14. Anterior to the aorta, gently insert the tip of a probe between the pericardium and the ascending aorta. Slowly advance the probe until it stops. This is the superior limit of the pericardial cavity.

15. Use your fingers to explore the lines of reflection of the serous pericardium where the great vessels (aorta, pulmonary trunk, superior vena cava, inferior vena cava, and four pulmonary veins) enter and exit the heart (Fig. 3.16).

16. Replace the anterior thoracic wall into its correct anatomical position. Use the cadaver and an illustration to project the outline of the heart to the surface of the thoracic wall. [G 26; L 172, 173; N 196; R 252; C 109]

Pericardium

Inflammatory diseases can cause fluid to accumulate in the pericardial cavity (pericardial effusion). Bleeding into the pericardial cavity (hemopericardium) may result from penetrating heart wounds or perforation of a weakened heart muscle following myocardial infarction. Because the pericardium is composed of fibrous connective tissue, it cannot stretch, and fluids collected in the pericardial cavity compress the heart (cardiac tamponade).

REMOVAL OF THE HEART

1. The heart will be detached from the great vessels along the lines of reflection of the serous pericardium (Fig. 3.16).

2. Place a probe through the transverse pericardial sinus.

3. Use scissors to cut the **ascending aorta** and the **pulmonary trunk** anterior to the probe, about 1.5

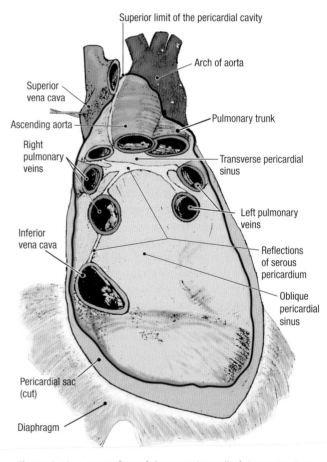

Figure 3.16. Inner surface of the posterior wall of the pericardium showing pericardial sinuses and serous reflections.

cm superior to the point where the aorta and pulmonary trunk emerge from the heart.

4. Use scissors to cut the **superior vena cava** about 1 cm superior to its junction with the right atrium.

5. Lift the apex of the heart superiorly and cut the **inferior vena cava** close to the surface of the diaphragm.

6. While lifting the apex of the heart, cut the **four pulmonary veins** where they form the boundary of the oblique pericardial sinus (Fig. 3.16). Cut the pulmonary veins very close to the inner surface of the pericardial sac.

7. The heart is now held in place only by reflections of serous pericardium from its posterior surface to the inner surface of the pericardial sac (Fig. 3.16). Cut these reflections and remove the heart.

8. Refer to Figure 3.16. Examine the posterior aspect of the pericardium and identify the openings of eight vessels and the lines of the pericardial reflections.

Dissection Review

1. Review the parts of the mediastinum and state their boundaries.

2. Review the attachments of the pericardium to the diaphragm and to the roots of the great vessels.

3. Review the embryonic origin of the transverse and oblique pericardial sinuses.

4. Compare the appearance and functional properties of the parietal serous pericardium to those of the parietal pleura.

EXTERNAL FEATURES OF THE HEART

Dissection Overview

Dissection of the heart will proceed in two stages. The external features of the heart will be studied, including its vascular supply. The internal features of each chamber of the heart will then be studied.

Dissection Instructions

SURFACE FEATURES

1. Examine the external surface of the heart. Identify the following (Fig. 3.15): [G 46, 47; L 180; N 214; R 252; C 136, 137]

- **Coronary (atrioventricular) sulcus** (L. *sulcus*, a groove; pl. sulci) – it runs around the heart, separating the atria from the ventricles.
- **Anterior interventricular sulcus** and the **posterior interventricular sulcus** – the interventricular sulci indicate the location of the interventricular septum. The interventricular sulci join the coronary sulcus at a right angle.

2. Identify the **surfaces of the heart**:
- **Sternocostal (anterior) surface** – formed mainly by the right ventricle.
- **Diaphragmatic (inferior) surface** – formed mainly by the left ventricle and a small part of the right ventricle.
- **Pulmonary (left) surface** – formed mainly by the left ventricle. The pulmonary surface of the heart is in contact with the cardiac impression of the left lung.

3. Note that the coronary sulcus and the interventricular sulci mark the boundaries of the four chambers of the heart.

4. On the surface of the heart, identify the chambers (Fig. 3.15):
- **Right atrium** and **right auricle**
- **Right ventricle**
- **Left ventricle**
- **Left atrium** and **left auricle**

5. Examine the heart in superior view. Identify:
- **Aorta** and **aortic valve**
- **Pulmonary trunk** and **pulmonary valve**
- **Superior vena cava**

6. Examine the diaphragmatic surface of the heart and identify:
- **Inferior vena cava**
- **Posterior interventricular sulcus**

7. Note that the cardiac veins and coronary arteries are located in the coronary and interventricular sulci.

CARDIAC VEINS [G 53; L 183; N 216; R 262; C 136, 137]

1. As you study the vessels of the heart, realize that they (and the fat that surrounds them) are located between the visceral pericardium (epicardium) and the muscular surface of the heart.

2. The **cardiac veins** course superficial to the **coronary arteries**, so they will be dissected first. The coronary sulcus and the interventricular sulci are filled with fat that must be removed to observe the vessels. Use blunt dissection to remove the fat.

3. Identify the **coronary sinus** on the diaphragmatic surface of the heart (Fig. 3.17). The coronary sinus is a dilated portion of the venous system of the heart that is located in the coronary sulcus.

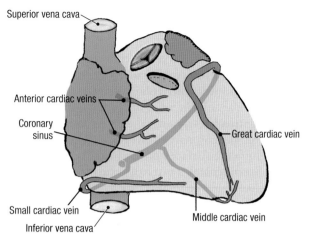

Figure 3.17. Cardiac veins.

The coronary sinus is about 2 to 2.5 cm in length and opens into the right atrium. Its opening will be seen when the internal features of the right atrium are dissected.

4. Use a probe to clean the surface of the coronary sinus (Fig. 3.17).
5. Follow the coronary sinus superiorly in the coronary sulcus to the point where it receives the **great cardiac vein**.
6. Use blunt dissection to follow the great cardiac vein onto the sternocostal surface of the heart. The great cardiac vein courses from the apex of the heart toward the coronary sinus in the anterior interventricular sulcus.
7. In the posterior interventricular sulcus, identify the **middle cardiac vein** and trace it to the coronary sinus.
8. Near the inferior end of the coronary sinus, identify the **small cardiac vein**. Use a probe to dissect the small cardiac vein and follow it to the anterior surface of the heart where it courses along the inferior border of the heart.
9. Note that most veins of the heart are tributaries to the coronary sinus. The anterior cardiac veins are the exceptions to this rule.
10. **Anterior cardiac veins** bridge the atrioventricular sulcus between the right atrium and right ventricle. The anterior cardiac veins drain the anterior wall of the right ventricle directly into the right atrium. Anterior cardiac veins pass superficial to the right coronary artery.

CORONARY ARTERIES [G 52; L 182; N 216; R 262; C 136]

1. Begin the dissection of the coronary arteries by observing the **aortic valve** in the lumen of the ascending aorta. Identify the **right**, **left**, and **posterior semilunar cusps** of the aortic valve. Behind

each valve cusp is a small pocket called an **aortic sinus** (**right**, **left**, and **posterior**, respectively).
2. In the left aortic sinus, identify the **opening of the left coronary artery**. Insert the tip of a probe into the opening. On the surface of the heart, palpate the tip of the probe between the left auricle and the pulmonary trunk. This is the initial portion of the left coronary artery.
3. Use blunt dissection to clean the left coronary artery. The left coronary artery is quite short. In the coronary sulcus, the left coronary artery divides into the **anterior interventricular branch** and the **circumflex branch** (Fig. 3.18).
4. Trace the **anterior interventricular branch** in the anterior interventricular sulcus to the apex of the heart. Clinicians call the anterior interventricular branch of the left coronary artery the **left anterior descending (LAD) artery**. Note that the anterior interventricular artery accompanies the great cardiac vein.
5. Follow the **circumflex branch of the left coronary artery** in the coronary sulcus and around the left border of the heart. The circumflex branch of the left coronary artery has several unnamed branches that supply the posterior wall of the left ventricle. The circumflex branch of the left coronary artery accompanies the coronary sinus in the coronary sulcus.
6. To begin the dissection of the **right coronary artery**, identify its opening in the right aortic sinus. Insert the tip of a probe into its opening. On the surface of the heart, palpate the tip of the probe in the coronary sulcus between the right auricle and the ascending aorta. This is the beginning of the right coronary artery.
7. Use blunt dissection to clean the right coronary artery and identify the **anterior right atrial**

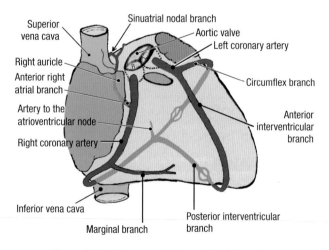

Figure 3.18. Coronary arteries and their branches.

branch (Fig. 3.18). The anterior right atrial branch arises close to the origin of the right coronary artery and ascends along the anterior wall of the right atrium toward the superior vena cava. The anterior right atrial branch gives rise to the **sinuatrial nodal branch**, which supplies the sinuatrial node.

8. Follow the right coronary artery in the coronary sulcus. Preserve the anterior cardiac veins. The **marginal branch** of the right coronary artery usually arises near the inferior border of the heart. The marginal branch accompanies the small cardiac vein along the inferior border of the heart.

9. Continue to follow the right coronary artery in the coronary sulcus onto the diaphragmatic surface of the heart. When the right coronary artery reaches the posterior interventricular sulcus, it gives rise to the **posterior interventricular branch**. The posterior interventricular branch courses along the posterior interventricular sulcus to the apex of the heart, where it anastomoses with the anterior interventricular branch of the left coronary artery. The posterior interventricular branch accompanies the middle cardiac vein.

10. Note that the **artery to the atrioventricular node** arises from the right coronary artery at the point where the posterior interventricular sulcus meets the coronary sulcus (Fig. 3.18).

CLINICAL CORRELATION

Coronary Arteries

In approximately 75% of hearts, the right coronary artery gives rise to the posterior interventricular branch and supplies the left ventricular wall and posterior portion of the interventricular septum. In approximately 15% of hearts, the left coronary artery gives rise to the posterior interventricular branch. Other variations account for 10%.

Dissection Review

1. Review the borders of the heart.
2. On the surface of the heart, review the boundaries of the four chambers.
3. Review the coronary sulcus and interventricular sulci of the heart and the vessels that course within these sulci.
4. Trace a drop of blood from the right aortic sinus to the coronary sinus, naming all vessels that are involved.

5. Trace a drop of blood from the left aortic sinus to the apex of the heart and its venous return to the coronary sinus, naming all vessels that are involved.

INTERNAL FEATURES OF THE HEART

Dissection Overview

The atria and ventricles of the heart will be opened and their internal features will be studied. The incisions that will be used are designed to preserve most of the vessels that you have previously dissected. The heart will contain clotted blood, which must be removed. The clots will be hard and may need to be broken before they can be extracted. The chambers will be dissected in the sequence that blood passes through the heart: **right atrium**, **right ventricle**, **left atrium**, and **left ventricle**. All descriptions are based on the heart in anatomical position.

Dissection Instructions

RIGHT ATRIUM [G 56; L 184; N 220; R 258; C 142]

1. The cuts used to open the right atrium are illustrated in Figure 3.19.
2. Use scissors to make a cut through the tip of the right auricle. Insert one blade of the scissors through the opening and make a short horizontal cut toward the right (Fig. 3.19, cut 1).
3. Turn the scissors and cut through the anterior wall of the right atrium in an inferior direction. Stop superior to the inferior vena cava (Fig. 3.19, cut 2).
4. Make a horizontal cut toward the left, stopping just short of the coronary sulcus (Fig. 3.19, cut 3).

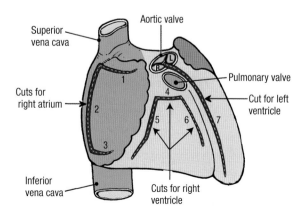

Figure 3.19. Cuts used to open the right atrium, right ventricle, and left ventricle of the heart.

5. Turn the flap of the atrial wall toward the left and open the right atrium widely (Fig. 3.20). Remove blood clots and take the heart to the sink to rinse it with water.

6. Observe the inner surface of the **anterior wall of the right atrium**. Identify (Fig. 3.20):
   • **Pectinate muscles** – horizontal ridges of muscle
   • **Crista terminalis** – a vertical ridge of muscle that connects the pectinate muscles

7. Observe the **posterior wall of the right atrium**. Identify (Fig. 3.20):
   • **Opening of the superior vena cava**
   • **Opening and valve of the inferior vena cava**
   • **Opening and valve of the coronary sinus**
   • **Fossa ovalis** and the **limbus fossa ovalis** (L. *limbus*, a border)

CLINICAL CORRELATION

Fossa Ovalis

The **fossa ovalis** is the remnant of the **foramen ovale**. In fetal life, blood from the placenta is delivered to the heart by way of the inferior vena cava. This oxygen-rich and nutrient-rich blood is directed toward the foramen ovale, which allows passage into the left atrium and out to the body without passing through the lungs.

---

8. Parts of the **conducting system of the heart** are located in the walls of the right atrium, but cannot be seen in dissection. Familiarize yourself with their approximate locations in the dissected specimen (Fig. 3.20). The **sinuatrial node** (SA node) lies at the superior end of the crista terminalis at the junction between the right atrium and the superior vena cava. The **atrioventricular node** (AV node) is located in the interatrial septum, above the opening of the coronary sinus.

9. Identify the opening of the **right atrioventricular valve**, which leads into the right ventricle.

RIGHT VENTRICLE [G 57; L 184; N 220; R 261; C 142]

1. The cuts used to open the right ventricle are illustrated in Figure 3.19.

2. Insert your finger into the pulmonary trunk and determine the level of the **pulmonary valve**. Immediately inferior to the level of the pulmonary valve, use scissors to make a short horizontal cut through the **anterior wall of the right ventricle** (Fig. 3.19, cut 4).

3. Insert one blade of the scissors into the right end of the cut 4 and make a cut parallel to the coronary sulcus (Fig. 3.19, cut 5). This cut should be about 1 cm from the coronary sulcus and end at the inferior border of the heart. Cut only the ventricular wall, not the atrioventricular valve cusp.

4. Insert your finger through the opening in the ventricular wall and palpate the **interventricular septum**. From the left end of cut 4 (Fig. 3.19), make a cut toward the inferior border of the heart (Fig. 3.19, cut 6). This cut should be about 2 cm to the right of the anterior interventricular sulcus and should parallel the right side of the interventricular septum.

5. Turn the flap of the right ventricular wall inferiorly (Fig. 3.21).

6. Remove blood clots. Use care to avoid damaging the **chordae tendineae**. Rinse the right ventricle with water.

7. Identify the **opening of the right atrioventricular valve**. Observe that the right atrioventricular valve has **three cusps: anterior, septal, and posterior** (Fig. 3.21). The right atrioventricular valve is also called the **tricuspid valve**.

8. Identify the **chordae tendineae**. Observe that these delicate tendons pass from the valve cusps to the apices of **papillary muscles**. The papillary muscles arise from the walls of the right ventricle.

9. Identify **three papillary muscles: anterior, septal, and posterior**. The anterior papillary muscle is the largest. The septal papillary muscle is very small and may be multiple. Note that the chordae tendineae of each papillary muscle attach to the adjacent sides of two valve cusps.

10. Observe that the inner surface of the wall of the right ventricle is roughened by muscular ridges called **trabeculae carneae** (L. *trabs*, wooden beam; *carneus*, fleshy).

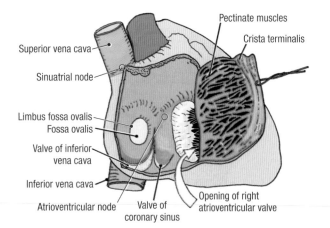

Pectinate muscles
Crista terminalis
Superior vena cava
Sinuatrial node
Limbus fossa ovalis
Fossa ovalis
Valve of inferior vena cava
Inferior vena cava
Atrioventricular node
Valve of coronary sinus
Opening of right atrioventricular valve

Figure 3.20. Interior of the right atrium with approximate locations of the sinuatrial and atrioventricular nodes.

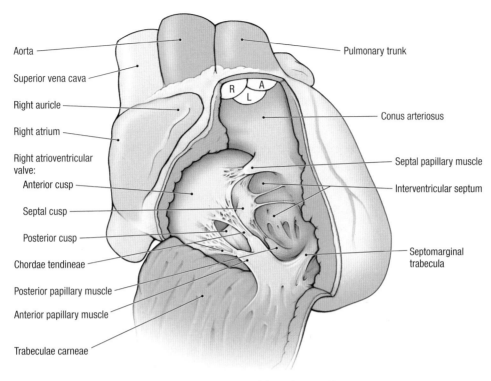

Aorta

Superior vena cava

Right auricle

Right atrium

Right atrioventricular valve:

Anterior cusp

Septal cusp

Posterior cusp

Chordae tendineae

Posterior papillary muscle

Anterior papillary muscle

Trabeculae carneae

Pulmonary trunk

R A L

Conus arteriosus

Septal papillary muscle

Interventricular septum

Septomarginal trabecula

Figure 3.21. Interior of the right ventricle.

11. Identify the **septomarginal trabecula (moderator band)**. The septomarginal trabecula extends from the interventricular septum to the base of the anterior papillary muscle. The septomarginal trabecula contains part of the right bundle of the conducting system, the part that stimulates the anterior papillary muscle.

12. Identify the **opening of the pulmonary trunk** (Fig. 3.21). The **conus arteriosus (infundibulum)** is the cone-shaped portion of the right ventricle inferior to the opening of the pulmonary trunk. The inner wall of the conus arteriosus is smooth.

13. Observe that the **pulmonary valve** consists of **three semilunar cusps: anterior, right,** and **left** (Fig. 3.21). [G 60, 63; L 184; N 222; R 259; C 136]

14. Look into the pulmonary trunk from above and examine the superior surface of the semilunar valve. Observe that each semilunar valve cusp has one fibrous **nodule** and two **lunules**. The nodule and lunules help to seal the valve cusps and prevent backflow of blood during diastole.

LEFT ATRIUM [G 58; L 185; N 221; R 258; C 144]

1. Examine the posterior surface of the heart. Observe the openings of the **four pulmonary veins** into the left atrium. The pulmonary veins

are usually arranged in pairs, two from the right lung and two from the left lung.

2. The cut used to open the left atrium is illustrated in Figure 3.22A.

3. Use scissors to make an inverted U-shaped incision through the posterior wall of the left atrium. Do not cut into the openings of the pulmonary veins; cut between them. Turn the flap inferiorly (Fig. 3.22B).

4. Remove blood clots and rinse with water.

5. Note that the inner surface of the wall of the left atrium is smooth except for its auricle, which has a rough inner surface.

6. Observe the following features in the left atrium (Fig. 3.22B):
   • **Valve of the foramen ovale** on the **interatrial septum**
   • **Opening into the left auricle**
   • **Opening of the left atrioventricular valve**

LEFT VENTRICLE [G 59; L 185; N 221; R 258; C 145]

1. The cut used to open the left ventricle is illustrated in Figure 3.19. Note that the following procedure will cut the anterior interventricular branch of the left coronary artery and the great cardiac vein.

2. Look into the aorta from above and identify the **aortic valve**. Identify **three semilunar valve**

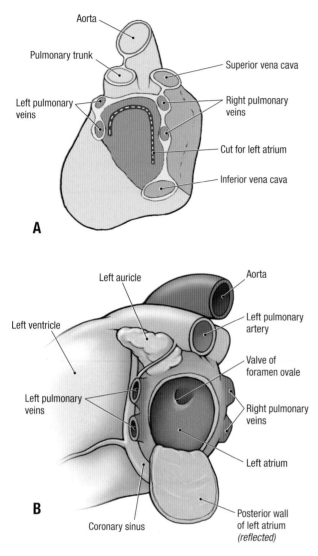

A

B

Figure 3.22. The left atrium of the heart. **A.** Cuts used to open the left atrium. **B.** Interior of the left atrium.

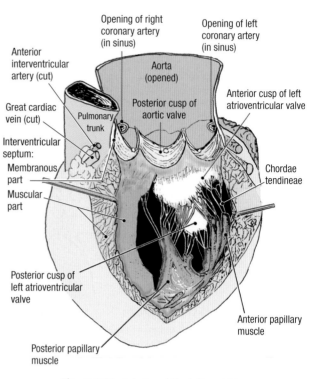

Figure 3.23. Interior of the left ventricle.

7. In the left ventricle, identify the **left atrioventricular valve (bicuspid valve, mitral valve)**. Identify the **anterior cusp** and the **posterior cusp** (Fig. 3.23).

8. Identify the **anterior papillary muscle** and the **posterior papillary muscle**. Observe that the **chordae tendineae** of each papillary muscle attach to both valve cusps.

9. Observe that the inner surface of the wall of the left ventricle is roughened by **trabeculae carneae**.

10. Examine the **aortic valve**. Again identify its **right, left**, and **posterior semilunar cusps**. Observe that each semilunar valve cusp has one nodule and two lunules.

11. Palpate the **muscular part of the interventricular septum**. Place the thumb of your right hand in the right ventricle and your index finger in the left ventricle and palpate the thickness of the muscular part of the interventricular septum.

12. Move your thumb and index finger superiorly along the interventricular septum and palpate the thin **membranous part of the interventricular septum**. It is located inferior to the attachment of the right cusp of the aortic valve.

13. In the aorta, observe the openings of the **coronary arteries** and study their relationship to the semilunar valve cusps and the **aortic sinuses**. The posterior cusp is also called the **noncoronary cusp** because there is no coronary artery arising from its sinus.

cusps: right, left, and **posterior**. [G 60, 63; L 185; N 222, 223; R 259; C 136]

3. Insert one blade of a scissors between the left and right semilunar cusps (Fig. 3.19).

4. Make a cut through the anterior wall of the ascending aorta between the left and right semilunar cusps (Fig. 3.19, cut 7). This cut should be anterior and parallel to the left coronary artery.

5. Continue the cut to the apex of the heart. The cut should be about 2 cm to the left of the anterior interventricular sulcus and should be parallel to the left side of the interventricular septum. The cut will cross the anterior interventricular branch of the left coronary artery and the great cardiac vein.

6. Open the left ventricle and the ascending aorta widely (Fig. 3.23). Remove blood clots and rinse with water.

14. Use an illustration to study the **conducting system of the heart.** [G 64; L 187; N 225; R 261; C 148, 149] Recall that the SA node is in the wall of the right atrium, at the superior end of the crista terminalis near the superior vena cava. Impulses from the SA node pass through the wall of the right atrium to the **AV node.** Impulses that originate in the AV node pass in the **AV bundle** through the membranous part of the interventricular septum. Subsequently, the AV bundle divides into **right and left bundles**, which lie on either side of the muscular part of the interventricular septum and stimulate the ventricles to contract. The right bundle is noteworthy because it carries impulses to the anterior papillary muscle through the **septomarginal trabecula.**

Dissection Review

1. Review the internal features of each of the chambers of the heart.
2. Replace the heart into the thorax in its correct anatomical position. Return the anterior thoracic wall to its anatomical position. Use an illustration, a textbook description, and the dissected specimen to project the heart valves to the surface of the anterior thoracic wall.
3. Read a description of the auscultation point used to listen to each heart valve. Locate each auscultation point on the anterior thoracic wall, and then lift the anterior thoracic wall to observe the location of the auscultation point relative to the heart.
4. Review the course of blood as it passes through the heart, beginning in the superior vena cava and ending in the ascending aorta. In the correct sequence, name all of the chambers and valves that the blood passes through.
5. Review the blood supply to the heart. Trace a drop of blood from the left coronary artery and the right coronary artery to the coronary sinus, naming all vessels traversed.
6. Review the connections of the great vessels to the heart.
7. Use an illustration to review the conducting system of the heart and relate the illustration to the dissected specimen.

SUPERIOR MEDIASTINUM

Dissection Overview

The superior mediastinum contains structures that pass between the thorax and the neck, or the thorax and the upper limb. These structures include several of the great vessels and their primary branches, the trachea, the esophagus, and the thoracic duct.

The order of dissection will be as follows: The brachiocephalic veins will be studied and reflected superiorly to expose the aortic arch. The aortic arch and its branches will be dissected. Note that only the proximal ends of some of the large vessels will be seen in this dissection. The distal parts of these vessels will be dissected with the neck or the upper limb. The trachea and its bifurcation will be studied. The upper part of the esophagus and the vagus nerves will be dissected.

Dissection Instructions

1. Study the **boundaries of the superior mediastinum** (Fig. 3.13).
   - **Superior** – superior thoracic aperture
   - **Posterior** – bodies of vertebrae T1 to T4
   - **Anterior** – manubrium of the sternum
   - **Lateral** – mediastinal pleurae (left and right)
   - **Inferior** – plane of the sternal angle
2. Remove the anterior thoracic wall.
3. Identify the **thymus**. In the adult, the thymus is a fatty remnant that lies immediately posterior to the manubrium of the sternum. [G 66–69; L 177; N 212; R 269]

CLINICAL CORRELATION

Thymus

In the newborn, the thymus is an active lymphatic organ that can be visualized on a chest radiograph. The thymus is replaced by connective tissue and fat after puberty. It may be difficult to recognize the thymus in the cadaver.

4. Remove the remnant of the thymus by blunt dissection.
5. Trace the superior vena cava superiorly until it bifurcates. Identify the **left brachiocephalic vein** (Fig. 3.24). Use blunt dissection to clean the anterior surface of the left brachiocephalic vein and to free it from the structures that lie posterior to it.
6. Identify the **right brachiocephalic vein**. The two **brachiocephalic veins** meet to form the **superior vena cava** posterior to the inferior border of the right first costal cartilage.
7. Follow the superior vena cava inferiorly. Note that the superior vena cava passes anterior to the root of the right lung. [G 80; L 179, 194; N 230; R 280; C 126]
8. Identify the **azygos vein** on the right side of the mediastinum. The **arch of the azygos vein** passes

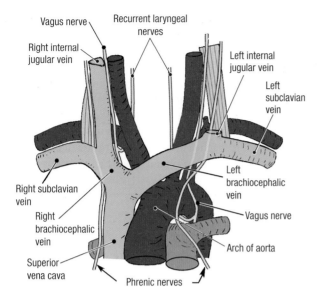

Figure 3.24. Relationships of the phrenic nerves and the vagus nerves to the great vessels.

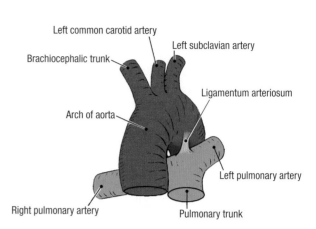

Figure 3.25. Branches of the arch of the aorta.

root of the left lung toward the esophagus. Review the relationship of the left recurrent laryngeal nerve to the ligamentum arteriosum.

superior to the root of the right lung and drains into the posterior surface of the superior vena cava.

9. Cut the superior vena cava just superior to the entrance of the azygos vein. Reflect the superior vena cava and the attached brachiocephalic veins superiorly.

10. Identify the **right phrenic nerve** and the **left phrenic nerve** that pass posterior to the brachiocephalic veins. The phrenic nerves were previously dissected in the middle mediastinum. Note that the right and left phrenic nerves pass anterior to the roots of the right and left lungs, respectively. Demonstrate that the phrenic nerves accompany the pericardiacophrenic vessels and that they enter the superior surface of the diaphragm.

11. Identify the **arch of the aorta** (Fig. 3.25). The arch of the aorta begins and ends at the level of the sternal angle. [G 81; L 179, 195; N 231; R 281; C 127]

12. Identify the three arteries that arise from the arch of the aorta (Fig. 3.25). From anterior to posterior these arteries are:
    • **Brachiocephalic trunk**
    • **Left common carotid artery**
    • **Left subclavian artery**

13. Identify the **ligamentum arteriosum**. The ligamentum arteriosum is a fibrous cord that connects the concavity of the arch of the aorta to the left pulmonary artery (Fig. 3.25).

14. Identify the **left vagus nerve** and the **left recurrent laryngeal nerve** on the left side of the arch of the aorta (Fig. 3.26). Follow the left vagus nerve inferiorly and note that it passes posterior to the

CLINICAL CORRELATION

Left Recurrent Laryngeal Nerve

The left recurrent laryngeal nerve has a close relationship to the aortic arch and passes through the superior mediastinum. In cases of mediastinal tumors or an aneurysm of the aortic arch, the left recurrent laryngeal nerve may be compressed, resulting in paralysis of the left vocal fold and hoarseness.

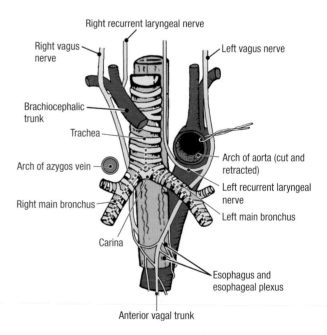

Figure 3.26. Course of the right and left vagus nerves.

15. On the right side note that the **right vagus nerve** passes posterior to the root of the right lung (Fig. 3.26). The **right recurrent laryngeal nerve** (a branch of the right vagus nerve) loops around the right subclavian artery.
16. Identify the **trachea**. Note that the esophagus lies posterior to the trachea in the superior mediastinum, but do not attempt to dissect it.
17. Identify the **bifurcation of the trachea**. The trachea bifurcates at the plane of the sternal angle to form the **right main bronchus** and the **left main bronchus**. Note that the arch of the azygos vein passes superior to the right main bronchus and the arch of the aorta passes superior to the left main bronchus (Fig. 3.26).
18. Observe that **tracheobronchial lymph nodes** are located around the trachea near its bifurcation.
19. Palpate the anterior and posterior surfaces of the trachea near its bifurcation. Observe that the **tracheal rings** are C-shaped and that the open part of the "C" is located posteriorly.
20. Observe that the esophagus is located posterior to the trachea in close relationship to the open part of the tracheal cartilages.
21. Use scissors to make a longitudinal cut through the anterior surface of the right and left main bronchi (Fig. 3.26, dashed lines). The cuts should meet anterior to the tracheal bifurcation. Make a third cut superiorly through the anterior surface of the trachea for a distance of 2.5 cm. Inside the tracheal bifurcation, identify the **carina** (L. *carina*, keel of a boat) (Fig. 3.26). The carina is a specialized piece of tracheal cartilage.
22. Compare the right and left main bronchi. Observe that the right main bronchus is larger in diameter, shorter, and oriented more vertically than the left main bronchus.

CLINICAL CORRELATION

Bifurcation of the Trachea

During bronchoscopy, the carina serves as an important landmark because it lies between the superior ends of the right and left main bronchi. The carina is usually positioned slightly to the left of the median plane of the trachea. When foreign bodies are aspirated, they usually enter the right main bronchus because it is wider and more vertically oriented than the left main bronchus.

Dissection Review

1. Replace the contents of the superior mediastinum into their correct anatomical positions.

2. Return the anterior thoracic wall to its correct anatomical position. Project the structures of the superior mediastinum to the surface of the thoracic wall.
3. Remove the anterior thoracic wall.
4. Review the formation of the superior vena cava and the position of the arch of the azygos vein.
5. Review the position of the ascending aorta and the position of the arch of the aorta.
6. Review the branches of the arch of the aorta.
7. Compare the positions of the phrenic and vagus nerves to the root of the lung.
8. Contrast the thoracic course of the left recurrent laryngeal nerve to the thoracic course of the right recurrent laryngeal nerve. Relate this difference to the embryonic origin of the arteries.

POSTERIOR MEDIASTINUM

Dissection Overview

The posterior mediastinum contains structures that course between the thorax and the abdomen. The posterior mediastinum lies posterior to the pericardium. To emphasize their close relationship to the heart, the structures in the posterior mediastinum will be approached through the **posterior wall of the pericardium**.

The order of dissection will be as follows: The pericardium will be reviewed and its posterior wall will be removed. The close relationship of the pericardium to the esophagus will be studied and then the pericardium will be removed. The esophagus will be studied. The azygos vein and its tributaries will be studied. The thoracic duct will be identified. Then, the descending aorta and its branches will be dissected. Finally, the thoracic portion of the sympathetic trunk and its branches will be dissected.

Dissection Instructions

1. Study the **boundaries of the posterior mediastinum** (Fig. 3.13):
    - **Superior** – plane of the sternal angle
    - **Posterior** – bodies of vertebrae T5 to T12
    - **Anterior** – pericardium
    - **Lateral** – mediastinal pleurae (left and right)
    - **Inferior** – diaphragm
2. Review the inner surface of the posterior wall of the pericardium (Fig. 3.16).
3. Place the heart back into the pericardium. From the right side of the thorax, examine the relationship of the heart to the esophagus. Note that the esophagus lies immediately posterior to the left atrium and part of the left ventricle. Remove the heart.

4. Remove the posterior wall of the pericardium in the **area of the oblique pericardial sinus** (Fig. 3.27). Identify the **esophagus**. The esophagus is a muscular tube that sits just to the right of the midline. To the left and slightly posterior to the esophagus is the **thoracic aorta**.

5. Use blunt dissection to remove the remainder of the posterior wall of the pericardium. Leave the portion adhering to the diaphragm undisturbed. Use scissors to cut the pericardium at its attachments to the great vessels and diaphragm and place the pericardium in the tissue container. [G 82; L 196; N 232; R 274; C 158]

6. Use blunt dissection to clean the **esophagus**. Note that the surface of the esophagus is covered by the **esophageal plexus of nerves** (Fig. 3.27). The esophageal plexus innervates the inferior portion of the esophagus.

7. Find the **right vagus nerve** in the angle formed by the arch of the azygos vein and the superior vena cava (Fig. 3.28). Follow it posterior to the root of the right lung. Confirm that the fibers of the right vagus nerve spread out on the surface of the esophagus.

8. Identify the **left vagus nerve** as it crosses the left side of the arch of the aorta. Follow the left vagus nerve posterior to the root of the left lung and confirm that its fibers contribute to the esophageal plexus.

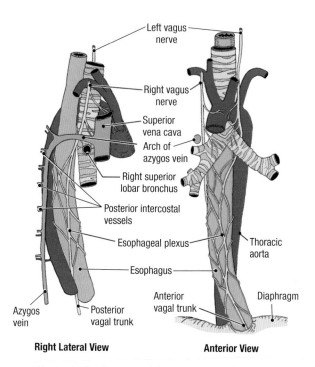

Figure 3.28. Contents of the posterior mediastinum.

9. Near the diaphragm, identify the **anterior vagal trunk** and the **posterior vagal trunk**. The vagal trunks are found on the inferior part of the esophagus, just before it passes through the diaphragm (Figs. 3.27 and 3.28). The vagal trunks pass through the diaphragm with the esophagus and innervate a large part of the gastrointestinal tract.

10. Identify the **azygos vein** where it arches superior to the root of the right lung (Fig. 3.28). Clean the azygos vein and follow it inferiorly to the level of the diaphragm. Note that the **posterior intercostal veins** on the right side are tributaries to the azygos vein. [G 78; L 194, 198; N 238; R 279; C 159]

11. Identify the **thoracic duct**. To find the thoracic duct, retract the esophagus to the left and explore the area between the **azygos vein** and the **thoracic aorta**. The thoracic duct lies immediately to the left of the azygos vein and it is posterior to the esophagus. The thoracic duct is thin-walled and easily torn. It has the appearance of a small vein without blood in it. [G 76; L 199; N 316; R 277; C 159]

12. Use a probe to free the thoracic duct from the surrounding connective tissue. The thoracic duct may be a network of several small ducts instead of a single duct. Inferiorly, the thoracic duct passes through the diaphragm with the thoracic aorta. Superiorly, the thoracic duct terminates by draining into the junction of the left internal jugular vein and left subclavian vein. Do not attempt to demonstrate its termination at this time.

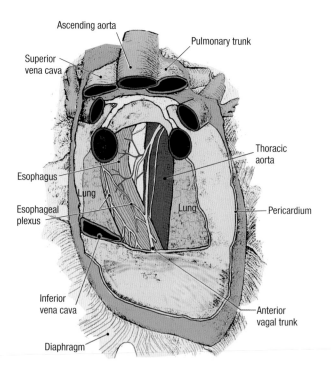

Figure 3.27. The relationship of the pericardium to the posterior mediastinum.

13. Note that the thoracic duct crosses the anterior surface of the **right posterior intercostal arteries**, the **hemiazygos vein,** and the **accessory hemiazygos vein**.

14. On the left side of the posterior mediastinum, observe that the left posterior intercostal veins drain into the **hemiazygos vein** or **accessory hemiazygos vein**. The hemiazygos and accessory hemiazygos veins cross the bodies of the ninth and eighth thoracic vertebrae, respectively, and terminate by draining into the azygos vein. Note that variations of the azygos system are common.

15. Identify the **thoracic aorta.** Use a probe to clean it from the surrounding connective tissue.

16. Identify **esophageal arteries** and the **left bronchial arteries.** These small arteries are unpaired vessels that arise from the anterior surface of the aorta. They are distinguished by their area of distribution.

17. Dissect one pair of **posterior intercostal arteries** (right and left). Follow them to their intercostal space. The right posterior intercostal arteries cross the midline on the anterior surface of the vertebral bodies. Note that the right posterior intercostal arteries pass posterior to all other contents of the posterior mediastinum.

18. On both sides of the thorax, identify and clean one **intercostal nerve.** Follow it laterally until it disappears posterior to the **innermost intercostal muscle**.

19. On both sides of the thorax, identify the **sympathetic trunk.** Starting high in the thorax, follow the sympathetic trunk inferiorly and observe that it crosses the heads of ribs 2 to 9. Inferior to rib 9, observe that the sympathetic trunk lies on the sides of the thoracic vertebral bodies. [G 82; L 194, 195; N 240; R 280; C 162]

20. Observe that the sympathetic trunk has one **sympathetic ganglion** for each thoracic vertebral level.

21. Demonstrate that two **rami communicantes** (**white ramus communicans, gray ramus communicans**) connect each intercostal nerve with its corresponding thoracic sympathetic ganglion. During dissection, it is impossible to distinguish white and gray rami from each other based on color. However, the more lateral of the two rami is the white ramus communicans.

22. Use a probe to dissect the **greater splanchnic nerve** on both the right and left sides. Note that the greater splanchnic nerve receives contributions from the fifth through the ninth thoracic sympathetic ganglia and that it is not completely formed until lower thoracic levels. As an aid to identification, observe that the greater splanchnic nerve is found on the sides of vertebral bodies T5 to T9, while the sympathetic trunk crosses the heads of ribs 5 to 9 (i.e., the sympathetic trunk is located posterior to the greater splanchnic nerve).

23. The **lesser splanchnic nerve** arises from the 10th and 11th thoracic sympathetic ganglia. The **least splanchnic nerve** arises from the 12th thoracic sympathetic ganglion. Due to the curvature of the diaphragm, these two nerves cannot be seen at this time.

Dissection Review

1. Review the boundaries of the anterior, middle, and posterior mediastina.

2. Study a transverse section through the midlevel of the thorax and identify the contents of the posterior mediastinum. Note the relationship of the contents of the posterior mediastinum to the heart and vertebral bodies.

3. Review the course and function of an intercostal nerve, naming all structures that it innervates.

4. Review the parts of the aorta (ascending, arch, thoracic), naming all branches and describing their distribution.

5. Review the origin and course of the right and left posterior intercostal arteries.

6. Name the structures in the posterior mediastinum that course anterior to the right posterior intercostal arteries.

CHAPTER 4

THE ABDOMEN

The abdomen is the portion of the trunk that lies between the thorax and the pelvis. The abdominal cavity is divided from the thoracic cavity by the diaphragm but it is continuous with the pelvic cavity. Viscera contained within the abdominal cavity are not bilaterally symmetrical. Therefore, it is worth noting that use of the words "right" and "left" in names and instructions refers to the right and left sides of the cadaver in the anatomical position.

SURFACE ANATOMY

Firm fixation of tissues in the cadaver may make it difficult to distinguish between bony landmarks and well-fixed soft tissue structures. Place the cadaver in the supine position and attempt to palpate the following structures (Fig. 4.1): [G 98; L 213; N 247]

- **Xiphoid process**
- **Costal margin**
- **Pubic symphysis**
- **Pubic crest**
- **Pubic tubercle**
- **Anterior superior iliac spine**
- **Tubercle of the iliac crest**

To prepare patient notes, you will need to understand the terminology used to describe the abdomen. The quadrant and regional systems are both in common use. The **quadrant system** divides the abdomen by means of the transumbilical plane and the median plane (Fig. 4.2). The quadrant system is suitable for general descriptions and will be used to describe the position of organs in this dissection guide. The **regional system** divides the abdomen based on the right and left midclavicular lines, the subcostal plane and the transtubercular plane (Fig. 4.3). Clinical complaints may be more specifically described using the regional system.

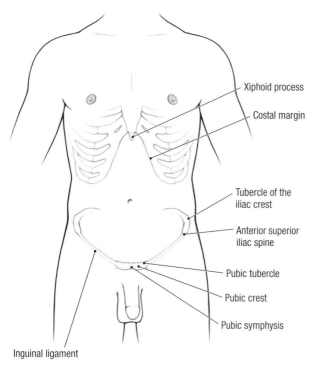

Figure 4.1. Surface anatomy of the abdomen.

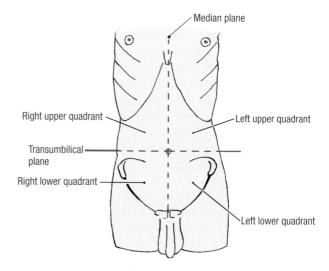

Figure 4.2. The four abdominal quadrants.

ATLAS REFERENCES
G = *Grant's Atlas,* 12th ed., page number
L = *LWW Atlas of Anatomy,* 1st ed., page number
N = *Netter's Atlas,* 4th ed., plate number
R = *Color Atlas of Anatomy,* 6th ed., page number
C = *Clemente's Atlas,* 5th ed., plate number

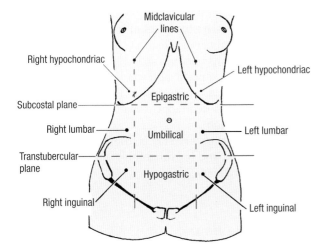

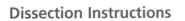

Figure 4.3. The nine abdominal regions.

SUPERFICIAL FASCIA OF THE ANTEROLATERAL ABDOMINAL WALL

Dissection Overview

The contents of the abdominal cavity are protected by the anterolateral abdominal wall. The organization of the layers forming the anterolateral abdominal wall is illustrated in Figure 4.4. The superficial fascia is unique in this region in that it has a superficial **fatty layer** called **Camper's fascia** and a deep **membranous layer** called **Scarpa's fascia**. The membranous layer is noteworthy, because it is continuous with named fascias in the perineum. [G 105; L 218; N 252; R 213; C 186]

Dissection Instructions

SKIN INCISIONS

1. Refer to Figure 4.5.
2. Make a midline skin incision from the xiphisternal junction (C) to the pubic symphysis (E), encircling the umbilicus.
3. Make an incision from the xiphoid process (C) along the costal margin to a point on the midaxillary line (V). If the thorax has been dissected previously, this incision has been made.
4. Make a skin incision beginning 3 cm below the pubic crest (E). Extend this incision laterally, 3 cm inferior to the inguinal ligament to a point 3 cm below the anterior superior iliac spine. Continue the incision posteriorly, 3 cm below the iliac crest to a point on the midaxillary line (F).
5. Make a vertical skin incision along the midaxillary line from point V to point F.
6. Make a transverse skin incision from the umbilicus to the midaxillary line.
7. Reflect the skin from medial to lateral, detach it along the midaxillary line, and place it in the tissue container.

SUPERFICIAL FASCIA

1. Use a probe to tear through the superficial fascia about 7.5 cm lateral to the midline (Fig. 4.6). The **superficial epigastric artery and vein** are in the superficial fascia in this area, but do not make a special effort to find them.
2. Dissect through the superficial fascia down to the aponeurosis of the external oblique muscle. On

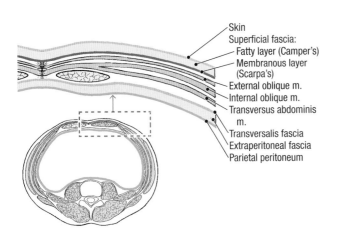

Figure 4.4. Layers of the anterior abdominal wall.

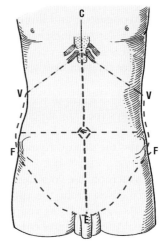

Figure 4.5. Skin incisions.

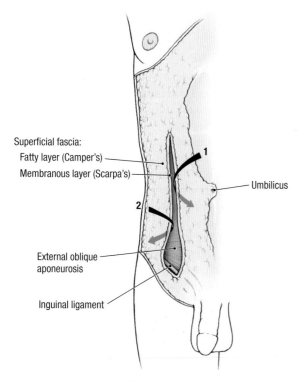

Superficial fascia:
Fatty layer (Camper's)
Membranous layer (Scarpa's)

Umbilicus

2

External oblique
aponeurosis

Inguinal ligament

Figure 4.6. Removal of the abdominal superficial fascia.

the medial side of the incision, use your fingers to separate the superficial fascia from the aponeurosis of the external oblique muscle (Fig. 4.6, arrow 1). As you remove the superficial fascia, observe that its deep surface is fibrous connective tissue containing relatively little fat (Scarpa's fascia) and the more superficial part is composed entirely of fat (Camper's fascia).

3. As you approach the midline, palpate the **anterior cutaneous nerves** that enter the superficial fascia about 2 to 3 cm lateral to the midline. Clean one anterior cutaneous nerve. The abdominal anterior cutaneous nerves are branches of **intercostal nerves (T7 to T11), the subcostal nerve (T12), and the iliohypogastric and ilioinguinal nerves (L1)**. Consult a dermatome chart and note that: [G 348; L 162; N 164; C 175]
    *   T7 innervates the skin overlying the tip of the xiphoid process.
    *   T10 innervates the skin of the umbilicus.
    *   T12 innervates the skin superior to the pubic symphysis.
    *   L1 innervates the skin overlying the pubic symphysis. [G 102; L 214; N 257; R 214; C 176]

4. Lateral to the incision, use your fingers to separate the superficial fascia from the external oblique muscle (Fig. 4.6, arrow 2). As you near the mid-axillary line, palpate the **lateral cutaneous nerves** entering the superficial fascia. The lateral cuta-

neous nerves are branches of intercostal nerves or the subcostal nerve. Clean the branches of one lateral cutaneous nerve.

5. Remove the superficial fascia in an inferior direction until the lower border of the external oblique muscle is exposed (approximately 2.5 cm into the proximal thigh).

6. Detach the superficial fascia from the midline, mid-axillary line, and proximal thigh and place it in the tissue container.

Dissection Review

1. Use an illustration to review the distribution of the superficial epigastric vessels.
2. Review the abdominal distribution of the ventral rami of spinal nerves T7 to L1.

CLINICAL CORRELATION

Superficial Veins of the Abdominal Wall

The superficial epigastric vein anastomoses with the lateral thoracic vein in the superficial fascia. This is an important collateral venous channel from the femoral vein to the axillary vein. In patients who have an obstruction of the inferior vena cava or hepatic portal vein, the superficial veins of the abdominal wall may be engorged, and may become visible around the umbilicus (**caput medusae**).

MUSCLES OF THE ANTEROLATERAL ABDOMINAL WALL

Dissection Overview

Three flat muscles (**external oblique, internal oblique, and transversus abdominis**) form most of the anterolateral abdominal wall. The rectus abdominis muscle completes the anterior abdominal wall near the midline. The three flat muscles have fleshy proximal attachments (to the ribs, vertebrae, and pelvis) and broad, aponeurotic distal attachments (to the ribs, linea alba, and pubis). Each of the three flat muscles contributes to the formation of the rectus sheath and the inguinal canal.

In the male, the testes are housed in the scrotum, which is an outpouching of the anterior abdominal wall. Each testis passes through the abdominal wall during development, dragging its ductus deferens behind it. This passage occurs through the **inguinal canal**. The inguinal canal is located superior to the medial half of the inguinal ligament and extends from the **superficial (external) inguinal ring** to the **deep (internal) inguinal ring**. In the female, the inguinal canal is smaller in diameter.

It must be noted that the structures forming the inguinal canal are identical in the two sexes, but the *contents* of the inguinal canal differ. In the male, the inguinal canal contains the **spermatic cord**, while in the female the inguinal canal contains the **round ligament of the uterus**. Dissection instructions are provided for male cadavers, but these instructions are applicable to female cadavers.

The order of dissection will be as follows: The three flat muscles of the abdominal wall will be studied, particularly in the inguinal region. The composition and contents of the rectus sheath will be explored. The anterior abdominal wall will be reflected.

SKELETON OF THE ABDOMINAL WALL

Use a skeleton to identify the following structures (Fig. 4.7): [G 10, 196; L 215; N 248; R 189; C 104, 266]

• **Xiphisternal junction**
• **Xiphoid process**
• **Costal margin**
• **Pubic symphysis**
• **Pubic crest**
• **Pubic tubercle**
• **Anterior superior iliac spine**
• **Iliac crest**
• **Tubercle of the iliac crest**

Dissection Instructions

EXTERNAL OBLIQUE MUSCLE [G 102; L 216; N 249; R 210; C 178]

1. Clean any remnants of the superficial fascia from the surface of the external oblique muscle and place them in the tissue container.
2. The **external oblique muscle** forms the most superficial portion of the inguinal canal (Fig. 4.8A). The proximal attachments of the external oblique muscle are the external surfaces of ribs 5 to 12. The distal attachments of the external oblique muscle are the linea alba, pubic tubercle, and anterior half of the iliac crest. Observe that the fibers of the external oblique muscle course from superolateral to inferomedial.
3. In the inguinal region, use blunt dissection to clean the aponeurosis of the external oblique mus-

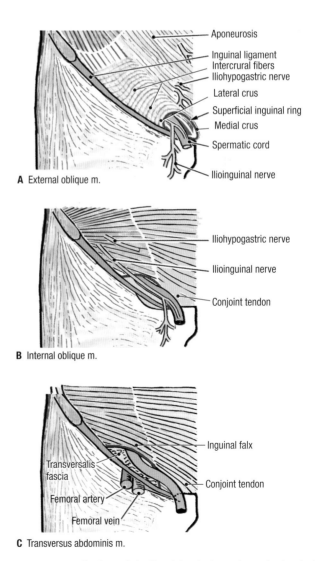

A External oblique m.

B Internal oblique m.

C Transversus abdominis m.

Figure 4.8. Contributions of the flat abdominal muscles to the inguinal canal.

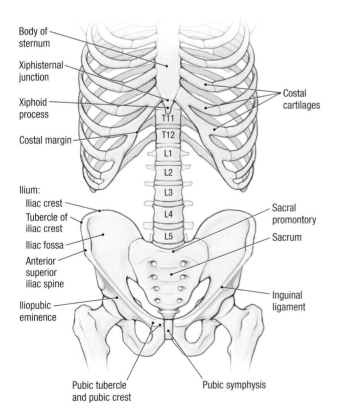

Figure 4.7. Skeleton of the anterior abdominal wall.

cle. Gentle scraping motions with a dull scalpel blade yield good results. Be careful not to damage the **spermatic cord** (or **round ligament of the uterus**) where it emerges from the superficial inguinal ring. [G 106, 110; L 216, 220; N 249; R 217, 220; C 179]

4. Identify the **superficial inguinal ring** (Fig. 4.8A), which is an opening in the external oblique aponeurosis.
5. Identify the **lateral (inferior) crus**. The lateral crus is the portion of the external oblique aponeurosis that forms the lateral margin of the superficial inguinal ring. It is attached to the pubic tubercle.
6. Identify the **medial (superior) crus**. The medial crus is the portion of the external oblique aponeurosis that forms the medial margin of the superficial inguinal ring. It is attached to the pubic crest.
7. Identify the **intercrural fibers**. Intercrural fibers span across the crura superolateral to the superficial inguinal ring. They prevent the crura from spreading apart.
8. At the margins of the superficial inguinal ring, observe the thin layer of fascia that extends from the external oblique aponeurosis onto the spermatic cord or round ligament of the uterus. This is the **external spermatic fascia,** which is the contribution of the external abdominal oblique muscle to the layers of the spermatic cord.

9. Note that the **ilioinguinal nerve** emerges from the inguinal canal at the superficial inguinal ring, anterior to the spermatic cord (or round ligament of the uterus). The ilioinguinal nerve supplies sensory fibers to the skin on the anterior surface of the external genitalia and the medial aspect of the thigh.
10. Identify the **inguinal ligament**. It is the inferior border of the aponeurosis of the external oblique muscle. Palpate the attachment of the inguinal ligament to the anterior superior iliac spine and to the pubic tubercle. Vessels and nerves exit the abdominal cavity and enter the lower limb by passing deep to the inguinal ligament.
11. Use an illustration to study the **lacunar ligament.** [G 106; L 220, 221; N 258; C 179] The lacunar ligament is formed by the medial fibers of the inguinal ligament that turn posteriorly to attach to the pecten pubis.

INTERNAL OBLIQUE MUSCLE [G 103; L 216; N 250; R 212; C 180]

The internal oblique muscle lies deep to the external oblique muscle. The internal oblique muscle forms the intermediate layer of the inguinal canal (Fig. 4.8B). To expose the internal oblique muscle, the external oblique muscle must be transected and reflected (Fig. 4.9). Perform this transection bilaterally.

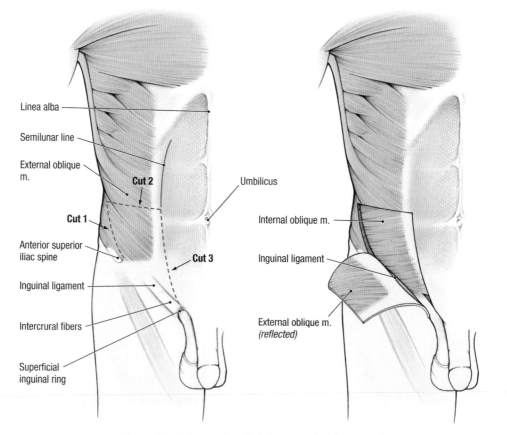

Figure 4.9. Cuts used to reflect the external oblique muscle.

1. Make a vertical cut through the external oblique muscle in the midaxillary line by the following method: Insert closed scissors between the fibers of the external oblique muscle at the level of the umbilicus. Open the scissors parallel to the muscle fiber direction to create an opening in the external oblique muscle. Insert your finger into the opening and direct it inferiorly, and then use scissors to make a vertical cut across the muscle fibers in the inferior direction (Fig. 4.9A, cut 1). Ex-tend cut 1 inferiorly as far as the anterior superior iliac spine.

2. Insert your fingers into cut 1 and use blunt dissection to separate the fibers of the external oblique muscle from the underlying internal oblique muscle. Note that your fingers cannot pass medial to the semilunar line because the external oblique aponeurosis is fused to the internal oblique aponeurosis.

3. In the transumbilical plane, use scissors to cut the external oblique muscle. Extend the cut as far medially as the semilunar line (Fig. 4.9A, cut 2).

4. Inferior to cut 2, use your fingers to separate the external oblique muscle from the internal oblique muscle. Be gentle as you approach the superficial inguinal ring.

5. Using scissors, make an incision from the medial end of cut 2 to the superior margin of the superficial inguinal ring (Fig. 4.9A, cut 3). Cut 3 should follow the lateral side of the semilunar line and cut only the external oblique aponeurosis.

6. Reflect the external oblique muscle in an inferior and lateral direction to reveal the lower half of the internal oblique muscle (Fig. 4.9B).

7. Identify the **internal oblique muscle**. The proximal attachments of the internal oblique muscle are the thoracolumbar fascia, the iliac crest, and the lateral half of the inguinal ligament. The distal attachments of the internal oblique muscle are the inferior borders of ribs 10 to 12, the linea alba, the pubic crest, and the pecten pubis. [G 107, 111; L 220; N 250; R 217, 220; C 181]

8. Observe the portion of the internal oblique muscle that arises from the lateral part of the inguinal ligament (Fig. 4.10). Note that this portion of the internal oblique muscle arches medially and attaches to the pecten pubis. It contributes to the roof of the inguinal canal.

9. Lateral to the spermatic cord (or round ligament of the uterus), observe muscle fibers connecting the internal oblique muscle to the spermatic cord (or round ligament) (Fig. 4.10). This is the layer of **cremaster muscle and fascia**, which is the contribution of the internal oblique muscle to the coverings of the spermatic cord. In the female, the

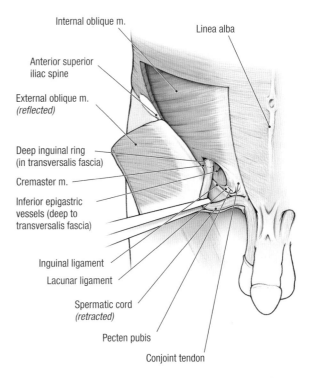

Figure 4.10. The internal oblique muscle in the inguinal region.

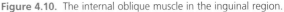

cremaster muscle and fascia surround the round ligament of the uterus.

10. In the intermuscular plane between the external oblique and the internal oblique muscles two nerves may be found (Fig. 4.8B):
   - **Ilioinguinal nerve** courses through the inguinal canal to emerge at the superficial inguinal ring.
   - **Iliohypogastric nerve** runs parallel to the ilioinguinal nerve and superior to it.

11. Just medial to the superficial inguinal ring the aponeurosis of the internal oblique becomes fused with the aponeurosis of the transversus abdominis muscle to form the **conjoint tendon** (Fig. 4.10).

TRANSVERSUS ABDOMINIS MUSCLE [G 103; L 217; N 251; R 215; C 183]

The transversus abdominis muscle lies deep to the internal oblique muscle. The transversus abdominis muscle contributes to the deepest layer of the inguinal canal (Fig. 4.8C). In the inguinal region the transversus abdominis muscle has attachments and fiber directions that are similar to the internal oblique muscle.

1. Use an illustration to study the proximal attachments, distal attachments, and fiber direction of the **transversus abdominis muscle**. The proximal attachments of the transversus abdominis muscle

are the internal surfaces of the costal cartilages of ribs 7 to 12, the thoracolumbar fascia, the iliac crest, and the lateral third of the inguinal ligament. The distal attachments of the transversus abdominis muscle are the linea alba, the pubic crest, and the pecten pubis. [G 108; L 217; N 251; R 218; C 183] **Dissection Note:** The transversus abdominis muscle is often difficult to separate from the internal oblique muscle because their tendons are fused near their distal attachments (conjoint tendon), and the muscle bellies adhere to each other laterally. If you are not required to separate the internal oblique muscle from the transversus abdominis muscle, go to the section entitled "Deep Inguinal Ring." If you are required to separate the internal oblique muscle from the transversus abdominis muscle, proceed with the next dissection step.

2. The ilioinguinal nerve may be traced laterally to find the plane of separation between the internal oblique muscle and the transversus abdominis muscle.

3. Locate the ilioinguinal nerve near the superficial inguinal ring and follow it laterally until it disappears into the surface of the internal oblique muscle (Fig. 4.8B).

4. To follow the ilioinguinal nerve, insert a pair of closed scissors into the internal oblique muscle superficial to the course of the ilioinguinal nerve and open the scissors parallel to the muscle fiber direction to split the muscle.

5. Insert your finger through the split and into the plane between the internal oblique and transversus abdominis muscles. Push your finger inferiorly and medially to separate the muscles. Proceed until you reach the arcuate line. Observe that the aponeuroses of the two muscles are inseparable near their attachment to the pecten pubis (conjoint tendon).

6. Note that the inferior free edge of the transversus abdominis muscle is slightly superior to the inferior free edge of the internal oblique muscle. Below the arch formed by these two muscles, the abdominal wall is unsupported by muscle. This weak point occurs directly posterior to the superficial inguinal ring.

DEEP INGUINAL RING [G 109; L 217, 219, 220; N 259; R 218; C 177]

Transversalis fascia lines the inner surface of the abdominal muscles (Fig. 4.4). The **deep inguinal ring** is the point at which the testis passed through the transversalis fascia during development. The deep inguinal ring is located superior to the midpoint of the inguinal ligament and it marks the deep extent of the inguinal

canal. In the male, the ductus deferens passes through the deep inguinal ring. In the female, the round ligament of the uterus passes through the deep inguinal ring.

1. Use a probe to lift the inferior margin of the fused internal oblique and transversus abdominis muscles.

2. Carefully use blunt dissection to separate the transversus abdominis muscle from the transversalis fascia.

3. Retract the spermatic cord (or round ligament of the uterus) inferiorly and observe the **inferior epigastric vessels** through the transversalis fascia (Fig. 4.10). The inferior epigastric vessels are located within the layer of extraperitoneal fascia.

4. The location of the deep inguinal ring is lateral to the inferior epigastric vessels, and is identified by the presence of the ductus deferens (or round ligament of the uterus).

5. To review, the **boundaries of the inguinal canal** are (Fig. 4.8):
   • **Deep** – deep inguinal ring
   • **Superficial** – superficial inguinal ring
   • **Anterior** – aponeurosis of the external oblique muscle
   • **Inferior** (floor) – inguinal ligament and lacunar ligament
   • **Superior** (roof) – the arching fibers of the internal oblique and the transversus abdominis muscles
   • **Posterior** – transversalis fascia, reinforced medially by the conjoint tendon

---

CLINICAL CORRELATION

Inguinal Hernias [L 223]

The inguinal canal is a weak area of the abdominal wall through which abdominal viscera may protrude (inguinal hernia). An inguinal hernia is classified according to its position relative to the inferior epigastric vessels. An **indirect inguinal hernia** exits the abdominal cavity through the deep inguinal ring *lateral* to the inferior epigastric vessels, and it follows the inguinal canal (an indirect course through the abdominal wall) (Fig. 4.11B). In contrast, a **direct inguinal hernia** exits the abdominal cavity *medial* to the inferior epigastric vessels and it follows a direct course through the abdominal wall (Fig. 4.11C).

RECTUS ABDOMINIS MUSCLE [G 102; L 217, 218; N 250; R 211; C 183]

The **rectus sheath** is formed by the aponeuroses of the three flat abdominal muscles. The rectus sheath

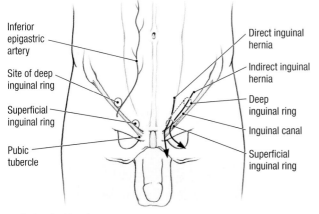

A Inguinal hernias

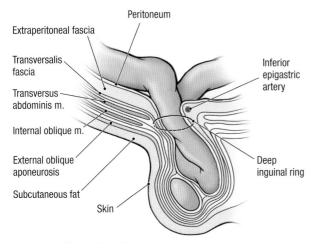

B Indirect inguinal hernia

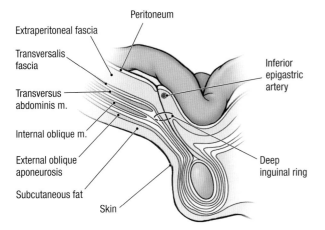

C Direct inguinal hernia

Figure 4.11. Inguinal hernias. **A.** Anatomical relationships and course through the abdominal wall. **B.** An indirect inguinal hernia leaves the abdominal cavity lateral to the inferior epigastric vessels and passes down the inguinal canal. **C.** A direct inguinal hernia leaves the abdominal cavity medial to the inferior epigastric vessels.

contains the **rectus abdominis muscle**, the **superior** and **inferior epigastric vessels**, the terminal ends of the ventral rami of spinal nerves T7 to T12, and the **pyramidalis muscle**.

1. Reposition the internal oblique and external oblique muscles. The following cuts should be made bilaterally.
2. Use scissors to make a transverse incision across the anterior surface of the rectus sheath at the level of the umbilicus (Fig. 4.12, cut 1). Begin the cut approximately 2.5 cm lateral to the umbilicus and continue it laterally as far as the semilunar line.
3. Use scissors to cut the rectus sheath along the medial border of the rectus abdominis muscle (Fig. 4.12, cut 2). This incision should extend in a superior direction, about 2.5 cm from the midline. Stop at the costal margin.
4. Extend the vertical incision inferiorly along the medial border of the rectus abdominis muscle (Fig. 4.12, cut 3). Cut 3 should be about 1.2 cm from the midline and stop at the pubic crest.
5. Insert your fingers into the vertical incision and bluntly dissect the anterior wall of the rectus sheath from the anterior surface of the rectus abdominis muscle. Observe that the anterior wall of

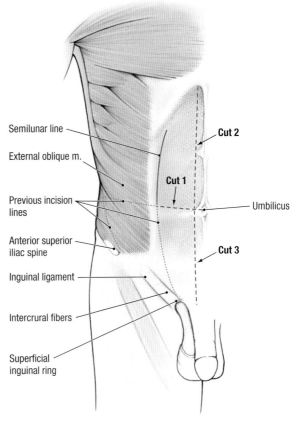

Figure 4.12. Cuts used to open the rectus sheath.

the rectus sheath is firmly attached to the anterior surface of the rectus muscle by several **tendinous intersections** (Fig. 4.13). Insert scissors between the rectus sheath and the anterior surface of the rectus abdominis muscle and cut the tendinous intersections to free the rectus sheath from the rectus abdominis muscle.

6. Observe the rectus abdominis muscle (Fig. 4.13). The inferior attachment of the rectus abdominis muscle is the symphysis and body of the pubis. The superior attachment of the rectus abdominis muscle is on the costal cartilages of ribs 5 to 7. The rectus abdominis muscle flexes the trunk.

7. Observe that the branches of six nerves (T7 to T12) enter the lateral side of the rectus sheath (Fig. 4.14). These nerves innervate the rectus abdominis muscle and then emerge as **anterior cutaneous branches**. [G 103; L 171, 214; N 257; R 216; C 176]

8. Use your fingers to mobilize the medial border of the rectus abdominis muscle. At the level of the umbilicus, transect the rectus abdominis muscle with scissors. Reflect the two halves superiorly and inferiorly, respectively. If the nerves prevent full reflection of the rectus abdominis muscle, cut them along the lateral border of the muscle.

9. Observe two sets of vessels on the deep surface of the rectus abdominis muscle: [G 103; L 217, 219; N 255; R 216; C 187]
   - **Superior epigastric artery and vein** − on the superior half of the rectus abdominis muscle
   - **Inferior epigastric artery and vein** − on the inferior half of the rectus abdominis muscle

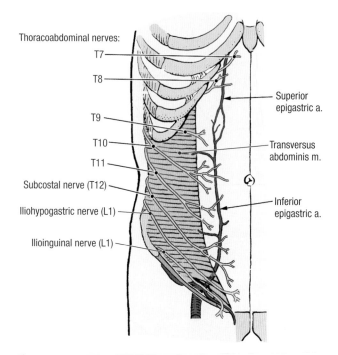

Figure 4.14. Nerves and arteries within the rectus sheath. The rectus abdominis muscle has been removed.

CLINICAL CORRELATION

Epigastric Anastomoses

The superior epigastric vessels anastomose with the inferior epigastric vessels within the rectus sheath (Fig. 4.14). If the inferior vena cava becomes obstructed, the anastomosis between the inferior epigastric and superior epigastric veins provides a collateral venous channel that drains into the superior vena cava. If the aorta is occluded, collateral arterial circulation to the lower part of the body occurs through the superior and inferior epigastric arteries.

10. Examine the posterior wall of the rectus sheath (Fig. 4.15). Identify the **arcuate line,** which is located midway between the pubic symphysis and the umbilicus. The arcuate line is the inferior limit of the posterior wall of the rectus sheath, and it may be indistinct. At the level of the arcuate line, the inferior epigastric vessels enter the rectus sheath.

11. Inferior to the arcuate line, observe the **transversalis fascia**. Deep to the transversalis fascia observe a thin layer of extraperitoneal fascia and the **parietal peritoneum** (Fig. 4.15).

12. In the midline, identify the **linea alba**. The linea alba is formed by the fusion of the aponeuroses of

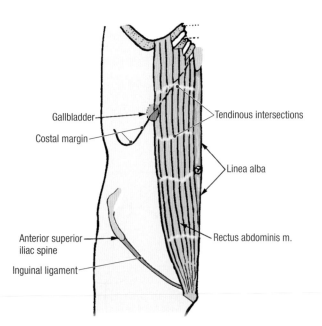

Figure 4.13. Rectus abdominis muscle.

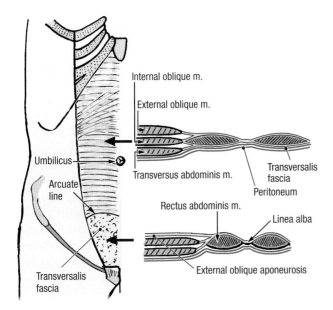

Figure 4.15. Posterior wall of the rectus sheath (*left*) and transverse sections of the rectus sheath at the two levels indicated by the arrows.

the right and left flat abdominal muscles (external oblique, internal oblique, and transversus abdominis).

13. Anterior to the inferior end of the rectus abdominis muscle, look for the **pyramidalis muscle**. It is frequently absent. When present, the pyramidalis muscle attaches to the anterior surface of the pubis and the linea alba, and it draws down on the linea alba.

Dissection Review

1. Replace the muscles of the anterior abdominal wall in their correct anatomical positions.
2. Review the proximal attachment, distal attachment, and action of each muscle.
3. Review the structures that form the nine layers of the abdominal wall (Fig. 4.4).
4. Use the dissected specimen to review the rectus sheath at the level of the umbilicus and just superior to the pubic symphysis (Fig. 4.15).
5. Review the nerve supply to the anterior abdominal wall. Review the blood supply to the anterior abdominal wall.

REFLECTION OF THE ABDOMINAL WALL

Dissection Overview

The anterior abdominal wall will be reflected in such a way that the contents of the abdominopelvic cavity can be ac-

cessed, but the abdominal wall can be repositioned for review. The incision lines will be similar to the quadrant lines illustrated in Figure 4.2. The incisions are designed to give direct reference to the position of the abdominal organs within the abdominal quadrants.

The order of dissection will be as follows: The anterior abdominal wall will be incised and opened. The inner surface of the anterior abdominal wall will be studied.

Dissection Instructions

1. Reflect the halves of the rectus abdominis muscles superiorly and inferiorly.
2. Refer to Figure 4.16. On the left side of the umbilicus, use scissors to create a small hole (2 cm) through the posterior wall of the rectus sheath, extraperitoneal fascia, and parietal peritoneum.
3. Insert your finger through the hole into the abdominal cavity. Pull the posterior wall of the rectus sheath anteriorly to create a space between the abdominal wall and the abdominal viscera.
4. Use scissors to make a vertical incision through the linea alba to the xiphoid process (Fig. 4.16, cut 1). Stay 1 cm to the left of the midline to preserve the falciform ligament.

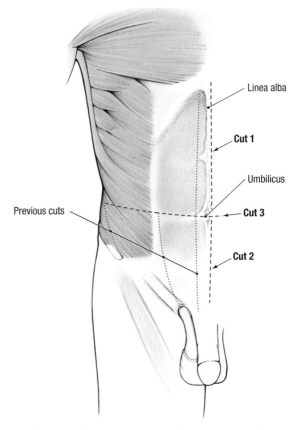

Figure 4.16. Cuts used to open the abdominal cavity.

5. Extend the incision inferiorly as far as the pubic symphysis (Fig. 4.16, cut 2). Stay 1 cm to the left of the midline to preserve the median umbilical fold.

6. Return the rectus abdominis muscle and the external oblique muscle to their correct anatomical positions.

7. At the level of the umbilicus, place one hand through the vertical incision and raise the abdominal wall from the abdominal contents.

8. On the right side of the abdomen, use scissors to incise the posterior wall of the rectus sheath, extraperitoneal fascia, and peritoneum in the transumbilical plane (Fig. 4.16, cut 3). The scissors should pass through the previous transverse cut that was made in the rectus abdominis muscle and the external oblique muscle. Extend the cut laterally through all three flat abdominal muscles as far as the midaxillary line. Repeat this transverse cut on the left side of the abdomen.

9. Open the flaps of the abdominal wall.

10. Identify the **falciform ligament** on the inner surface of the right upper quadrant flap. The falciform ligament connects the anterior abdominal wall to the surface of the liver. [G 118; L 219, 224; N 253; R 293; C 204]

11. On the inner surface of the lower abdominal wall, identify three folds:
    - **Median umbilical fold** – in the midline inferior to the umbilicus. It is attached to the right lower quadrant flap, but may have been cut longitudinally. The median umbilical fold contains the urachus (obliterated allantoic duct).
    - **Medial umbilical fold** – located lateral to the median umbilical fold. The medial umbilical fold contains the obliterated umbilical artery.
    - **Lateral umbilical fold** – located lateral to the medial umbilical fold. The lateral umbilical fold overlies the inferior epigastric artery and vein.

12. Lateral to the lateral umbilical fold, observe a small depression that marks the location of the **deep inguinal ring**.

PERITONEUM AND PERITONEAL CAVITY

Dissection Overview

All body cavities (thoracic cavity, pericardial cavity, and abdominopelvic cavity) are lined by serous membranes, which secrete a small amount of fluid to lubricate the movements of organs. In the abdominal cavity and pelvic cavity this membrane is called the **peritoneum**. There are two types of peritoneum: **Parietal peritoneum** lines the inner surfaces of the abdominal and pelvic walls, and **visceral peritoneum** covers the surfaces of the abdominal and pelvic organs. Between these two types of peritoneum is a potential space called the **peritoneal cavity**.

During development, some organs develop in the peritoneal cavity and are called **intraperitoneal (peritoneal) organs**. Examples of intraperitoneal organs include the stomach, small intestine, liver, and spleen. Some organs develop behind the peritoneum and are called **retroperitoneal (extraperitoneal) organs**: The ureters, suprarenal glands, and kidneys are examples. Some parts of the gastrointestinal tract begin as intraperitoneal organs and then become attached to the abdominal wall during development. These organs are **secondarily retroperitoneal**. Examples of secondarily retroperitoneal organs include the duodenum, pancreas, ascending colon, and descending colon.

The order of dissection will be as follows: The abdominal viscera will be identified and localized by abdominal quadrant. The named specializations of the peritoneum will be studied. For a more complete understanding, review the development of the gastrointestinal tract before examining the peritoneal specializations.

Dissection Instructions

ABDOMINAL VISCERA [G 119, 128; L 224, 225; N 269; R 291, 292; C 198, 199]

1. Use your hands to inspect the abdominal cavity. As you perform the inspection, you may encounter adhesions. If adhesions are present, tear them with your fingers to mobilize the organs.

2. Open the flaps of the abdominal wall. The incision lines correlate to the abdominal quadrant lines. As you examine the organs, you should close and open the flaps to help you relate the organs to the abdominal quadrants. Most of the organs to be identified are parts of the **gastrointestinal tract**.

3. Identify the **liver** (Fig. 4.17). It is an intraperitoneal organ. The liver occupies the right upper quadrant and extends across the midline into the left upper quadrant. The liver lies against the inferior surface of the diaphragm. The attachment of the falciform ligament divides the liver into **right** and **left lobes**.

4. The **gallbladder**, an intraperitoneal organ, is also in the right upper quadrant. The gallbladder extends below the inferior border of the liver. It is usually found at the tip of the right ninth costal cartilage in the midclavicular line. Confirm this relationship.

5. Identify the **stomach**. It is an intraperitoneal organ and lies in the left upper quadrant. It is con-

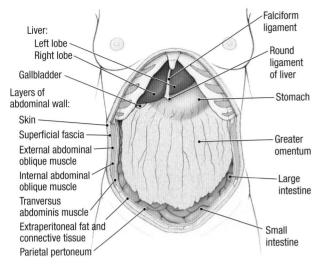

Figure 4.17. The relationship of the greater omentum to the abdominal viscera.

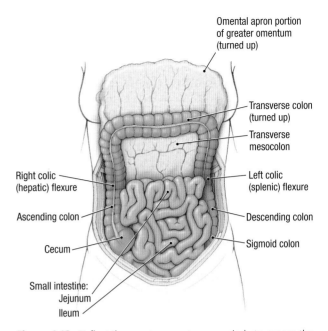

Figure 4.18. Reflect the greater omentum superiorly to expose the small intestine and large intestine.

tinuous with the esophagus proximally and the duodenum distally. The liver partially covers the anterior surface of the stomach.

6. Find the **spleen**. It is an intraperitoneal organ that lies in the left upper quadrant. It is found posterior to the stomach and may be difficult to find unless it is enlarged. Reach around the left side of the stomach with your right hand and palpate the spleen.

7. Identify the **greater omentum** (Fig. 4.17). The greater omentum is attached to the greater curvature of the stomach. Reflect the greater omentum superiorly over the costal margin (Fig. 4.18).

8. Identify the **small intestine** (Figs. 4.18 and 4.19). The small intestine begins at the pyloric end of the stomach. It has three parts:
   • **Duodenum**
   • **Jejunum**
   • **Ileum**

9. Most of the duodenum is secondarily retroperitoneal. It will be studied with the pancreas.

10. The **jejunum** and **ileum** are intraperitoneal organs that extend from the left upper quadrant to the right lower quadrant, but due to their length and mobility, they occupy all four quadrants. Beginning in the left upper quadrant, pass the jejunum and ileum between your hands and appreciate their length, position, and termination.

11. Identify the **large intestine**. The large intestine begins in the right lower quadrant at the ileocecal junction (Figs. 4.18 and 4.19). It has six parts:
   • **Cecum** − located in the right lower quadrant. The **appendix** is attached to the inferior end of the cecum.
   • **Ascending colon** extends from the right lower quadrant to the right upper quadrant. It ends at

the **right colic (hepatic) flexure**. The ascending colon is secondarily retroperitoneal.
• **Transverse colon** extends from the right upper quadrant to the left upper quadrant. The

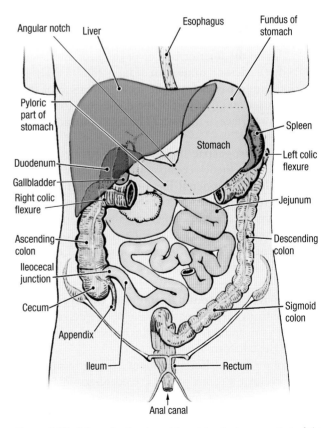

Figure 4.19. Schematic drawing of the abdominal organs. Part of the transverse colon has been removed.

transverse colon ends at the **left colic (splenic) flexure**. The transverse colon is intraperitoneal.

- **Descending colon** extends from the left upper quadrant to the left lower quadrant. The descending colon is secondarily retroperitoneal.
- **Sigmoid colon** – located in the left lower quadrant. The sigmoid colon ends in the pelvic cavity at the level of the third sacral vertebral level. The sigmoid colon is an intraperitoneal organ.
- **Rectum** – located in the pelvis. The rectum will be dissected with the pelvic viscera.

12. Use your hands to trace the large intestine from the right lower quadrant to the left lower quadrant. Note the position (quadrant) and mobility of each of its parts.

PERITONEUM [G 119; L 224–226; N 269; R 306; C 204]

1. Observe the **visceral peritoneum** on the surface of the stomach or small intestine (Fig. 4.20). Note that visceral peritoneum is smooth and slippery.
2. Observe the **parietal peritoneum** on the inner surface of the abdominal wall (Fig. 4.20). Note that parietal peritoneum is also smooth and slippery.
3. Observe the **greater omentum** (Fig. 4.17). Spread this apron-like structure to appreciate its size. The greater omentum normally lies between the intestines and the anterior abdominal wall (Fig. 4.20). [G 124; L 224; N 275; R 311; C 212]
4. Elevate the inferior border of the liver and identify the **lesser omentum** (Fig. 4.20). The lesser omentum passes from the lesser curvature of the stomach and first part of the duodenum to the inferior surface of the liver. The lesser omentum has two parts:
   - **Hepatogastric ligament** extends from the liver to the lesser curvature of the stomach.
   - **Hepatoduodenal ligament** extends from the liver to the first part of the duodenum.
5. Return the right upper quadrant flap to its anatomical position and review the **falciform ligament**. The falciform ligament passes from the parietal peritoneum on the anterior abdominal wall to the visceral peritoneum on the surface of the liver. The **round ligament of the liver (ligamentum teres hepatis)** is the obliterated umbilical vein, and it is found in the inferior free margin of the falciform ligament.
6. Follow the falciform ligament superiorly and observe that it is one part of the **coronary ligament** that attaches the liver to the diaphragm. Two additional peritoneal ligaments are also parts of the coronary ligament:

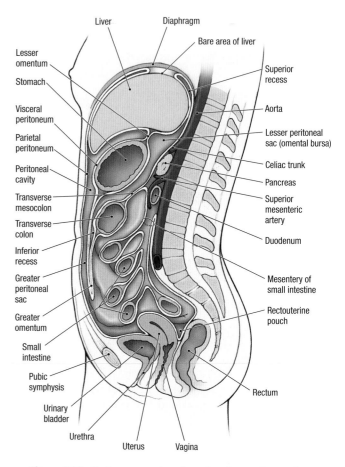

Figure 4.20. Peritoneum and peritoneal cavity, median section.

- **Left triangular ligament** – located between the left lobe of the liver and the diaphragm
- **Right triangular ligament** – located between the right lobe of the liver and the diaphragm
7. The **gastrophrenic ligament** connects the superior part of the greater curvature of the stomach to the diaphragm. Slide your hand superiorly to the left of the stomach to feel this ligament.
8. The **gastrosplenic (gastrolienal) ligament** passes from the greater curvature of the stomach to the spleen, and the **splenorenal (lienorenal) ligament** connects the spleen to the posterior abdominal wall over the left kidney (Fig. 4.21).
9. Reflect the greater omentum superiorly over the costal margin and identify the **transverse mesocolon** (Figs. 4.18 and 4.20). The transverse mesocolon attaches the transverse colon to the posterior abdominal wall. At the left end of the transverse mesocolon is the **phrenicocolic ligament**, which attaches the left colic flexure to the diaphragm. [L 224; N 271; R 306; C 226]
10. Identify the **mesentery** (Fig. 4.20). The mesentery suspends the jejunum and ileum from the pos-

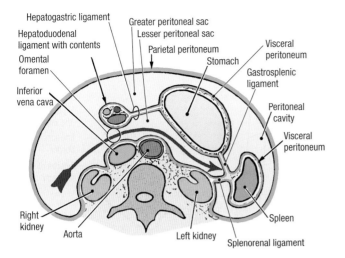

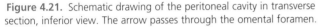

Hepatogastric ligament
Hepatoduodenal ligament with contents
Omental foramen
Inferior vena cava
Greater peritoneal sac
Lesser peritoneal sac
Parietal peritoneum
Stomach
Visceral peritoneum
Gastrosplenic ligament
Peritoneal cavity
Visceral peritoneum
Right kidney
Aorta
Left kidney
Splenorenal ligament
Spleen

Figure 4.21. Schematic drawing of the peritoneal cavity in transverse section, inferior view. The arrow passes through the omental foramen.

terior abdominal wall. The root of the mesentery attaches to the posterior abdominal wall from the left upper quadrant to the right lower quadrant.

11. Observe the **mesoappendix**. The mesoappendix attaches the appendix to the posterior abdominal wall and it contains the appendicular artery.

12. Identify the **sigmoid mesocolon** in the lower left quadrant. The sigmoid mesocolon suspends the sigmoid colon from the posterior abdominal wall.

13. Note that these peritoneal structures are all related to a subdivision of the peritoneal cavity called the **greater peritoneal sac** (Fig. 4.20). Posterior to the stomach and lesser omentum is a smaller subdivision of the peritoneal cavity called the **lesser peritoneal sac (omental bursa)** (Figs. 4.20 and 4.21).

14. The **omental foramen (epiploic foramen)** connects the greater and lesser peritoneal sacs. The omental foramen lies posterior to the hepatoduodenal ligament (Fig. 4.21). [G 124; L 230; N 275; R 311; C 235]

15. Insert your finger into the omental foramen and review its **four boundaries**:
    - **Anterior** – hepatic portal vein, hepatic artery proper, and bile duct contained within the hepatoduodenal ligament (Fig. 4.21)
    - **Posterior** – inferior vena cava and right crus of the diaphragm covered with parietal peritoneum
    - **Superior** – caudate lobe of the liver covered with visceral peritoneum
    - **Inferior** – first part of the duodenum covered with visceral peritoneum

16. Study a diagram of the **lesser peritoneal sac** (Fig. 4.20). The lowest part of the lesser peritoneal sac is called the **inferior recess** and it extends inferi-

orly as far as the greater omentum. During development, the inferior recess extended between the layers of the greater omentum (review an embryology text). The highest part of the lesser peritoneal sac is the **superior recess**. The diaphragm lies posterior to the superior recess and the caudate lobe of the liver is anterior to the superior recess. [G 120; L 230; N 172; R 313; C 203]

17. Posterior to the main part of the lesser peritoneal sac is the pancreas (Fig. 4.20). The peritoneum that covers the pancreas forms part of the posterior wall of the lesser peritoneal sac.

Dissection Review

1. Use the cadaver specimen to review all parts of the gastrointestinal tract in proximal to distal order. State the quadrant(s) in which each abdominal organ normally is found.

2. Review all parts and specializations of the peritoneum listed on the preceding pages.

3. Review the embryology of the gut tube and mesenteries.

CELIAC TRUNK, STOMACH, SPLEEN, LIVER, AND GALLBLADDER

Dissection Overview

The order of dissection will be as follows: The ribs and diaphragm will be cut to allow the liver to be retracted superiorly, exposing the lesser omentum. The surface features of the stomach will be studied. The vessels and ducts in the hepatoduodenal ligament will be demonstrated. The branches of the celiac trunk that supply the stomach, spleen, liver, and gallbladder will be dissected. The remainder of the field of supply of the celiac trunk (to the duodenum and pancreas) will be dissected later. The hepatic portal vein will be studied. The spleen, liver, and gallbladder will be studied.

Dissection Instructions

1. Place the greater omentum in its correct anatomical position.

2. Identify the parts of the stomach (Fig. 4.22): [G 129; L 231; N 275; R 294; C 208]
    - **Anterior surface**
    - **Greater curvature**

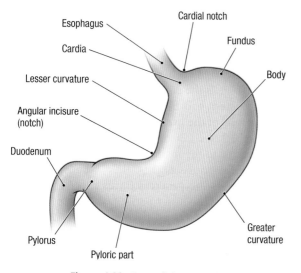

Figure 4.22. Parts of the stomach.

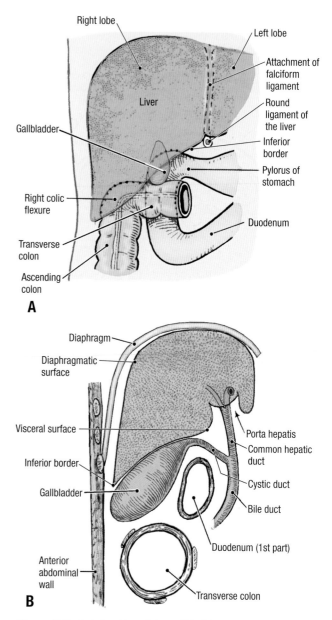

Figure 4.23. Relationships of the gallbladder. **A.** Anterior view. **B.** Sagittal view.

- **Lesser curvature**
- **Cardia**
- **Cardial notch**
- **Fundus**
- **Body**
- **Angular incisure (notch)**
- **Pyloric part**
- **Pylorus**

3. Identify the following features of the liver (Fig. 4.23A, B): [G 146; L 233; N 287; R 298; C 217]
    - **Right lobe**
    - **Left lobe**
    - **Diaphragmatic surface**
    - **Inferior border**

4. Use your hand to raise the inferior border of the liver. Identify the **visceral surface of the liver** (Fig. 4.23B). The visceral surface is in contact with the gallbladder and the peritoneum covering the stomach, duodenum, colon, right kidney, and right suprarenal gland.

5. Identify the **porta hepatis** on the visceral surface of the liver. It is the fissure through which vessels, ducts, lymphatics, and nerves enter the liver (Fig. 4.23B). [G 147; L 233; N 287; R 299; C 217]

6. Identify the **gallbladder** (Fig. 4.23B). The gallbladder may have been surgically removed.

CELIAC TRUNK [G 130; L 231; N 301; R 315; C 206]

As you dissect the branches of the celiac trunk, realize that *arteries are named by their region of distribution, not by their origin or branching pattern.*

1. On the left side only, use bone cutters to detach the costal cartilages of ribs 6 and 7 from the xiphisternal junction and lateral border of the ster-

num. Working through the opening just created, use scissors to make a vertical cut through the diaphragm. Extend this cut to the level of the coronary ligament on the superior surface of the liver. Retract the ribs, diaphragm, and liver superiorly to expose the lesser omentum.

2. Insert the index finger of your left hand into the omental foramen. Anterior to your finger is the **hepatoduodenal ligament** and its contents: **bile ducts, hepatic artery proper, hepatic portal vein, autonomic nerves,** and **lymphatics**.

3. To aid dissection, place a strip of white paper into the omental foramen (Fig. 4.24).

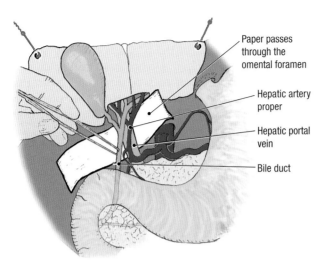

Figure 4.24. Structures contained within the hepatoduodenal ligament.

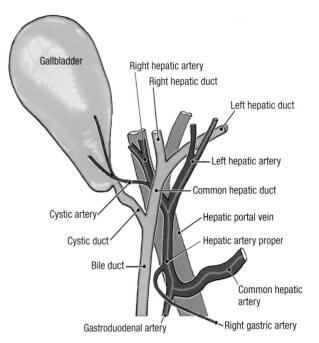

Figure 4.25. Structures contained within the hepatoduodenal ligament. Tributaries of the (common) bile duct and branches of the common hepatic artery.

4. Use blunt dissection to remove the peritoneum from the anterior surface of the hepatoduodenal ligament (anterior to the vessels and ducts).

5. Identify the three large structures that are contained within the hepatoduodenal ligament: **bile duct**, **hepatic artery proper**, and **hepatic portal vein** (Fig. 4.24). The bile duct is the most lateral of the three.

6. Use a probe to trace the bile duct superiorly. Identify the **cystic duct** and the **common hepatic duct** (Fig. 4.25).

7. Follow the common hepatic duct superiorly until it receives its tributaries, the **right hepatic duct** and the **left hepatic duct**. The right and left hepatic ducts exit the **porta hepatis**.

8. Clean the **hepatic artery proper**. The tough "connective tissue" around these vessels contains an **autonomic nerve plexus**. To clear the dissection field, remove the autonomic nerves. [G 130; L 231; N 300; R 315; C 206]

9. Follow the hepatic artery proper toward the liver through the hepatoduodenal ligament. At the porta hepatis the hepatic artery proper branches into the **left hepatic artery** and the **right hepatic artery** (Fig. 4.25).

10. Two other arteries arise in the hepatoduodenal ligament (Fig. 4.25):
    • **Cystic artery** arises from the right hepatic artery. Follow it to the gallbladder.
    • **Right gastric artery** arises from the hepatic artery proper. Follow it to the lesser curvature of the stomach.

11. **Lymphatics** are also contained within the hepatoduodenal ligament. The lymphatic vessels are too small to dissect but **hepatic lymph nodes** can be seen. The lymph nodes may be removed to clear the dissection field.

12. Follow the hepatic artery proper inferiorly and confirm that it is the continuation of the **common hepatic artery** (Fig. 4.25).

13. Observe that the common hepatic artery gives rise to the **gastroduodenal artery**. The gastroduodenal artery passes posterior to the first part of the duodenum (Fig. 4.26). Follow the gastroduodenal artery until it divides to give rise to the **right gastro-omental (gastroepiploic) artery** and the **anterior superior pancreaticoduodenal artery**.

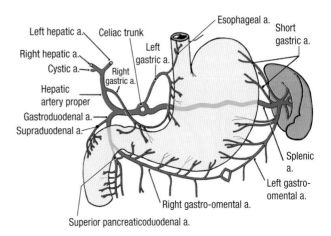

Figure 4.26. Schematic drawing of the branches of the celiac trunk.

Anatomical Variation in Arteries

In about 12% of cases the right hepatic artery arises from the superior mesenteric artery. An aberrant left hepatic artery may arise from the left gastric artery. During surgical removal of the stomach (gastrectomy), blood flow to an aberrant left hepatic artery could be interrupted, endangering the left lobe of the liver.

The cystic artery usually arises from the right hepatic artery, but other origins are possible. The cystic artery may pass posterior (75%) or anterior (24%) to the common hepatic duct (Fig. 4.27).

14. Follow the common hepatic artery to the left toward the **celiac trunk** (Fig. 4.26). Note that the celiac trunk arises from the anterior surface of the abdominal aorta at the level of the 12th thoracic vertebra. The celiac trunk is very short (less than 2 cm in most cases) and divides into three branches:
    - **Common hepatic artery** (already dissected)
    - **Left gastric artery**
    - **Splenic artery**
15. Use blunt dissection to follow the **left gastric artery** toward the esophagus and stomach (Fig. 4.26). The left gastric artery reaches the stomach near the esophagus and then follows the lesser curvature of the stomach within the lesser omentum. The left gastric artery forms an anastomosis with the right gastric artery along the lesser curvature of the stomach. Branches of the gastric arteries distribute to the anterior and posterior surfaces of the stomach.
16. Follow the **splenic artery** to the left for about 5 cm and verify that it lies against the posterior abdominal wall. The splenic artery courses along the superior border of the pancreas and may be partially imbedded in it. Do not dissect the splenic artery from the pancreas at this time. Note that **short gastric arteries** arise from the splenic artery to supply the fundus of the stomach (Fig. 4.26).
17. Find the **left gastro-omental (gastroepiploic) artery** in the greater omentum about 2 cm from the greater curvature of the stomach (Fig. 4.26). The left gastro-omental artery is a branch of the splenic artery.
18. Find the **right gastro-omental artery** in the greater omentum near the right end of the greater curvature of the stomach. The right gastro-omental artery anastomoses with the left gastro-omental artery. Follow the right gastro-omental artery to the right to find its origin from the gastroduodenal branch of the common hepatic artery. [G 130; L 231; N 301; R 314; C 206]
19. Return to the hepatoduodenal ligament and identify the **hepatic portal vein**. The hepatic portal vein lies posterior to both the hepatic artery proper and the bile duct (Fig. 4.24). Follow the hepatic portal vein superiorly and observe that it passes into the porta hepatis, where it divides into **right and left portal veins**. The hepatic portal vein usually receives the **left and right gastric veins** as tributaries. Inferiorly, the hepatic portal vein passes posterior to the first part of the duodenum.

SPLEEN [G 131; L 232; N 299; R 317; C 212]

The spleen is the largest hematopoietic organ in the body. Its size and weight may vary considerably depending upon the blood volume that it contains. The spleen is covered by visceral peritoneum except at the hilum where the splenic vessels enter and leave.

1. Use your left hand to retract the fundus of the stomach to the right. Use your right hand to gently pull the spleen anteriorly.
2. Observe that the spleen has a smooth diaphragmatic surface. The spleen has sharp anterior, inferior, and superior borders. The superior border of the spleen is often notched.
3. The **visceral surface of the spleen** is related to four organs:
   - **Stomach**
   - **Left kidney**
   - **Transverse colon (left colic flexure)**
   - **Pancreas**
4. The diaphragmatic surface of the spleen **is related (through the diaphragm) to ribs 9, 10, and 11** (Fig. 4.28).

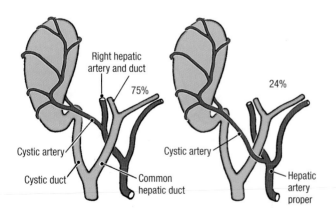

Figure 4.27. The two most common branching patterns of the cystic artery.

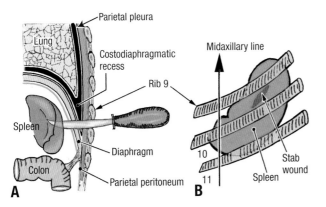

Figure 4.28. Relationships of the spleen to the thoracic wall. **A.** Frontal section. **B.** Lateral view. A penetrating wound through the ninth intercostal space, just posterior to the midaxillary line, will penetrate the pleural cavity, diaphragm, peritoneal cavity, and spleen.

CLINICAL CORRELATION

Spleen

The relationship of the spleen to ribs 9, 10, and 11 is of clinical importance in evaluating rib fractures and penetrating wounds. A lacerated spleen bleeds profusely into the abdominal cavity and may have to be removed surgically (splenectomy). It must be emphasized that there is a risk of puncturing the spleen during pleural tap (thoracocentesis).

An enlarged spleen (splenomegaly) may be encountered during physical examination. The spleen is considered enlarged when it can be palpated inferior to the costal margin.

LIVER [G 146; L 233; N 287; R 298; C 216, 217]

The **liver** is the largest gland in the body, comprising about 2.5% of the body weight of an adult. To study the surface features of the liver, it must be detached from the diaphragm.

1. Review the falciform ligament and the coronary ligament of the liver.
2. Use scissors to cut the falciform ligament along its attachment to the anterior abdominal wall. Extend the cut superiorly and cut the right and left triangular ligaments along the inferior surface of the diaphragm.
3. Insert your fingers between the liver and the diaphragm and tear the connective tissue that attaches the liver to the diaphragm. Cut the posterior layer of the coronary ligament.
4. Use scissors to cut the inferior vena cava between the liver and the diaphragm. Elevate the inferior border of the liver and cut the inferior vena cava again, as close to the inferior surface of the liver as

possible. These two cuts will leave a short segment of the inferior vena cava within the liver (Fig. 4.29B).

5. The liver should now be freely mobile but attached to the other abdominal viscera by the bile duct, hepatic artery proper, and hepatic portal vein. Move the liver carefully to avoid tearing these structures.
6. Examine the **liver** and note that the **right lobe** is six times larger than the **left lobe**. The sharp **inferior border** of the liver separates the **visceral surface** from the **diaphragmatic surface**.
7. Identify the **bare area** on the posterior aspect of the diaphragmatic surface. Here, the liver was adjacent to the diaphragm and not covered by peritoneum. Around the bare area, note the cut edges of the **coronary ligament**.

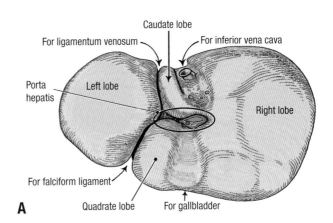

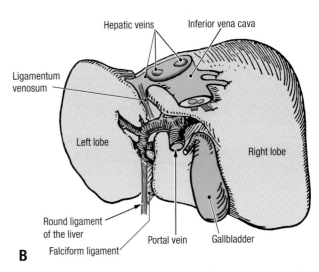

Figure 4.29. Posterior views of the liver. **A.** Fissures and sulci define the four lobes of the liver (right, left, quadrate, and caudate). **B.** Structures located in the H-shaped fissures.

8. Examine the **visceral surface** of the liver (Fig. 4.29A). An H-shaped set of fissures and fossae defines four lobes. Identify the **right lobe**, **left lobe**, **caudate lobe**, and **quadrate lobe**. [G 147, 154; L 233; N 287; R 299; C 217]

9. Observe that the **ligamentum venosum** and **falciform ligament** occupy the left fissure of the "H" (Fig. 4.29B). The **gallbladder** and **inferior vena cava** occupy the fossae that form the right side of the "H."

10. Identify the **porta hepatis**. It forms the horizontal bar of the "H." The structures passing through the hepatoduodenal ligament (bile ducts, hepatic arteries, hepatic portal vein, lymphatics, and autonomic nerves) enter or leave the liver at the porta hepatis.

11. Examine the small segment of the **inferior vena cava** that is attached to the liver. Note that several **hepatic veins** drain directly into the inferior vena cava (Fig. 4.29B).

12. Use a textbook to study the two conventions by which the liver may be divided into lobes. The falciform ligament divides the liver into **right and left anatomical lobes**. The pattern of its bile drainage and vascular supply are used to divide the liver into **right and left functional lobes**. [G 150; L 234, 235; N 289; R 299]

13. The liver has a substantial lymphatic drainage. At the porta hepatis, small lymph vessels drain into **hepatic lymph nodes**. From the hepatic lymph nodes, lymphatic vessels follow the hepatic arteries to **celiac lymph nodes** located around the celiac trunk.

CLINICAL CORRELATION

Liver

The liver may undergo pathologic changes that could be encountered during dissection. The liver may be enlarged. This happens in liver congestion due to cardiac insufficiency (cardiac liver). In contrast, the liver may be small and have fibrous nodules. Such a finding may indicate cirrhosis of the liver. Because the liver is essentially a capillary bed downstream from the gastrointestinal tract, metastatic tumor cells are often trapped within it, resulting in secondary tumors.

GALLBLADDER [G 154; L 236; N 294; R 297; C 221]

The gallbladder is a reservoir for the storage and concentration of bile. The gallbladder occupies a shallow fossa on the visceral surface of the liver (Fig. 4.29B).

The gallbladder is usually stained dark green by bile, which leaks through the wall of the gallbladder after death.

1. Replace the liver into its correct anatomical position.

2. Confirm that the gallbladder is located near the tip of the ninth costal cartilage in the midclavicular line.

3. Reposition the liver to expose the visceral surface. Use blunt dissection to remove the gallbladder from its fossa.

4. Identify the parts of the gallbladder (Fig. 4.30):
   • **Neck**
   • **Body**
   • **Fundus**

5. Review the course of the **cystic artery**. The cystic artery is stained green by bile and is often fragile and difficult to dissect.

6. Use scissors to make a longitudinal incision through the wall of the gallbladder, beginning at the fundus and continuing through the neck. If gallstones are present, remove them. Look for the **spiral fold**, which is a fold in the mucosal lining of the neck that continues into the **cystic duct**.

Dissection Review

1. Replace the organs in their correct anatomical positions.

2. Close and open the flaps of the abdominal wall and review the location of each organ relative to the abdominal quadrant system.

3. Use an illustration and the dissected specimen to trace the branches of the celiac trunk.

4. Review the relationships of the structures in the hepatoduodenal ligament.

5. Review the boundaries of the omental foramen.

6. Review the parts of the organs dissected and their relationships to surrounding structures.

7. Use an embryology textbook to review the development of the liver and the ventral mesogastrium.

8. Review the derivatives of the embryonic foregut.

SUPERIOR MESENTERIC ARTERY AND SMALL INTESTINE

Dissection Overview

The order of dissection will be as follows: The mesentery will be examined. The branches of the superior mesenteric artery that supply the jejunum, ileum, cecum, ascending colon, and transverse colon will be dissected. The remain-

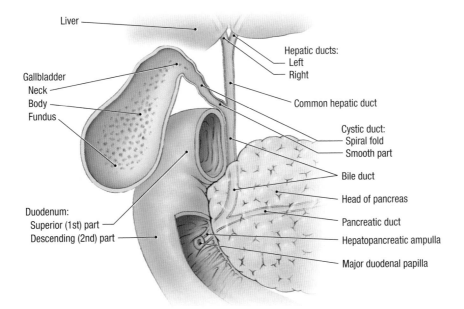

Figure 4.30. Gallbladder and extrahepatic bile ducts.

der of the field of supply of the superior mesenteric artery (to the duodenum and pancreas) will be dissected later, since these structures lie behind the attachment of the transverse mesocolon. The external features of the jejunum and ileum will be studied.

Dissection Instructions

SUPERIOR MESENTERIC ARTERY [G 140; L 225; N 306, 307; R 303; C 230]

The superior mesenteric artery arises from the anterior surface of the abdominal aorta about 1 cm inferior to the celiac trunk (L1 vertebral level). At its origin, the superior mesenteric artery lies posterior to the neck of the pancreas. When the superior mesenteric artery emerges from posterior to the neck of the pancreas, it passes anterior to the uncinate process, third part of the duodenum, and left renal vein. The superior mesenteric artery then enters the mesentery. Within the mesentery the superior mesenteric artery courses toward the terminal end of the ileum.

1. Return the liver to its correct anatomical position.
2. Turn the transverse colon and greater omentum superiorly over the costal margin. The posterior surface of the transverse mesocolon should face anteriorly (Fig. 4.31).
3. Move the coils of the **jejunum** and **ileum** to the left side of the abdomen so that the right side of the mesentery faces anteriorly (Fig. 4.31). Observe that the root of the mesentery is attached to the posterior abdominal wall along a line from the left upper quadrant to the right lower quadrant.

4. Remove the peritoneum on the right side of the mesentery to expose the branches of the superior mesenteric artery. To do this, use a probe to tear the peritoneum, and then grasp it between your thumb and index finger. Peel it slowly, using the handle of a forceps to scrape the peritoneum free from deeper structures.
5. Remove the parietal peritoneum from the posterior abdominal wall on the right side of the mesentery. Remove the peritoneum as far laterally as the ascending colon.

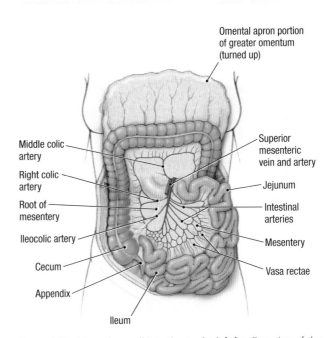

Figure 4.31. Move the small intestine to the left for dissection of the superior mesenteric artery.

6. Identify the **superior mesenteric artery.** Use blunt dissection to trace the superior mesenteric artery proximally and observe that it crosses anterior to the third part of the duodenum. Note that the third part of the duodenum and the left renal vein can become compressed between the superior mesenteric vessels and the abdominal aorta.

7. Use blunt dissection to clean the branches of the superior mesenteric artery. As you dissect, note the dense autonomic nerve network surrounding the vessels. This is the **superior mesenteric plexus of nerves.** Remove the nerves as necessary to clear the dissection field.

8. Identify the **branches of the superior mesenteric artery** (Fig. 4.31):

   • **Inferior pancreaticoduodenal artery** is the first branch of the superior mesenteric artery. The inferior pancreaticoduodenal artery will be dissected with the duodenum.

   • **Intestinal arteries** – 15 to 18 arteries to the jejunum and the ileum. Intestinal arteries end in straight terminal branches called **vasa rectae** (Fig. 4.32). **Arcades** connect the intestinal arteries. Observe the blood supply to the proximal jejunum and note that only one or two arcades are found between adjacent intestinal arteries, resulting in relatively long vasa recta (Fig. 4.32A). Examine the distal ileum and note that four or five arcades occur between adjacent intestinal arteries, resulting in relatively short vasa rectae (Fig. 4.32B).

   • **Ileocolic artery** supplies the cecum. The ileocolic artery gives rise to the **appendicular artery** (Fig. 4.33). The ileocolic artery anasto-

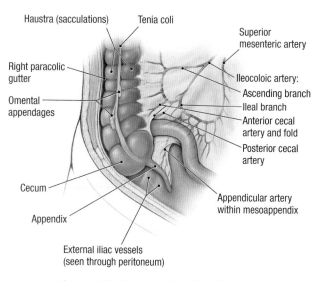

Figure 4.33. Branches of the ileocolic artery.

moses with intestinal branches and with the right colic artery.

   • **Right colic artery** supplies the ascending colon. The right colic artery arises from the right side of the superior mesenteric artery and passes to the right in a retroperitoneal position. It divides into a superior branch and an inferior branch.

   • **Middle colic artery** supplies the transverse colon. The middle colic artery arises from the anterior surface of the superior mesenteric artery and courses through the transverse mesocolon. It divides into a right branch and a left branch.

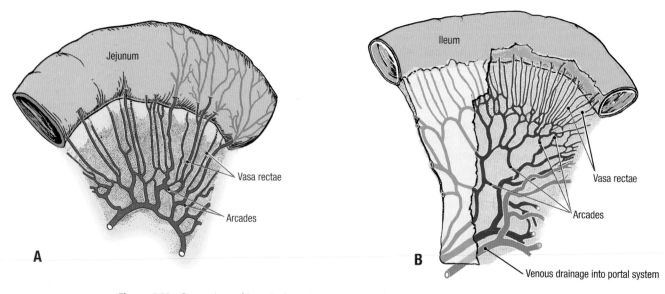

Figure 4.32. Comparison of intestinal arteries. **A.** Arteries of the jejunum. **B.** Arteries of the ileum.

9. Identify the **superior mesenteric vein**. The superior mesenteric vein courses along the right side of the superior mesenteric artery. The superior mesenteric vein is formed by branches that correspond in name and position to the branches of the superior mesenteric artery. Posterior to the pancreas, the superior mesenteric vein joins the splenic vein to form the **hepatic portal vein**.

10. The mesentery may contain up to 200 **mesenteric lymph nodes**. Identify one or two of these lymph nodes along the branches of the superior mesenteric vessels. The **superior mesenteric lymph nodes** are located near the origin of the superior mesenteric artery from the abdominal aorta. Lymph nodes may be removed to clear the dissection field.

SMALL INTESTINE [G 136, 137; L 225, 228; N 270; R 310; C 232]

The small intestine consists of the duodenum, jejunum, and ileum. The function of the small intestine is to absorb nutrients from food. It has elaborate folds of mucosa that increase surface area and a rich blood supply to transport the absorbed nutrients. The **jejunum** (proximal two-fifths) and **ileum** (distal three-fifths) will be studied together since their transition is not obvious.

1. Move the small intestine to the left side of the abdominal cavity and follow the jejunum proximally (Fig. 4.34). Find the **duodenojejunal junction**.
2. Note that the **suspensory ligament of the duodenum** is a fibromuscular ligament that arises from the right crus of the diaphragm and anchors the intestine at the duodenojejunal junction (Fig. 4.34, inset).
3. Palpate the small intestine and note that the wall of the jejunum is thicker than the wall of the ileum.
4. Identify the termination of the ileum where it empties into the **cecum** at the **ileocecal junction** (Fig. 4.34).
5. Verify that the **root of the mesentery** crosses the posterior abdominal wall from the duodenojejunal junction to the ileocecal junction (Fig. 4.34). The root of the mesentery is about 15 cm long. The **intestinal attachment of the mesentery** is nearly 6 m long.

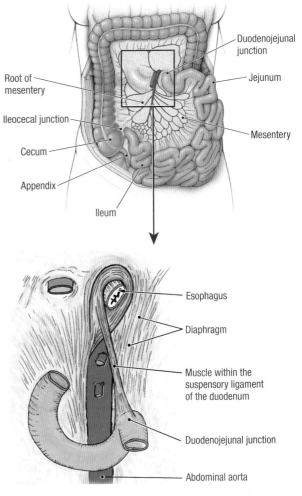

Figure 4.34. Move the small intestine to the left side to find the duodenojejunal junction. *Inset:* The duodenojejunal junction is suspended by the suspensory muscle (ligament) of the duodenum.

3. Review the relationships of the jejunum and ileum to surrounding structures.
4. Use an illustration and the dissected specimen to review the branches of the superior mesenteric artery.
5. Use an embryology textbook to review the derivatives of the embryonic midgut.

INFERIOR MESENTERIC ARTERY AND LARGE INTESTINE

Dissection Overview

The **inferior mesenteric artery** arises from the anterior surface of the abdominal aorta at the level of the intervertebral disc between vertebrae L2 and L3. The objective is to demonstrate the field of supply of the inferior mesenteric artery (left half of the transverse colon, descending colon, sigmoid colon, and most of the rectum). Except for the branches that pass through the sigmoid mesocolon to

Dissection Review

1. Replace the small intestine in its correct anatomical position.
2. Close and open the flaps of the abdominal wall and review the location of the jejunum and ileum relative to the abdominal quadrant system.

supply the sigmoid colon, the inferior mesenteric artery and its branches lie retroperitoneally.

The order of dissection will be as follows: The inferior mesenteric artery and its branches will be dissected. The external features of the large intestine will be studied.

Dissection Instructions

INFERIOR MESENTERIC ARTERY [G 142; L 226; N 307; R 305; C 232]

1. Turn the transverse colon and greater omentum superiorly over the costal margin to expose the posterior surface of the transverse mesocolon.
2. Move the small intestine to the right so that the descending colon is visible from the left colic flexure to the sigmoid colon (Fig. 4.35).
3. The origin of the inferior mesenteric artery lies posterior to the third part of the duodenum. If you have trouble finding it, find one of its branches in the sigmoid mesocolon and trace the branch back to the main vessel. Then proceed with the dissection of the peripheral branches.

   Dissection note: The left ureter could be mistaken for the inferior mesenteric artery or one of its branches. The inferior mesenteric artery and vein and the ureter all lie in the retroperitoneal space, but the vessels pass anterior to the ureter.
4. Use a probe to clean the **branches of the inferior mesenteric artery** (Fig. 4.35):
   - **Left colic artery** supplies the descending colon and the left third of the transverse colon. The left colic artery anastomoses with the middle colic branch of the superior mesenteric artery.
   - **Sigmoid arteries** – three or four arteries that supply the sigmoid colon. Sigmoid arteries pass through the sigmoid mesocolon. Note that they form arcades similar to those of the intestinal arteries.
   - **Superior rectal artery** supplies the proximal part of the rectum. The superior rectal artery divides into a **right branch** and a **left branch**. The right and left branches of the superior rectal artery descend into the pelvis on either side of the rectum. Do not follow them into the pelvis.
5. Observe the tributaries of the **inferior mesenteric vein**. The tributaries of the inferior mesenteric vein correspond to the branches of the inferior mesenteric artery. The inferior mesenteric vein is a tributary of the hepatic portal vein. The inferior mesenteric vein ascends on the left side of the inferior mesenteric artery, passes posterior to the pancreas, and joins either the **splenic vein** or (less frequently) the **superior mesenteric vein**.
6. The inferior mesenteric artery and vein are accompanied by lymph vessels that drain into the **inferior mesenteric nodes** around the origin of the inferior mesenteric artery.

LARGE INTESTINE [G 136, 137; L 224, 226; N 284; R 307; C 226, 228]

The large intestine consists of the **cecum** (with attached **appendix**), **colon** (ascending, transverse, descending, and sigmoid), **rectum**, and **anal canal**. Absorption of water from fecal material is a major function of the large intestine. The relatively smooth mucosal surface of the large intestine is well suited for this function, as a smooth surface is less likely to impede the movement of progressively more solid fecal matter.

1. Return the small intestine and transverse colon to their correct anatomical positions.
2. In the right lower quadrant, identify the **cecum** (L. *caecus*, blind) (Fig. 4.33). The length of its mesentery and the degree of its mobility vary considerably from individual to individual.
3. The **appendix (vermiform appendix)** (L. *appendere*, to hang on) is attached to the end of the cecum. The appendix may be found in one of several positions (Fig. 4.36). Recall that the appendix is suspended on a mesentery called the **mesoappendix**. The **appendicular artery** is found within the mesoappendix (Fig. 4.33).
4. Identify the **ascending colon**. The ascending colon extends from the cecum to the **right colic flexure** (Fig. 4.19).

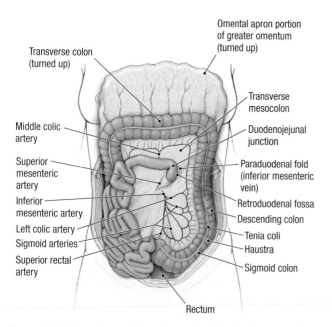

Figure 4.35. Move the small intestine to the right for dissection of the inferior mesenteric artery.

Labels in figure:
Transverse colon (turned up)
Omental apron portion of greater omentum (turned up)
Transverse mesocolon
Duodenojejunal junction
Middle colic artery
Superior mesenteric artery
Paraduodenal fold (inferior mesenteric vein)
Inferior mesenteric artery
Retroduodenal fossa
Left colic artery
Descending colon
Sigmoid arteries
Tenia coli
Superior rectal artery
Haustra
Sigmoid colon
Rectum

4/ THE ABDOMEN 101

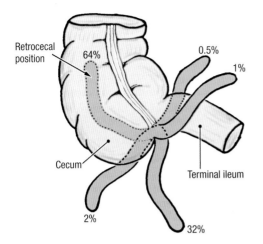

Figure 4.36. Variations in the position of the appendix.

2. Review the relationship of each part of the large intestine to surrounding structures.
3. Use an illustration and the dissected specimen to trace the branches of the inferior mesenteric artery.
4. Use an embryology textbook to review the derivatives of the embryonic hindgut.

DUODENUM, PANCREAS, AND HEPATIC PORTAL VEIN

Dissection Overview

The duodenum is the part of the small intestine between the stomach and the jejunum. The duodenum is the drainage point for the ducts of the liver and pancreas. The pancreas lies within the bend of the duodenum. The pancreas is both an endocrine and an exocrine organ and has a rich blood supply arising from the celiac trunk and the superior mesenteric artery.

The order of dissection will be as follows: The parts of the duodenum will be studied. The pancreas will be dissected. The formation of the hepatic portal vein will be demonstrated.

5. Identify the **transverse colon**. The transverse colon extends from the **right colic flexure** to the **left colic flexure**. Observe that the left colic flexure is at a more superior level than the right colic flexure. Between the two flexures, the transverse colon is freely movable.
6. Observe the **descending colon.** It is a secondarily retroperitoneal organ. The descending colon descends from the left colic flexure to the left lower quadrant (Fig. 4.19).
7. In the left lower quadrant, find the **sigmoid colon**. Observe that the sigmoid colon has a mesentery (**sigmoid mesocolon**) and is mobile. The sigmoid colon ends in the pelvis at the level of the third sacral segment, where it becomes continuous with the rectum.
8. The **rectum** is contained entirely within the pelvic cavity and will be dissected with the pelvic viscera.
9. Observe the external surface of the large intestine and note three features that distinguish it from the small intestine (Fig. 4.35):
   • **Teniae coli** – three narrow bands of longitudinal muscle
   • **Haustra** – outpouchings of the wall of the colon
   • **Omental appendices (epiploic appendages)** – small accumulations of fat covered by visceral peritoneum
10. Review the branches of the superior mesenteric artery and inferior mesenteric artery that supply the large intestine. [G 145; L 226; N 307; R 308; C 230, 232]

Dissection Review

1. Close and open the flaps of the abdominal wall to review the location of each part of the large intestine relative to the abdominal quadrant system.

Dissection Instructions

DUODENUM [G 133, 134; L 238, 239; N 278; R 316; C 223]

1. Turn the transverse colon and greater omentum superiorly over the costal margin.
2. Use blunt dissection to remove the remaining connective tissue and peritoneum from the anterior surface of the duodenum and pancreas.
3. Observe the **four parts of the duodenum** (Fig. 4.37):
   • **Superior (first) part** – at the level of vertebra L1. The superior part of the duodenum lies in the transverse plane and the hepatoduodenal ligament is attached to it. It is mostly intraperitoneal.
   • **Descending (second) part** – at the level of vertebra L2. The descending part of the duodenum is positioned to the right of the midline and anterior to the right kidney, right renal vessels, and inferior vena cava. It is retroperitoneal. The bile duct and the pancreatic duct drain into the descending part of the duodenum.
   • **Horizontal (third) part** – at the level of vertebra L3. The horizontal part of the duodenum lies anterior to the inferior vena cava and the abdominal aorta. It is retroperitoneal. The horizontal part of the duodenum is crossed anteri-

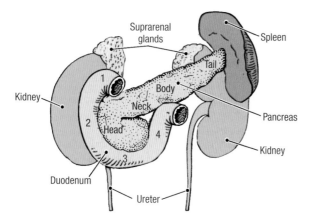

Figure 4.37. Relationships of the spleen, pancreas, duodenum, and kidneys.

orly by the superior mesenteric vessels and posteriorly by the inferior mesenteric vessels.

- **Ascending (fourth) part** – ascends to the level of vertebra L2. The ascending part of the duodenum is retroperitoneal throughout most of its length. The ascending part of the duodenum turns anteriorly to join the jejunum at the duodenojejunal junction.

PANCREAS [G 133, 156; L 239; N 298; R 317; C 224]

1. Identify the **pancreas** within the bend of the duodenum. Note that it is a secondarily retroperitoneal organ that lies across the midline and that it is positioned against vertebral bodies L1 to L3.
2. Identify the parts of the pancreas (Fig. 4.37):
   - **Head** – lies within the curve of the duodenum. The **uncinate process** is a small projection from the inferior margin of the head that passes posterior to the superior mesenteric vessels. The inferior vena cava lies posterior to the head of the pancreas.
   - **Neck** – a short portion that lies anterior to the superior mesenteric vessels and connects the head of the pancreas to the body.
   - **Body** – extends from right to left and slightly superiorly as it crosses the posterior abdominal wall. The abdominal aorta lies posterior to the body of the pancreas.
   - **Tail** – the narrow left end of the gland. The tip of the tail lies in the splenorenal ligament and contacts the hilum of the spleen.
3. Use a probe to dissect into the anterior surface of the head of the pancreas and find the **main pancreatic duct**. Trace the main pancreatic duct through the neck and into the body. The **accessory pancreatic duct** joins the superior side of the main pancreatic duct.

4. Follow the main pancreatic duct toward the descending part of the duodenum. Observe that the main pancreatic duct is joined by the bile duct.
5. Identify the **posterior superior** and **anterior superior pancreaticoduodenal arteries** (Fig. 4.38). Both are branches of the gastroduodenal artery. [G 135; L 239; N 301; R 316; C 223]
6. The **inferior pancreaticoduodenal artery** is usually the most proximal branch of the superior mesenteric artery, although its origin is variable (Fig. 4.38). The inferior pancreaticoduodenal artery enters the inferior portion of the head of the pancreas.
7. Return to the celiac trunk and follow the splenic artery as it passes to the left along the superior margin of the pancreas (Fig. 4.38). Up to 10 small branches of the splenic artery supply the body and tail of the pancreas. Identify only two:
   - **Dorsal pancreatic artery** – enters the neck of the pancreas
   - **Greater pancreatic (pancreatica magna) artery** – enters the pancreas at the junction of the medial two-thirds and lateral one-third of the gland
8. Follow the splenic artery to the hilum of the spleen and identify the **left gastro-omental artery**. Complete the dissection of the left gastro-omental artery by following it through the greater omentum to its anastomosis with the right gastro-omental artery.
9. The veins of the pancreas correspond to the arteries. They drain into the superior mesenteric and splenic veins and ultimately are tributary to the hepatic portal vein.

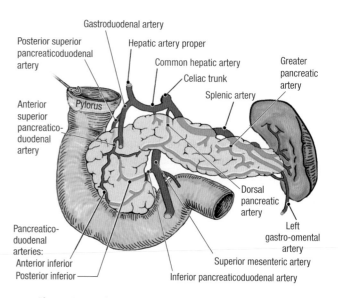

Figure 4.38. Blood supply of the duodenum and pancreas.

HEPATIC PORTAL VEIN [G 160; L 240; N 311; R 300; C 207]

Use an illustration to review the hepatic portal venous system. The **superior mesenteric vein** and the **splenic vein** join to form the hepatic portal vein posterior to the neck of the pancreas. The **hepatic portal vein** carries venous blood to the liver from the abdominal portion of the gastrointestinal tract, the spleen, and the pancreas.

1. The **splenic vein** courses posterior to the pancreas, inferior to the splenic artery. Use a probe to dissect posterior to the body of the pancreas and find the splenic vein.
2. Follow the splenic vein to the right, where it is joined by the superior mesenteric vein. This is the origin of the **hepatic portal vein**. Recall that the hepatic portal vein ascends in the hepatoduodenal ligament to the porta hepatis.
3. Return to the field of distribution of the inferior mesenteric vein. Find it and follow it superiorly. The inferior mesenteric vein usually joins the splenic vein, but it may join the superior mesenteric vein or the junction of the superior mesenteric and splenic veins.
4. Use a textbook or atlas to review the portal-systemic (portal-caval) anastomoses:
   • **Gastroesophageal** – left gastric vein/esophageal veins/azygos vein
   • **Anorectal** – superior rectal vein/middle and inferior rectal veins
   • **Paraumbilical** – paraumbilical veins/superficial epigastric veins
   • **Retroperitoneal** – colic veins/retroperitoneal veins

CLINICAL CORRELATION

Portal Hypertension

The hepatic portal system of veins has no valves. When the hepatic portal vein becomes blocked, blood pressure increases in the hepatic portal system (portal hypertension) and its tributaries become engorged. Portal hypertension causes hemorrhoids and varicose gastric and esophageal veins. Bleeding from ruptured gastroesophageal varices is a dangerous complication of portal hypertension.

Dissection Review

1. Review the relationship of each part of the duodenum to surrounding structures.
2. Review the branches of the celiac trunk and superior mesenteric artery.

3. Use an illustration and the dissected specimen to reconstruct the blood supply to the pancreas and duodenum.
4. Review the formation and field of drainage of the hepatic portal vein.
5. Trace a drop of blood from the small intestine to the inferior vena cava, naming all veins that are encountered along the way.
6. Use an embryology textbook to review the development of the liver, pancreas, and duodenum.

REMOVAL OF THE GASTROINTESTINAL TRACT

Dissection Overview

The order of dissection will be as follows: The arteries to the gastrointestinal tract (celiac trunk, superior mesenteric artery, and inferior mesenteric artery) will be cut close to the aorta. The esophagus and rectum will be cut, using ligatures to prevent spilling their contents. The gastrointestinal tract will then be removed and reviewed outside of the body. The gastrointestinal tract will be taken to a sink and selected areas will be opened and rinsed in order to study their internal features.

Dissection Instructions

1. Tie two strings 4 cm apart around the superior end of the rectum. Use scissors to cut the rectum *between the strings*. Cut the superior rectal artery.
2. Inferior to the diaphragm, tie one string around the esophagus and cut the esophagus superior to the string. Cut the vagus nerve trunks at the same level.
3. Use scissors to cut the celiac trunk close to the aorta, leaving no stump.
4. Use scissors to cut the superior mesenteric artery near the aorta, leaving a 1-cm stump.
5. Use scissors to cut the inferior mesenteric artery near the aorta, leaving a 1-cm stump.
6. Free the stomach from any peritoneal attachments it may still have to the posterior abdominal wall.
7. Grasp the spleen and gently pull medially. Insert your fingers posterior to the spleen and carefully free the splenic vessels, tail of the pancreas, and body of the pancreas from the posterior abdominal wall.
8. Use scissors to cut the suspensory ligament of the duodenum close to the duodenojejunal junction.
9. Insert your fingers posterior to the duodenum and free it from the posterior abdominal wall.

10. Use scissors to cut the parietal peritoneum lateral to the ascending colon and use your fingers to free the ascending colon from the posterior abdominal wall. Roll the ascending colon toward the midline and use your fingers to loosen its blood vessels from the posterior abdominal wall.

11. Cut the parietal peritoneum lateral to the descending colon and use your fingers to free the descending colon from the posterior abdominal wall. Roll the descending colon toward the midline and use your fingers to loosen its blood vessels from the posterior abdominal wall.

12. The gastrointestinal tract, liver, pancreas, and spleen should now be free of attachments. Remove them from the abdominal cavity. Be careful not to twist or tear the structures in the hepatoduodenal ligament.

13. Arrange the abdominal viscera on the dissecting table in anatomical position and study the parts from the anterior view:
    • Trace the branches of the celiac trunk, superior mesenteric artery, and inferior mesenteric artery to their areas of distribution.
    • Observe the formation and termination of the hepatic portal vein.
    • Note the differences between the branching pattern of the arteries and the veins.
    • Turn the viscera and repeat the exercise from the posterior view.

14. Carry the viscera to a sink to examine their internal features.

15. Use scissors to open the stomach along its anterior surface. Extend the cut into the first part of the duodenum. Rinse the mucosa and observe the following features (Fig. 4.39): [G 129; L 231; N 276; R 294; C 209]
    • **Gastric folds (rugae)**
    • **Pyloric antrum**
    • **Pyloric canal**
    • **Pyloric sphincter**
    • **Pyloric orifice**

16. Use scissors to make a longitudinal incision in the anterior wall of the duodenum. In the second part of the duodenum identify the following (Fig. 4.40): [G 133; L 238; N 279; R 297; C 224]
    • **Circular folds (plicae circulares)**
    • **Major (greater) duodenal papilla** – an elevation of mucosa on the medial wall of the second part of the duodenum. The major duodenal papilla is the shared opening of the main pancreatic duct and bile duct.
    • **Minor (lesser) duodenal papilla** – the site of drainage of the accessory pancreatic duct. If present, it will be approximately 2 cm superior to the major duodenal papilla.

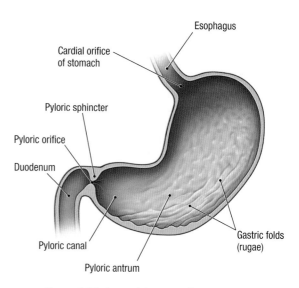

Figure 4.39. Internal features of the stomach.

17. Use scissors to make one 5-cm longitudinal incision in the **proximal jejunum** and another in the **distal ileum**. Rinse the mucosa and compare features. Note that the circular folds are larger and closer together in the jejunum (Fig. 4.41). [G 136; N 280]

18. Use scissors to make an incision approximately 7.5 cm long in the anterior wall of the **cecum**. Rinse the mucosa and identify the following (Fig. 4.42): [G 139; L 227; N 282; R 310; C 236]
    • **Ileocecal orifice**
    • **Superior and inferior lips of the ileocecal valve**
    • **Opening of the appendix**

19. Make an incision approximately 5 cm long in the anterior surface of the transverse colon. Note the

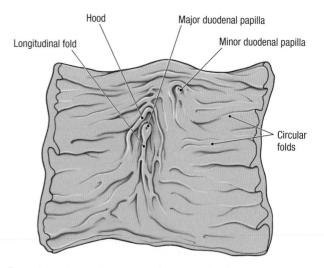

Figure 4.40. Mucosal features in the descending (second) part of the duodenum.

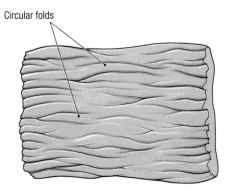

Circular folds

Proximal jejunum

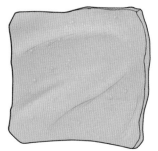

Distal ileum

Figure 4.41. Comparison of mucosal features in the proximal jejunum and distal ileum.

semilunar folds (plicae semilunares) between adjacent **haustra**. Observe the relative smoothness of the mucosa. [G 137; N 284; C 238]

20. The viscera may be stored in a large plastic bag or in the abdominal cavity. Wet these specimens frequently with mold-inhibiting solution.

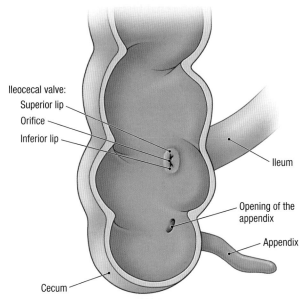

Ileocecal valve:
Superior lip
Orifice
Inferior lip

Ileum

Opening of the appendix

Appendix

Cecum

Figure 4.42. Interior of the cecum, from an anterior view.

Dissection Review

1. Review the features of the gastrointestinal mucosa.
2. Compare the quantity and complexity of circular folds in the proximal and distal parts of the small intestine. Compare this arrangement to the mucosal features seen in the stomach and large intestine. Correlate your findings to the function of the organs dissected.
3. Recall the locations of valves in the gastrointestinal tract.

POSTERIOR ABDOMINAL VISCERA

Dissection Overview

The posterior abdominal viscera are located in an area that is referred to as the **retroperitoneal space**. The retroperitoneal space is not a real space. It is that part of the body between the parietal peritoneum and the muscles and bones of the posterior abdominal wall (Fig. 4.43). The retroperitoneal space contains the kidneys, ureters, suprarenal glands, aorta, inferior vena cava, and abdominal portions of the sympathetic trunks. [G 171; L 243; N 342; R 324; C 260]

The order of dissection will be as follows: The posterior abdominal viscera will be palpated. The kidneys and suprarenal glands will be removed from the renal fascia and studied. The abdominal aorta and the inferior vena cava will be dissected. The muscles of the posterior abdominal wall will be studied. The lumbar plexus of nerves will be examined. Finally, the diaphragm will be studied.

Dissection Instructions

1. Use a sponge or paper towels to clean the posterior abdominal wall.
2. Palpate the **kidneys** and the **suprarenal (adrenal) glands**. They lie lateral to the vertebral column at vertebral levels T12 to L3. [G 163; L 242; N 329; R 331; C 243]
3. Palpate the abdominal aorta.
4. To the right of the abdominal aorta, palpate the inferior vena cava.
5. Remove any remaining parietal peritoneum from the posterior abdominal wall.
6. If you are dissecting a female cadaver, go to step 10.
7. Identify the **testicular artery and vein** at the deep inguinal ring. The testicular artery is quite small and delicate. Follow the testicular vessels superiorly and note that they cross anterior to the ureter. Do not damage the ureter.

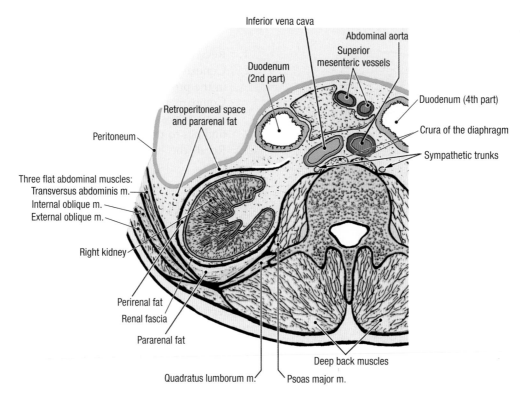

Figure 4.43. Transverse section through the posterior abdominal wall at the level of the kidneys.

8. The **right** and **left testicular arteries** branch directly from the aorta at about vertebral level L2. This origin is inferior to the origin of the renal arteries.

9. Observe that the left testicular vein drains into the left renal vein. The right testicular vein drains directly into the inferior vena cava.

CLINICAL CORRELATION

Testicular Varicocele

Varicocele is a varicose condition of the pampiniform plexus of veins. Varicocele is more common on the left side because the left testicular vein drains into the left renal vein, and the left renal vein is subject to compression where it passes inferior to the superior mesenteric artery.

---

10. In the **female cadaver**, identify the **ovarian vessels**. Their origin is comparable to that of the testicular vessels in the male. Note that the ovarian vessels cross anterior to the ureter.

11. Inferiorly, the ovarian vessels end in the pelvic cavity. Follow the ovarian vessels inferiorly until they cross the external iliac vessels. Do not follow them into the pelvis at this time.

KIDNEYS [G 163; L 243, 244; N 329; R 331; C 243]

The retroperitoneal position of the kidneys is well illustrated on transverse section (Fig. 4.43). The kidneys are well protected by their position within the body as well as by a cushioning layer of fat.

1. Note that the kidney lies against the posterior abdominal wall. The anterior surface of the kidney faces anterolaterally (Fig. 4.43).

2. Use your fingers to separate the **kidney** from the **perirenal fat** and **renal fascia** (Fig. 4.43).

3. Observe that the **superior pole** of the kidney is separated from the suprarenal gland by a thin layer of renal fascia. Carefully insert your fingers between the kidney and the suprarenal gland and separate the two organs. Be careful not to remove the suprarenal gland with the fat.

4. Note the size and shape of the kidney.

5. Identify the **left renal vein**. Use a probe to trace the left renal vein from the left kidney to the inferior vena cava. Observe that it crosses anterior to the renal arteries and aorta.

6. Identify and clean the tributaries of the left renal vein:
   • **Left testicular** (or **ovarian**) **vein**
   • **Left suprarenal vein**

7. Use scissors to cut the left renal vein close to the inferior vena cava. Reflect the left renal vein toward the left. Do not detach the testicular (or

ovarian) vein or the left suprarenal vein from the left renal vein.

8. Identify the **left renal artery**, which lies posterior to the left renal vein. Follow the left renal artery to the hilum of the kidney. The renal artery usually divides before it enters the kidney, and accessory renal arteries are common.

9. Observe small branches of the left renal artery to the ureter and left suprarenal gland.

10. Using the left renal artery as a hinge, turn the left kidney toward the right. At the most posterior part of the hilum, identify the **renal pelvis** and its inferior continuation, the **ureter**.

11. Use blunt dissection to follow the ureter inferiorly. Observe that the abdominal part of the ureter passes posterior to the testicular (or ovarian) vessels and crosses the anterior surface of the psoas major muscle. The pelvic part of the ureter will be dissected with the pelvic viscera.

12. Return the left kidney to its correct anatomical position.

13. Clean the relatively short right renal vein. Note that it has no tributaries.

14. Reflect the inferior vena cava inferiorly and slightly toward the right. Identify the **right renal artery**, which lies posterior to the right renal vein and inferior vena cava. Note that the right renal artery is longer than the left renal artery. The right renal pelvis lies posterior to the right renal artery.

15. Follow the right ureter inferiorly and observe its relationship to the right testicular (ovarian) vessels.

16. Use an illustration to review the relationships of the kidneys: [G 162; L 241; N 329; R 318; C 244, 246]
    - The suprarenal gland is superior to the kidney.
    - Through the peritoneum, the right kidney is in contact with the right colic flexure, the visceral surface of the liver, and the second part of the duodenum.
    - Through the peritoneum, the left kidney is in contact with the tail of the pancreas, the left colic flexure, the stomach, and the spleen.

17. Divide the left kidney into anterior and posterior halves by splitting it longitudinally along its lateral border. Open the two halves of the kidney like a book.

18. Identify (Fig. 4.44): [G 166; L 244; N 334; R 326; C 247]
    - **Renal capsule** – a fibrous capsule that can be stripped off the surface of the kidney.
    - **Renal cortex** – the outer zone of the kidney (about one-third of its depth).
    - **Renal medulla** – the inner zone of the kidney consisting of **renal pyramids** and **renal columns** (about two-thirds of its depth).
    - **Renal sinus** – the space within the kidney that is occupied by the renal pelvis, calices, vessels, nerves, and fat.

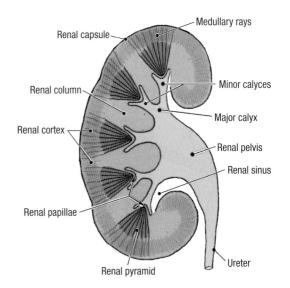

Figure 4.44. Internal features of the kidney in longitudinal section.

- **Renal papilla** – the apex of the renal pyramid that projects into a minor calyx.
- **Minor calyx** – a cup-like chamber that is the beginning of the extrarenal duct system. Several minor calyces combine to form a major calyx.
- **Major calyx** – two or three per kidney that combine to form the renal pelvis.
- **Renal pelvis** – the funnel-like end of the ureter that lies within the renal sinus.
- **Ureter** – the muscular duct that carries urine from the kidney to the urinary bladder.

CLINICAL CORRELATION

Kidney Stones

Kidney stones (renal calculi) may form in the calyces and renal pelvis. Small kidney stones may spontaneously pass through the ureter into the bladder. Larger kidney stones may lodge at one of three natural constrictions of the ureter: (1) where the renal pelvis joins the ureter; (2) where the ureter crosses the pelvic brim; and (3) at the entrance of the ureter into the urinary bladder.

SUPRARENAL GLANDS [G 163; L 243, 244; N 332, 347; R 326; C 245]

The **suprarenal (adrenal) glands** are fragile and easily torn. They are closely related to the superior poles of the kidneys (Fig. 4.45). The suprarenal glands are highly vascularized endocrine glands.

1. Observe that the **right suprarenal gland** is triangular in shape. Part of the right suprarenal gland lies posterior to the inferior vena cava.

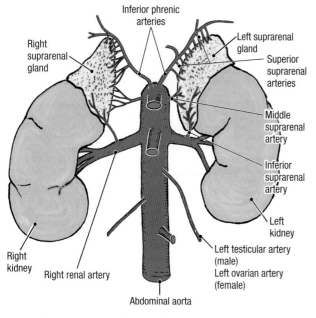

Figure 4.45. Blood supply of the suprarenal glands.

2. Observe that the **left suprarenal gland** is semilunar in shape.
3. The suprarenal gland receives multiple arteries (Fig. 4.45). Identify:
    *   **Superior suprarenal arteries** arise from the inferior phrenic artery.
    *   **Middle suprarenal artery** arises from the aorta near the celiac trunk.
    *   **Inferior suprarenal artery** arises from the renal artery.
4. Note that the left suprarenal vein empties into the left renal vein. The right suprarenal vein drains directly into the inferior vena cava.
5. The suprarenal glands receive numerous sympathetic nerve fibers.

CLINICAL CORRELATION

Suprarenal Glands

The kidneys and suprarenal glands have different embryonic origins. If the kidney fails to ascend to its normal position during development, the suprarenal gland develops in its normal position lateral to the celiac trunk.

ABDOMINAL AORTA AND INFERIOR VENA CAVA
[G 175; L 246; N 329; R 333; C 253]

1. Use an illustration to study the abdominal aorta. Observe that the abdominal aorta has three types of branches:

*   **Unpaired arteries to the gastrointestinal tract** (celiac trunk and superior mesenteric and inferior mesenteric arteries)
*   **Paired arteries to the three paired abdominal organs** (suprarenal, renal, and testicular or ovarian arteries)
*   **Paired arteries to the abdominal wall** (inferior phrenic and lumbar arteries)

2. Identify at least one **lumbar artery** (Fig. 4.46). Four pairs of lumbar arteries supply the posterior abdominal wall. Trace one lumbar artery to its origin from the posterior aspect of the abdominal aorta. Note that the lumbar arteries pass deep to the psoas major muscle.
3. Observe the **bifurcation of the abdominal aorta** at vertebral level L4 (Fig. 4.46). In a thin person, the umbilicus projects superior to the bifurcation of the aorta.
4. Identify the **common iliac arteries**, which arise at the bifurcation of the aorta. The common iliac arteries supply blood to the pelvis and lower limbs.
5. Review the **inferior vena cava** and its tributaries. Recall that a segment of the inferior vena cava was removed with the liver. Note that the inferior vena cava has no unpaired visceral tributaries because the hepatic portal system collects blood from the gastrointestinal tract. Review the hepatic portal vein. Recall that the hepatic portal vein drains into the liver, and that the hepatic veins drain into the inferior vena cava.

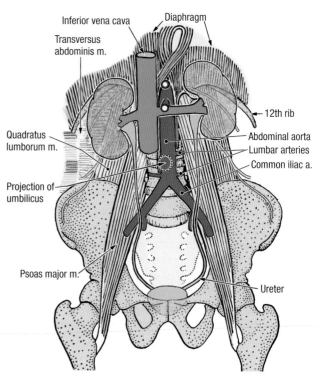

Figure 4.46. Posterior relationships of the kidneys.

Dissection Review

1. Replace the kidneys in their correct anatomical positions.
2. Use an illustration and the dissected specimen to review the relationships of each kidney to surrounding structures.
3. Trace the path taken by a drop of urine from the renal papilla to the ureter.
4. Review the position, relationships, and blood supply of each suprarenal gland.
5. Review the branches of the abdominal aorta.

POSTERIOR ABDOMINAL WALL

Dissection Overview

The posterior abdominal wall is composed of the vertebral column, muscles that move the vertebral column, muscles that move the lower limb, and the diaphragm. The nerves that supply the abdominal wall and the lumbar plexus of nerves that supply the lower limb will be dissected with the posterior abdominal wall.

The order of dissection will be as follows: The branches of the lumbar plexus will be studied. Muscles that form the posterior abdominal wall will be dissected. The abdominal part of the sympathetic trunk will be studied.

Dissection Instructions

1. Move the kidney and suprarenal gland toward the midline (don't cut their vessels) and use your hands to remove the remaining fat and the renal fascia from the posterior abdominal wall.
2. Identify the **psoas major muscle** (Fig. 4.47). The proximal attachments of the psoas major muscle are the lumbar vertebrae (bodies, intervertebral discs, and transverse processes). Its distal attachment is the lesser trochanter of the femur. The psoas major muscle is a strong flexor of the thigh and vertebral column. [G 172; L 245; N 263; R 333; C 250]
3. Look for the **psoas minor muscle**. The psoas minor muscle is absent in approximately 40% of cases and may be present on only one side of the cadaver. The psoas minor muscle has a long flat tendon that passes down the anterior surface of the psoas major muscle to its distal attachment on the iliopubic eminence and arcuate line of the ilium.
4. Identify the **iliacus muscle** (Fig. 4.47). The proximal attachment of the iliacus muscle is the iliac fossa. Its distal attachment is on the lesser trochanter of the femur. The iliacus muscle flexes the thigh. The iliacus and psoas major muscles

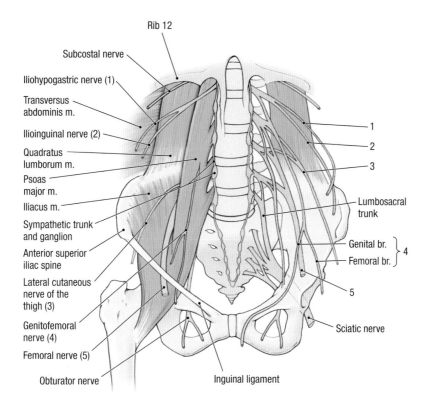

Figure 4.47. Lumbar plexus of nerves.

form a functional unit and together they are called the **iliopsoas muscle**.

5. Identify the **quadratus lumborum muscle** (Fig. 4.47). The proximal attachments of the quadratus lumborum muscle are the 12th rib and lumbar transverse processes. Its distal attachments are the iliolumbar ligament and iliac crest. The quadratus lumborum muscle flexes the vertebral column laterally and anchors the inferior end of the rib cage during respiration.

6. Review the **transversus abdominis muscle.** The transversus abdominis muscle forms the lateral part of the posterior abdominal wall. The transversus abdominis muscle lies posterior to the quadratus lumborum muscle.

7. Use an illustration and the dissected specimen to study the relationships between the kidneys and the posterior abdominal wall (Fig. 4.46). Verify that the dorsal surface of each kidney is related, through the renal fat and fascia, to the diaphragm, psoas major muscle, quadratus lumborum muscle, and transversus abdominis muscle. The superior pole of the right kidney is at the level of the 12th rib. The superior pole of the left kidney is slightly higher, at the level of the 11th rib.

LUMBAR PLEXUS [G 172, 173; L 250; N 267; R 333; C 253]

The nerves of the posterior abdominal wall arise from the ventral rami of spinal nerves T12 to L4. The **lumbar plexus** (L1 to L4) is formed within the psoas major muscle and its branches can be seen as they emerge from the lateral border of this muscle. The lumbar plexus can be seen only after removal of the psoas major muscle.

Dissect the lumbar plexus on the left side only. Since each branch of the lumbar plexus passes through the psoas major muscle at a different depth, it is necessary to follow each nerve proximally into the psoas major muscle, removing the muscle piece by piece. The nerves of the lumbar plexus are variable in their branching. Use the peripheral relationships of the nerves (their region of distribution or a point of exit from the abdominal cavity) for positive identification.

1. Identify the **genitofemoral nerve**. It is found on the anterior surface of the psoas major muscle (Fig. 4.47). It is the motor nerve to the cremaster muscle (genital part) and supplies a small area of skin inferior and medial to the inguinal ligament (genital and femoral parts). The two parts of the genitofemoral nerve divide on the anterior surface of the psoas major muscle superior to the inguinal ligament.

2. Use blunt dissection to remove the extraperitoneal fascia from the posterior abdominal wall lateral to the psoas major muscle. The branches of the lumbar plexus are in the extraperitoneal fascia and care must be taken to move the dissection instrument parallel to the course of the nerves (Fig. 4.47).

3. To find the **subcostal nerve**, palpate rib 12 and look for the subcostal nerve about 1 cm inferior to it.

4. Find the **iliohypogastric** and **ilioinguinal nerves**. They descend steeply across the anterior surface of the quadratus lumborum muscle. Frequently, these two nerves arise from a common trunk and do not separate until they reach the transversus abdominis muscle. To positively identify the ilioinguinal nerve, follow it to the superficial inguinal ring.

5. Identify the **lateral cutaneous nerve of the thigh**. The lateral cutaneous nerve of the thigh passes deep to the inguinal ligament near the anterior superior iliac spine. The lateral cutaneous nerve of the thigh supplies the skin on the lateral aspect of the thigh.

6. Identify the **femoral nerve**. The femoral nerve lies on the lateral side of the psoas major muscle in the groove between the psoas major and iliacus muscles. The femoral nerve innervates these two muscles. The femoral nerve passes deep to the inguinal ligament and provides motor and sensory branches to the anterior thigh.

7. To find the **obturator nerve**, insert your finger into the extraperitoneal fascia on the medial side of the psoas major muscle and move your finger parallel to the muscle, creating a gap between the psoas major muscle and the common iliac vessels. The obturator nerve supplies motor and sensory innervation to the medial thigh.

8. Identify the **lumbosacral trunk**. The lumbosacral trunk is a large nerve that is formed by a contribution from the ventral ramus of L4 and all of the ventral ramus of L5. The lumbosacral trunk passes into the pelvis to join the sacral plexus.

ABDOMINAL PART OF THE SYMPATHETIC TRUNK
[G 176; L 251–253; N 318; R 334; C 255]

1. Study the location of the **sympathetic trunk** on a transverse section of the abdomen (Fig. 4.43). Note that the sympathetic trunk is found on the vertebral body between the crus of the diaphragm and the psoas major muscle.

2. Identify **lumbar splanchnic nerves** that pass anteriorly from the sympathetic trunk to the aortic autonomic nerve plexus.

3. Identify **rami communicantes** that pass posteriorly from the sympathetic ganglia to lumbar ventral rami. Note that each ramus communicans passes deeply between the psoas major muscle and

the vertebral body. The gray rami of the lower lumbar region are the longest in the body because the sympathetic trunk crosses the anterolateral surface of the lumbar vertebral bodies.

4. Use an illustration to review the autonomic nerve supply of the abdominal viscera.

Dissection Review

1. Use the dissected specimen to review the proximal and distal attachments, as well as the action of each of the muscles of the posterior abdominal wall.
2. Review the three muscles that form the anterolateral abdominal wall (external oblique, internal oblique, and transversus abdominis).
3. Follow each branch of the lumbar plexus peripherally. Review the region of innervation of each of these nerves.
4. Use an atlas drawing to review the sympathetic trunk.

DIAPHRAGM

Dissection Overview

The **diaphragm** forms the roof of the abdominal cavity and the floor of the thoracic cavity. It is the principal muscle of respiration. The diaphragm has a right half and a left half (the **hemidiaphragms**).

The order of dissection will be as follows: The parts of the diaphragm will be identified. The phrenic nerve will be reviewed. The greater splanchnic nerves that pass through the diaphragm will be studied.

Dissection Instructions

1. Use blunt dissection to strip the parietal peritoneum and connective tissue off the abdominal surface of the diaphragm. [G 174; L 245; N 263; R 282, 283; C 251]
2. Identify the parts of the diaphragm (Fig. 4.48):
   • **Central tendon** − the aponeurotic center of the diaphragm, which is the distal attachment of all of its muscular parts
   • **Sternal part** − two small bundles of muscle fibers that attach to the posterior surface of the xiphoid process
   • **Costal part** − the muscle fibers that attach to the inferior six ribs and their costal cartilages
   • **Lumbar part** − formed by two crura (right and left)
3. Identify the **right crus** (Fig. 4.48). The proximal attachments of the right crus of the diaphragm are

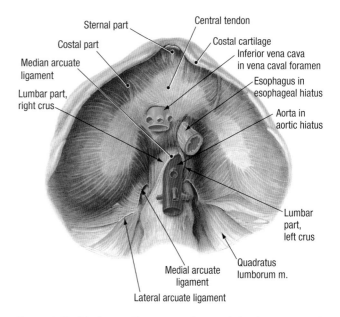

Figure 4.48. Diaphragm. The psoas major muscle has been removed.

the bodies of vertebrae L1 to L3. The **esophageal hiatus** is an opening in the right crus.

4. Observe the **left crus** (Fig. 4.48). The proximal attachments of the left crus of the diaphragm are the bodies of vertebrae L1 to L2.
5. Identify the **arcuate ligaments**. The arcuate ligaments are thickenings of fascia that serve as proximal attachments for some of the muscle fibers of the diaphragm.
   • **Lateral arcuate ligament** bridges the anterior surface of the quadratus lumborum muscle.
   • **Medial arcuate ligament** bridges the anterior surface of the psoas major muscle.
   • **Median arcuate ligament** (unpaired) bridges the anterior surface of the aorta at the aortic hiatus.
6. There are three large openings in the diaphragm (Fig. 4.48). Identify:
   • **Vena caval foramen** passes through the central tendon (vertebral level T8).
   • **Esophageal hiatus** passes through the right crus (vertebral level T10).
   • **Aortic hiatus** passes behind the diaphragm (vertebral level T12).
7. The **right** and **left phrenic nerves** innervate the diaphragm. Each phrenic nerve provides motor innervation to one half of the diaphragm (one hemidiaphragm). The phrenic nerves supply most of the sensory innervation to the abdominal (parietal peritoneum) and thoracic (parietal pleura) surfaces of the diaphragm. The pleural and peritoneal coverings of the peripheral part of the diaphragm receive sensory fibers from the lower intercostal nerves (T5 to T11) and the subcostal nerve.

CLINICAL CORRELATION

Diaphragm

The phrenic nerves arise from cervical spinal cord segments (C3 to C5). Therefore, pain from the diaphragm is referred to the shoulder region (supraclavicular nerve territory).

The diaphragm is paralyzed in cases of high cervical spinal cord injuries, but is spared in low cervical spinal cord injuries. A paralyzed hemidiaphragm cannot contract (descend), so it will appear high in the thorax on a chest radiograph.

8. Identify the **greater splanchnic nerve** in the thorax and follow it to the superior surface of the diaphragm. [G 176; L 251–253; N 267; C 253]
9. Push a probe through the diaphragm parallel to the greater splanchnic nerve. Note that the greater splanchnic nerve penetrates the crus to enter the abdominal cavity.
10. Observe that the main portion of the greater splanchnic nerve distributes to the celiac ganglion where its sympathetic axons will synapse. The greater splanchnic nerve also innervates the suprarenal gland.

11. Find the **celiac ganglia**. The celiac ganglia are found on the left and right sides of the celiac trunk near its origin from the aorta. The celiac ganglia are the largest of the sympathetic ganglia that are located on the surface of the aorta.
12. Use an illustration or textbook description to review the autonomic nerve supply of the abdominal viscera.

Dissection Review

1. Review the attachments of the diaphragm to the skeleton of the thoracic wall.
2. Trace the course of the thoracic aorta as it passes through the aortic hiatus to become the abdominal aorta.
3. Review the course of the esophagus and the vagus nerve trunks through the esophageal hiatus.
4. Recall the position of the heart on the superior surface of the diaphragm and review the course of the inferior vena cava.
5. Study an illustration and observe that the thoracic duct passes through the aortic hiatus and that the splanchnic nerves (greater, lesser, and least) penetrate the crura.

CHAPTER 5

THE PELVIS AND PERINEUM

The pelvis is the area of transition between the trunk and the lower limbs. The bony pelvis serves as the foundation for the pelvic region and provides strong support for the vertebral column upon the lower limbs. The pelvic cavity is continuous with the abdominal cavity, the transition occurring at the plane of the **pelvic inlet** (Fig. 5.1). The pelvic cavity contains the rectum, the urinary bladder, and the internal genitalia. [G 196]

The perineum is the region of the trunk that is located between the thighs. The **pelvic diaphragm** separates the pelvic cavity from the perineum (Fig. 5.1). The perineum contains the anal canal, the urethra, and the external genitalia (penis and scrotum in the male, vulva in the female).

This chapter begins with the dissection of structures in the anal triangle that are common to both sexes. Dissection of internal and external genitalia is divided into two sections, one for male cadavers and one for female cadavers. Students will be expected to demonstrate knowledge of both male and female anatomy in the pelvis and perineum. Each dissection team should partner with another dissection team that is working on a cadaver of the opposite sex.

SKELETON OF THE PELVIS

Refer to an articulated bony pelvis. The **pelvis** (L. *pelvis*, basin) is formed by two **hip bones (os coxae)** joined posteriorly by the **sacrum** (Fig. 5.2A). Each hip bone is formed by three fused bones: **pubis**, **ischium**, and **ilium**. The point of fusion of these three bones is the **acetabulum**. The **coccyx** is attached to the sacrum. [G 196; L 261; N 353; R 436; C 266]

On the hip bone, identify: [G 197; L 260; N 352; R 433; C 266]

- **Iliac fossa**
- **Iliopubic eminence**
- **Arcuate line**
- **Pecten pubis**
- **Superior pubic ramus**
- **Pubic symphysis**
- **Pubic arch**
- **Ischiopubic ramus** – formed by the ischial ramus and the inferior pubic ramus
- **Obturator foramen**
- **Ischial tuberosity**
- **Ischial spine**

On the sacrum, identify: [G 196; L 261; N 353; R 434; C 353]

- **Sacral promontory**
- **Anterior sacral foramina**

Identify the **coccyx**.

The hip bone and sacrum are connected by strong ligaments. On a model with pelvic ligaments, identify (Fig. 5.2A, B): [G 200, 201; L 263; N 352; R 444; C 271, 273]

- **Sacrotuberous ligament**
- **Sacrospinous ligament**
- **Greater sciatic foramen**
- **Lesser sciatic foramen**

Note that the sacrotuberous ligament and sacrospinous ligament convert the **greater and lesser sciatic notches** into the **greater and lesser sciatic foramina**.

The sacroiliac articulation is a synovial joint between the auricular surfaces of the sacrum and the ilium. It is strengthened by an **anterior sacroiliac ligament** and a **posterior sacroiliac ligament** (Fig. 5.2A, B). The articulation between the ilium and the L5 vertebra is strengthened by the **iliolumbar ligament**.

Identify the **pubic arch**. Note that the **subpubic angle** (angle of the pubic arch) is wider in females than males. [G 198, 199; L 262; N 354; R 436; C 270, 271]

ATLAS REFERENCES:
G = *Grant's Atlas,* 12th ed., page number
L = *LWW Atlas of Anatomy,* 1st ed., page number
N = *Netter's Atlas,* 4th ed., plate number
R = *Color Atlas of Anatomy,* 6th ed., page number
C = *Clemente's Atlas,* 5th ed., plate number

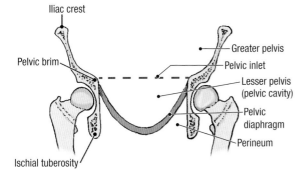

Figure 5.1. The pelvis on coronal section.

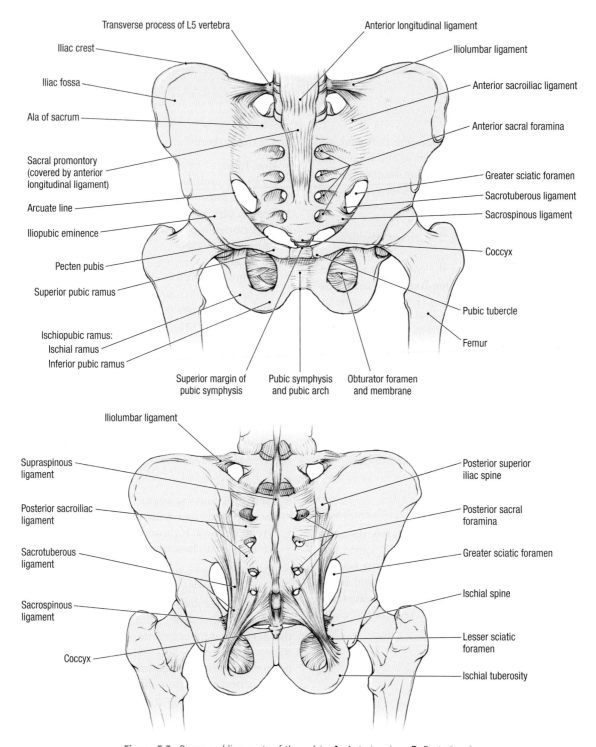

Figure 5.2. Bones and ligaments of the pelvis. **A.** Anterior view. **B.** Posterior view.

Identify the **pelvic inlet (superior pelvic aperture)**. The bony rim of the pelvic inlet is called the **pelvic brim**. From anterior to posterior, identify the structures that form the pelvic brim: [G 199; L 261; N 353; R 435; C 270]

- **Superior margin of the pubic symphysis**
- **Posterior border of the pubic crest**
- **Pecten pubis**

- **Arcuate line of the ilium**
- **Anterior border of the ala (wing) of the sacrum**
- **Sacral promontory**

Identify the **pelvic outlet**. The pelvic outlet is bounded on each side by: [G 202; L 260, 263; N 352; R 444; C 272]

- **Inferior margin of the pubic symphysis**
- **Ischiopubic ramus**

- **Ischial tuberosity**
- **Sacrotuberous ligament**
- **Tip of the coccyx**

The pelvic inlet divides the pelvis into the **greater (false) pelvis** and **lesser (true) pelvis** (Fig. 5.1). The greater pelvis is situated superior to the pelvic brim and is bounded bilaterally by the ala of the ilium. The lesser pelvis is located inferior to the pelvic brim. The inferior border of the lesser pelvis is the pelvic diaphragm. [G 196]

In the **erect posture** (anatomical position), the anterior superior iliac spines and the anterior aspect of the pubis are in the same vertical plane. In this position, the plane of the pelvic inlet forms an angle of approximately 55° to the horizontal. [G 197; L 262; N 352; R 439]

ANAL TRIANGLE

Dissection Overview

The **perineum** is a diamond-shaped area between the thighs that is divided for descriptive purposes into two triangles (Fig. 5.3). The **anal triangle** is the posterior part of the perineum and it contains the anal canal and anus. The **urogenital triangle** is the anterior part of the perineum and contains the urethra and the external genitalia. At the outset of dissection, it is important to understand that the *pelvic diaphragm separates the pelvic cavity from the perineum* (Fig. 5.1).

The order of dissection will be as follows: Dissection of the anal triangle will begin with removal of skin from the gluteal region and retraction of the gluteus maximus muscle. The nerves and vessels of the ischioanal fossa will be dissected. The fat will be removed from the ischioanal fossa to reveal the inferior surface of the pelvic diaphragm.

Dissection Instructions

SKIN AND SUPERFICIAL FASCIA REMOVAL

1. If the lower limb has been dissected previously, reflect the gluteus maximus muscle laterally and move ahead to the dissection of the *Ischioanal Fossa*. If the lower limb has not been dissected, continue with step 2.
2. Place the cadaver in the prone position.
3. Refer to Figure 5.4.
4. Make an incision that follows the lateral border of the sacrum and the iliac crest from the tip of the coccyx (S) to the midaxillary line (T). If the back has been skinned, this incision has been made previously.
5. Make a midline skin incision from S to the posterior edge of the anus.
6. Make an incision that encircles the anus.
7. Make an incision from the anterior edge of the anus down the medial surface of the thigh to point D (about 7.5 cm down the medial surface of the thigh).
8. Make a skin incision from D obliquely across the posterior surface of the thigh to point E on the lateral surface of the thigh. Point E should be approximately 30 cm inferior to the iliac crest.
9. Make a skin incision along the lateral side of the thigh from T to E.
10. Remove the skin from medial to lateral and place it in the tissue container.
11. Remove the superficial fascia from the surface of the gluteus maximus muscle and place it in the tissue container.

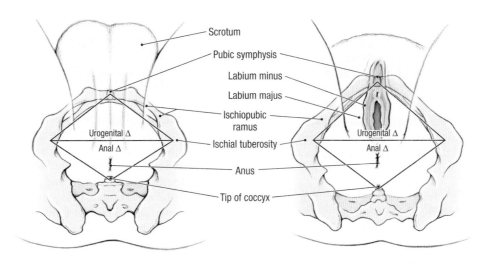

Figure 5.3. Boundaries of the urogenital and anal triangles in the male and female.

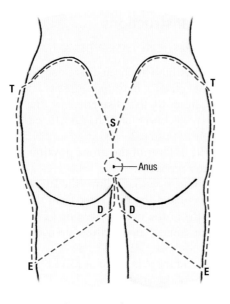

Figure 5.4. Skin incisions.

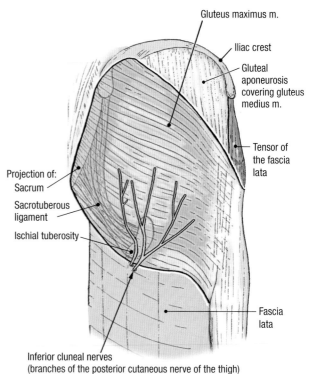

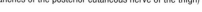
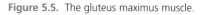

Figure 5.5. The gluteus maximus muscle.

12. Clean the inferior border of the **gluteus maximus muscle** (Fig. 5.5). Do not save the **inferior cluneal nerves**, but take care not to cut the fascia lata (deep fascia) of the posterior thigh.
13. Use your hands to define the inferior margin of the gluteus maximus muscle and separate it from the deeper fat and connective tissue.
14. Use your fingers to retract the inferior border of the gluteus maximus muscle and palpate the **sacrotuberous ligament**. Note that the gluteus maximus muscle is attached to the **sacrotuberous ligament** and also to the sacrum.
15. Retract the gluteus maximus muscle superiorly to broaden the dissection field and expose the fat of the ischioanal fossa.

ISCHIOANAL FOSSA

The **ischioanal (ischiorectal) fossa** is a wedge-shaped area on either side of the anus. The apex of the wedge is directed superiorly and the base is beneath the skin. The ischioanal fossa is filled with fat that helps accommodate the fetus during childbirth or the distended anal canal during the passage of feces. The ischioanal fat is part of the superficial fascia of this region. The goal of this dissection is to remove the fat and identify the nerves and vessels that pass through the ischioanal fossa. [G 261; L 283, 286; N 411; R 351; C 318]

1. Lateral to the anus, insert closed scissors into the ischioanal fat to a depth of 3 cm. Open the scissors in the transverse direction to tear the fat (Fig. 5.6, Incision).
2. Insert your finger into the incision and move it back and forth (medial to lateral) to enlarge the opening.

3. Palpate the **inferior rectal (anal) nerve** and **vessels** (Fig. 5.6). Preserve the branches of the inferior rectal nerve and vessels but use blunt dissection to remove the fat that surrounds them. Dry the area with paper towels if necessary.
4. Use blunt dissection to clean the **external anal sphincter muscle** (Fig. 5.6). The external anal sphincter muscle has three parts:
   • **Subcutaneous** – encircling the anus (not visible in dissection)
   • **Superficial** – anchoring the anus to the perineal body and coccyx
   • **Deep** – a circular band that is fused with the pelvic diaphragm
5. Use blunt dissection to clean the **inferior surface of the pelvic diaphragm** (medial boundary of the ischioanal fossa).
6. Use blunt dissection to clean the **fascia of the obturator internus muscle** (the lateral boundary of the ischioanal fossa).
7. Observe that the inferior rectal nerve and vessels penetrate the fascia of the obturator internus muscle. The inferior rectal vessels and nerve exit the **pudendal canal** to enter the ischioanal fossa.
8. Place gentle traction on the inferior rectal vessels and nerve and observe that a ridge is raised in the obturator internus fascia. Carefully incise the obturator fascia along this ridge to open the pudendal canal.
9. Use a probe to elevate the contents of the pudendal canal. The pudendal canal contains the **pudendal nerve** and the **internal pudendal artery** and **vein**.

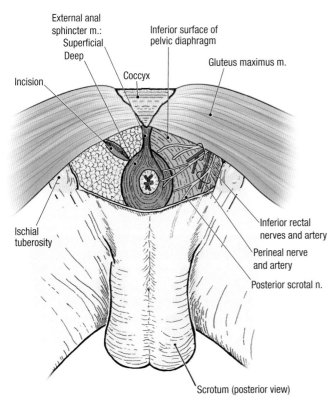

Figure 5.6. Initial incision used to begin the dissection of the ischioanal fossa.

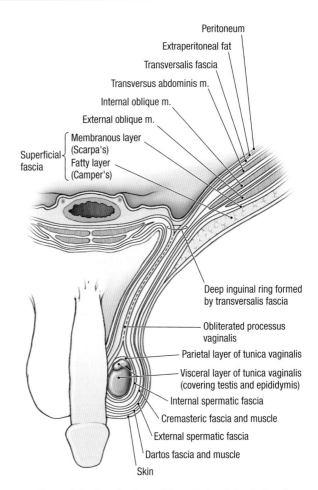

Figure 5.7. Contributions of the anterior abdominal wall to the coverings of the spermatic cord and testis.

Dissection Review

1. Review the boundaries of the true pelvis and the concept that the pelvic diaphragm separates the pelvic cavity from the perineum.
2. In the dissected specimen, review the inferior surface of the pelvic diaphragm and understand that this is the "roof" of the perineum.
3. Use the dissected specimen to review the lateral and medial walls of the ischioanal fossa. 4. Review the external anal sphincter muscle and its blood and nerve supply. Understand that the external anal sphincter muscle is skeletal muscle under voluntary control.

MALE EXTERNAL GENITALIA AND PERINEUM

Dissection Overview

If you are dissecting a female cadaver, go to the section entitled "Female External Genitalia and Perineum" located on page 133.

The **scrotum** is an outpouching of the anterior abdominal wall, and most layers of the abdominal wall are represented in its structure (Fig. 5.7). The superficial fascia of the scrotum contains no fat. Instead, the superficial fascia is represented by **dartos fascia**, which contains smooth muscle fibers (**dartos muscle**).

The order of dissection will be as follows: The scrotum will be opened by a vertical incision along its anterior surface. The spermatic cord will be followed from the superficial inguinal ring into the scrotum. The testis will be removed from the scrotum. The spermatic cord will be dissected. The testis will be studied.

Scrotum Dissection Instructions [G 112; L 282, 288; R 220; C 190]

1. Partner with a dissection team that has a female cadaver for the following dissection. You are expected to know the anatomical details for both sexes.
2. Inferior to the superficial inguinal ring, insert your finger deep to the subcutaneous tissue of the lower anterior abdominal wall and push your finger into the scrotum.
3. Use scissors to make an incision down the anterior surface of the scrotum through the skin, dartos, and superficial fascia.
4. Use your fingers to free the testis and spermatic cord from the scrotum.
5. Observe a band of tissue that anchors the inferior pole of the testis to the scrotum. This is the **scro-**

tal ligament (the remnant of the gubernaculum testis). [G 112; N 387; R 341; C 192]

6. Use scissors to cut the scrotal ligament. Use your fingers to remove the testis from the scrotum, but leave the testis attached to the spermatic cord.
7. Observe that the **scrotal septum** divides the scrotum into two compartments.

SPERMATIC CORD [G 116; L 288; N 387; R 341; C 192]

The spermatic cord contains the ductus deferens, testicular vessels, lymphatics, and nerves. The contents of the spermatic cord are surrounded by three fascial layers, the **coverings of the spermatic cord**, that are derived from layers of the anterior abdominal wall (Fig. 5.7). These coverings are added to the spermatic cord as it passes through the inguinal canal.

1. Study an illustration of a transverse section through the spermatic cord (Fig. 5.8).
2. Palpate the **ductus deferens (vas deferens)** within the spermatic cord. It is hard and cord-like.
3. Use a probe to longitudinally incise the **coverings of the spermatic cord**. The three coverings are fixed to each other at the time of embalming and cannot be separated. The coverings of the spermatic cord are (Fig. 5.8):
   • **External spermatic fascia** – derived from the external oblique muscle
   • **Cremasteric muscle and fascia** – derived from the internal oblique muscle
   • **Internal spermatic fascia** – derived from the transversalis fascia
4. Use a probe to separate the ductus deferens from the **pampiniform plexus of veins**.
5. Observe the **artery of the ductus deferens**, a small vessel located on the surface of the ductus deferens (Fig. 5.8)
6. Follow the ductus deferens superiorly into the inguinal canal and toward the deep inguinal ring.

Note that the ductus deferens passes through the deep inguinal ring lateral to the inferior epigastric vessels.

7. Use a probe to separate the **testicular artery** from the pampiniform plexus of veins. The testicular artery can be distinguished from the veins by its slightly thicker wall.
8. Note that sensory nerve fibers, autonomic nerve fibers, and lymphatic vessels accompany the blood vessels in the spermatic cord (Fig. 5.8), but they are too small to dissect.

CLINICAL CORRELATION

Vasectomy

The ductus deferens can be surgically interrupted in the superior part of the scrotum (vasectomy). Sperm production in the testis continues but the spermatozoa cannot reach the urethra.

TESTIS [G 117; L 289; N 390; R 341; C 193]

1. The testis is covered by the **tunica vaginalis**, a serous sac that is derived from the parietal peritoneum (Fig. 5.7). The tunica vaginalis has a **visceral layer** and a **parietal layer** (Fig. 5.9). The **cavity of the tunica vaginalis** is only a potential space

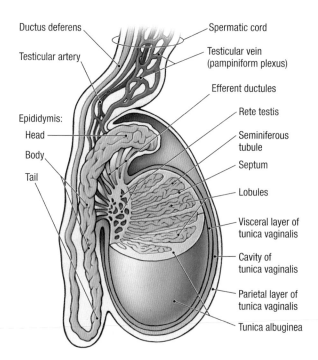

Figure 5.9. Parts of the testis and epididymis, right testis in lateral view.

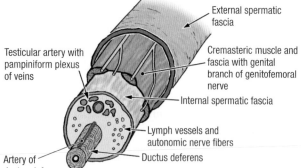

Figure 5.8. Transverse section through the spermatic cord.

that contains a very small amount of serous fluid.

2. Use scissors to incise the parietal layer of the tunica vaginalis along its anterior surface and open it widely. Observe that the visceral layer of the tunica vaginalis covers the anterior, medial, and lateral surfaces of the testis, but not its posterior surface.

3. Use a probe to trace the ductus deferens inferiorly until it joins the epididymis. Identify the **tail**, **body**, and **head of the epididymis** (Fig. 5.9).

4. Use a scalpel to section the testis longitudinally from its superior pole to its inferior pole. Make the cut along its anterior surface. Use the epididymis as a hinge, and open the halves of the testis like opening a book.

5. Note the thickness of the **tunica albuginea**, which is the fibrous capsule of the testis. Observe the **septa** that divide the interior of the testis into **lobules** (Fig. 5.9).

6. Use a needle or fine-tipped forceps to tease some of the **seminiferous tubules** out of one lobule.

CLINICAL CORRELATION

Lymphatic Drainage of the Testis

Lymphatics from the scrotum drain to the superficial inguinal lymph nodes. Inflammation of the scrotum may cause tender, enlarged superficial inguinal lymph nodes. In contrast, lymphatics from the testis follow the testicular vessels through the inguinal canal and into the abdominal cavity where they drain into lumbar (lateral aortic) nodes and preaortic lymph nodes. Testicular tumors may metastasize to lumbar and preaortic lymph nodes, not to superficial inguinal lymph nodes.

Dissection Review

1. Review the course of the ductus deferens from the abdominal wall to the testis.

2. Review the coverings of the spermatic cord and recall the layers of the abdominal wall from which they are derived.

3. Use an illustration to trace the route of spermatozoa from their origin in the seminiferous tubule to the ejaculatory duct.

4. Visit a dissection table with a female cadaver and complete the dissection review that follows the dissection of the labium majus located on page 133.

MALE UROGENITAL TRIANGLE

Dissection Overview

The order of dissection of the male urogenital triangle will be as follows: The skin will be removed from the urogenital triangle. The superficial perineal fascia will be removed and the contents of the superficial perineal pouch will be identified. The skin will be removed from the penis and its parts will be studied. The contents of the deep perineal pouch will be described, but not dissected.

Dissection Instructions

SKIN REMOVAL

1. Place the cadaver in the supine position. Stretch the thighs widely apart and brace them. Usually, only one student can work on the urogenital triangle at a time. The dissector should be positioned between the thighs with the cadaver pulled to the end of the dissection table.

2. Make a skin incision that encircles the proximal end of the penis (Fig. 5.10, blue dashed lines). The skin is very thin.

3. Make a midline skin incision posterior to the proximal end of the penis that splits the scrotum along the scrotal septum. Carry the cut posteriorly as far as the anus (Fig. 5.10).

4. Make an incision in the midline superior to the penis. Stop where the skin of the abdomen was removed previously.

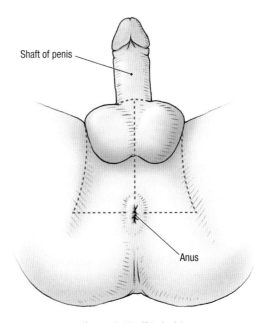

Shaft of penis

Anus

Figure 5.10. Skin incisions.

5. Reflect the skin flaps from medial to lateral. Detach the scrotum and skin flaps along the medial thigh (Fig. 5.10, red dashed lines) and place them in the tissue container.

6. If the cadaver has a large amount of fat in the superficial fascia of the medial thighs, remove a portion of the superficial fascia starting at the ischiopubic ramus and extending down the medial thigh about 7 cm. Stay superficial to the deep fascia when removing the superficial fascia.

7. Note that the **posterior scrotal nerve and vessels** enter the urogenital triangle by passing lateral to the external anal sphincter muscle. The posterior scrotal nerve and vessels supply the posterior part of the scrotum.

SUPERFICIAL PERINEAL POUCH [G 261, 257; L 284; N 381; R 350; C 318]

The superficial perineal fascia has a superficial fatty layer and a deep membranous layer. The superficial fatty layer is continuous with the superficial fatty layer of the lower abdominal wall, ischioanal fossa, and thigh. The **membranous layer of the superficial perineal fascia (Colles' fascia)** is continuous with the membranous layer of the superficial fascia of the anterior abdominal wall (Scarpa's fascia) and the **dartos fascia** of the penis and scrotum (Fig. 5.11A). The membranous layer of the superficial perineal fascia is attached to the ischiopubic ramus as far posteriorly as the ischial tuberosity and to the posterior edge of the **perineal membrane**. The membranous layer of the superficial perineal fascia forms the superficial boundary of the **superficial perineal pouch (space)**.

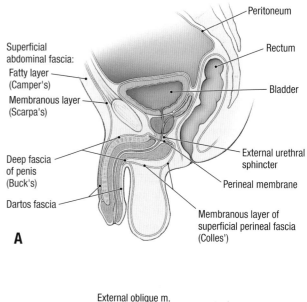

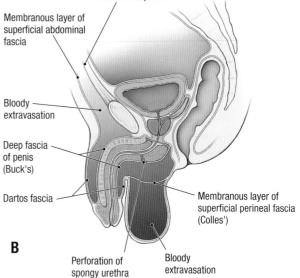

Figure 5.11. Fasciae of the perineum. **A.** The membranous layer of the superficial perineal fascia (Colles' fascia) is continuous with the superficial fascia (dartos fascia) of the scrotum and the penis. It is also continuous with the membranous layer of superficial fascia of the lower abdominal wall (Scarpa's fascia) and is attached to the posterior border of the perineal membrane. **B.** Following injury to the urethra in the perineum, extravasated urine is contained in the superficial perineal pouch and spreads into the lower abdominal wall.

CLINICAL CORRELATION

Superficial Perineal Pouch

If the urethra is injured in the perineum, urine may escape into the superficial perineal pouch. The urine may spread into the scrotum and penis, and upward into the lower abdominal wall between the membranous layer of the abdominal superficial fascia (Scarpa's fascia) and the aponeurosis of the external oblique muscle (Fig. 5.11B). The urine does not enter the thigh because the membranous layer of the superficial fascia attaches to the fascia lata, ischiopubic ramus, and posterior edge of the perineal membrane.

1. The **contents of the superficial perineal pouch in the male** are **three paired muscles (superficial transverse perineal, bulbospongiosus, and ischiocavernosus)**, the **crura of the penis**, and the **bulb of the penis** (Fig. 5.12A, B). The superficial perineal pouch also contains the arteries, veins, and nerves that supply these structures.

2. It is not necessary to identify the membranous layer of the superficial perineal fascia to complete the dissection. Use a probe to dissect through the superficial perineal fascia in the midline.

3. Use blunt dissection to find the **bulbospongiosus muscle** in the midline of the urogenital triangle (Fig. 5.12A). The bulbospongiosus muscle covers the superficial surface of the bulb of the penis. The posterior attachments of the bulbospongiosus

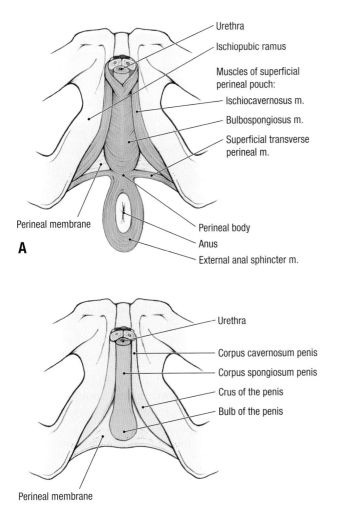

A

Urethra
Ischiopubic ramus
Muscles of superficial perineal pouch:
Ischiocavernosus m.
Bulbospongiosus m.
Superficial transverse perineal m.
Perineal membrane
Perineal body
Anus
External anal sphincter m.

B

Urethra
Corpus cavernosum penis
Corpus spongiosum penis
Crus of the penis
Bulb of the penis
Perineal membrane

Figure 5.12. Contents of the superficial perineal pouch in the male. **A.** Muscles. **B.** Erectile bodies.

muscle are the bulbospongiosus muscle of the opposite side (in a midline raphe) and the perineal body. The anterior attachment of the bulbospongiosus muscle is the corpus cavernosum penis. The bulbospongiosus muscle compresses the bulb of the penis to expel urine or semen.

4. Lateral to the bulbospongiosus muscle, use a probe to clean the surface of the **ischiocavernosus muscle** (Fig. 5.12A). The ischiocavernosus muscle covers the superficial surface of the crus of the penis. The proximal attachment of the ischiocavernosus muscle is the ischial tuberosity and the ischiopubic ramus. The distal attachment of the ischiocavernosus muscle is the crus of the penis. The ischiocavernosus muscle forces blood from the crus of the penis into the distal part of the corpus cavernosum penis.

5. Using blunt dissection, attempt to find the **superficial transverse perineal muscle** at the posterior border of the urogenital triangle (Fig. 5.12A). The

superficial transverse perineal muscle may be delicate and difficult to find; limit the time spent looking for it. The lateral attachments of the superficial transverse perineal muscle are the ischial tuberosity and the ischiopubic ramus. The medial attachment of the superficial transverse perineal muscle is the **perineal body**. The perineal body is a fibromuscular mass located anterior to the anal canal and posterior to the perineal membrane that serves as an attachment for several muscles. The superficial transverse perineal muscle helps to support the perineal body.

6. Use a probe to dissect between the three muscles of the superficial perineal pouch until a small triangular opening is created (Fig. 5.12A). The membrane that becomes visible through this opening is the **perineal membrane**. The perineal membrane is the deep boundary of the superficial perineal pouch and the bulb of the penis and crura are attached to it.

7. Use a scalpel to divide the bulbospongiosus muscles along their midline raphe. On the right side of the cadaver, remove the bulbospongiosus muscle.

8. Identify the **bulb of the penis** (Fig. 5.12B). The bulb of the penis is continuous with the corpus spongiosum penis and contains a portion of the spongy urethra.

9. On the right side of the cadaver, use blunt dissection to remove the ischiocavernosus muscle from the **crus of the penis** (Fig. 5.12B) (L. *crus*, a leglike part; pl. *crura*). The crus of the penis is the proximal part of the corpus cavernosum penis.

PENIS [G 265; L 288, 289; N 381, 382; R 336, 339; C 192, 320]

In the anatomical position, the penis is erect. The surface of the penis that is closest to the anterior abdominal wall is the **dorsal surface of the penis**.

Study a drawing of a transverse section of the **penis** (L. *penis*, tail) (Fig. 5.13). The **superficial fascia of the penis (dartos fascia)** has no fat, and contains the **superficial dorsal vein of the penis**. The **deep fascia of the penis (Buck's fascia)** is an investing fascia. Contained within the deep fascia of the penis are the **corpus spongiosum, corpus cavernosum (paired), deep dorsal vein of the penis (unpaired), dorsal artery of the penis (paired), and dorsal nerve of the penis (paired)**.

1. Identify the parts of the penis:
   • **Root (bulb and crura)**
   • **Body (shaft)**
   • **Glans penis**
   • **Corona of the glans**
   • **Prepuce**
   • **Frenulum**
   • **External urethral orifice**

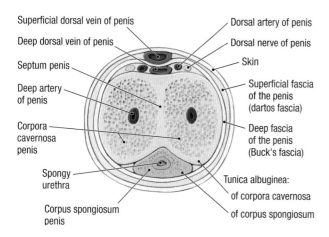

Figure 5.13. Transverse section through the body of the penis.

2. Use a scalpel to make a midline skin incision down the ventral surface of the penis. Remove the skin from the body of the penis, detaching it around the corona of the glans. Do not skin the glans.

3. Use a probe to dissect the **superficial dorsal vein** of the penis. The superficial dorsal vein of the penis drains into the **superficial external pudendal vein** of the inguinal region.

4. On the dorsum of the penis, use a probe to dissect through the **deep fascia of the penis** and identify (Fig. 5.14): [G 264; L 288; R 349; C 320]

   - **Deep dorsal vein of the penis** – a single vein in the midline. Most of the blood from the penis drains through the deep dorsal vein into the **prostatic venous plexus**.
   - **Dorsal artery of the penis (2)** – one artery on each side of the deep dorsal vein. The dorsal ar-

tery of the penis is a terminal branch of the internal pudendal artery.

   - **Dorsal nerve of the penis (2)** – one nerve on each side of the midline, lateral to the deep dorsal artery. The dorsal nerve of the penis is a branch of the pudendal nerve.

5. Use a probe to trace the vessels and nerves of the penis proximally. Use an illustration to study the course of the pudendal nerve and the internal pudendal artery (Fig. 5.14). Observe that the dorsal artery and nerve of the penis course deep to the perineal membrane before they emerge onto the dorsum of the penis. The deep dorsal vein passes between the inferior pubic ligament and the anterior edge of the perineal membrane to enter the pelvis. Note that the deep dorsal vein does not accompany the deep dorsal artery and dorsal nerve proximal to the body of the penis. [G 264, 267; N 403, 410; R 348; C 303]

SPONGY URETHRA [G 268; L 266; N 385; R 338, 339; C 306]

The male urethra consists of three portions: **prostatic urethra, membranous urethra,** and **spongy urethra** (Fig. 5.15). The spongy urethra is the portion that is located within the corpus spongiosum penis. The next objective is to longitudinally open the spongy urethra.

1. Examine the **external urethral orifice** at the tip of the glans penis. Push a probe into the external

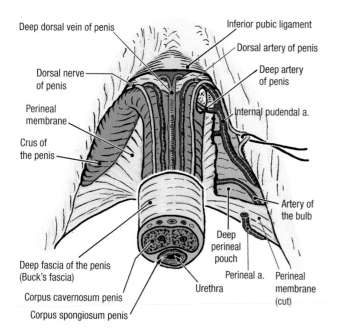

Figure 5.14. Arteries and nerves of the penis.

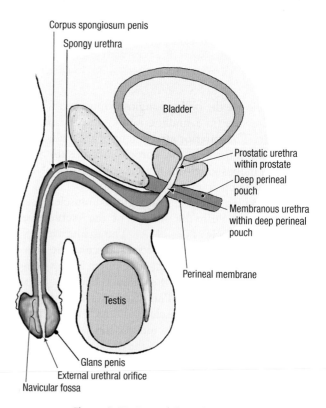

Figure 5.15. Parts of the male urethra.

urethral orifice, and then use a scalpel to cut down to the probe from both the dorsal and ventral surfaces of the penis. Cut in the median plane *of the penis* (it may not be a straight line).

2. Advance the probe proximally, and continue to divide the penis. Dorsal to the probe, the cut should pass between the corpora cavernosa and may split the deep dorsal vein longitudinally. Stop inferior to the pubic symphysis where the two corpora cavernosa separate. Ventral to the probe the cut should divide the corpus spongiosum into equal halves. Stop at the bulb of the penis.

3. In the bulb of the penis, the urethra bends at a sharp angle and passes through the perineal membrane (Fig. 5.15). Carefully complete the cut through the bulb posterior to the urethra but do not cut through the perineal membrane.

4. Note that the **glans penis** (L. *glans*, acorn) is the distal expansion of the corpus spongiosum and that it caps the two corpora cavernosa penis. The spongy urethra terminates by passing through the glans.

5. Examine the interior of the spongy urethra. Identify the **navicular fossa**, a widening of the urethra in the glans penis.

6. The openings of the ducts of the **bulbourethral glands** are in the proximal part of the spongy urethra, but may be too small to see.

7. On the right side of the penis, make a transverse cut through the body of the penis about midway down its length.

8. On the cut surface of the transverse section of the penis, study the relationship of the **corpus cavernosum penis** and **corpus spongiosum penis**. Identify (Fig. 5.13): [G 267; L 289; N 381; R 339; C 192]
    • **Tunica albuginea of the corpora cavernosa penis**
    • **Tunica albuginea of the corpus spongiosum penis**
    • **Septum penis**

9. Study the erectile tissue within the corpus spongiosum penis. Observe that the corpus spongiosum penis surrounds the spongy urethra.

10. Study the erectile tissue within the corpus cavernosum penis (Fig. 5.13). Identify the **deep artery of the penis** near the center of the erectile tissue. Review the origin of the deep artery of the penis from the internal pudendal artery.

DEEP PERINEAL POUCH

The deep perineal pouch (space) will not be dissected. The deep perineal pouch lies superior (deep) to the perineal membrane (Fig. 5.15). The **contents of the deep perineal pouch in the male** are the **membranous urethra, external urethral sphincter muscle, bulbourethral glands, branches of the internal pu-**

dendal vessels,** and **branches of the pudendal nerve** (Fig. 5.16).

1. Use an illustration to study the following: [G 257; L 285; N 383; C 308]
    • **Membranous urethra** − extends from the perineal membrane to the prostate gland (Fig. 5.15). This is the shortest (about 1 cm), thinnest, narrowest, and least distensible part of the urethra.
    • **External urethral sphincter (sphincter urethrae) muscle** − a voluntary muscle that surrounds the membranous urethra (Fig. 5.16). When the external urethral sphincter muscle contracts, it compresses the membranous urethra and stops the flow of urine.
    • **Deep transverse perineal muscle** − has a lateral attachment to the ischial tuberosity and the ischiopubic ramus and a medial attachment to the perineal body (Fig. 5.16). Its fiber direction and function are identical to those of the superficial transverse perineal muscle, which is a content of the superficial perineal pouch.

2. The **bulbourethral glands** are located in the deep perineal pouch. The duct of the bulbourethral gland passes through the perineal membrane and drains into the proximal portion of the spongy urethra.

3. The deep perineal pouch contains branches of the **pudendal nerve** and **internal pudendal artery**. These structures supply the external urethral sphincter muscle, the deep transverse perineal muscle, and the penis (Fig. 5.16).

4. Collectively, the muscles within the deep perineal pouch plus the perineal membrane are known as the **urogenital diaphragm**. This older anatomical nomenclature is still in clinical use.

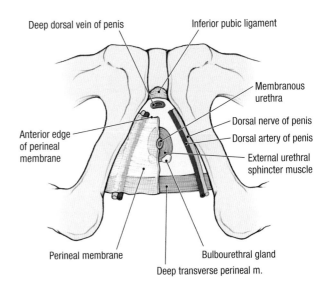

Figure 5.16. Contents of the deep perineal pouch in the male.

Dissection Review

1. Return the muscles of the urogenital triangle to their correct anatomical positions.
2. Review the contents of the male superficial perineal pouch. Visit a dissection table with a female cadaver and view the contents of the superficial perineal pouch.
3. Use an illustration to review the course of the internal pudendal artery from its origin in the pelvis to the dorsum of the penis.
4. Use an illustration to review the course and branches of the pudendal nerve.
5. Study an illustration showing the course of the deep dorsal vein of the penis into the pelvis to join the prostatic venous plexus.
6. Draw a cross section of the penis showing the erectile bodies, superficial fascia, deep fascia, vessels, and nerves.
7. Obtain an illustration that shows the entire male urethra and review its parts.

MALE PELVIC CAVITY

Dissection Overview

The male pelvic cavity contains the urinary bladder anteriorly, male internal genitalia, and the rectum posteriorly (Fig. 5.17). The order of dissection will be as follows: The peritoneum will be studied in the male pelvic cavity. The pelvis will be sectioned in the midline and the cut surface of the sectioned pelvis will be studied. The ductus deferens will be traced from the anterior abdominal wall to the region between the urinary bladder and rectum. The seminal vesicles and prostate gland will be studied.

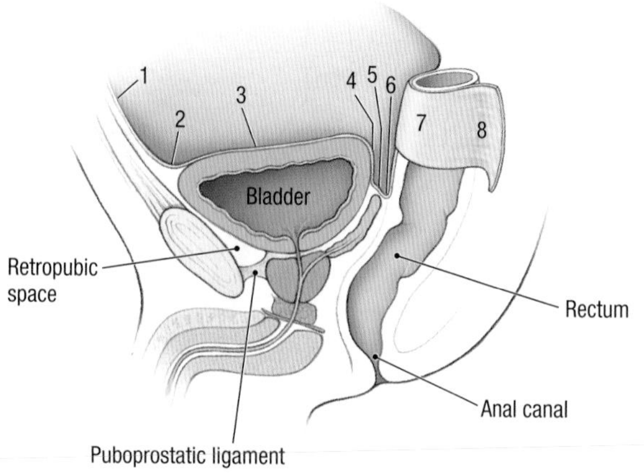

Figure 5.17. Peritoneum in the male pelvis. The numbered features of the peritoneum are explained in the text.

Dissection Instructions

PERITONEUM [G 209, 215; L 265; N 361; R 336; C 302]

1. Using Figure 5.17 as a reference, examine the **peritoneum** in the male pelvis. Note that the peritoneum:

   (1, 2) Passes from the anterior abdominal wall superior to the pubis

   (3) Covers the superior surface of the urinary bladder

   (4) Passes inferiorly along the posterior surface of the urinary bladder

   (5) Has a close relationship to the superior ends of the seminal vesicles

   (6) Passes inferiorly between the urinary bladder and the rectum to form the **rectovesical pouch**

   (7) Contacts the anterior surface and sides of the rectum

   (8) Forms the sigmoid mesocolon beginning at the level of the third sacral vertebra

2. Laterally, a **paravesical fossa** is apparent on each side of the urinary bladder. Further posteriorly, a **pararectal fossa** is apparent on each side of the rectum.

CLINICAL CORRELATION

Pelvic Peritoneum

As the urinary bladder fills, the peritoneal reflection is elevated above the level of the pubis and is raised from the anterior abdominal wall. A filled urinary bladder can be approached with a needle just superior to the pubis without entering the peritoneal cavity.

SECTION OF THE PELVIS

The pelvis will be divided in the midline. First, the pelvic viscera and the soft tissues of the perineum will be cut in the midline with a scalpel. The pubic symphysis and vertebral column (up to vertebral level L3) will be cut in the midline with a saw. Subsequently, the right side of the body will be transected at vertebral level L3. The left lower limb and left side of the pelvis will remain attached to the trunk.

Both halves of the pelvis will be used to dissect the pelvic viscera, pelvic vasculature, and nerves of the pelvis. One half of the pelvis will be used to demonstrate the muscles of the pelvic diaphragm.

1. Begin this dissection with a new scalpel blade.
2. In the pelvic cavity make a midline cut, beginning posterior to the pubic symphysis. Carry this mid-

line cut through the superior surface of the urinary bladder. Open the bladder and sponge the interior, if necessary.

3. Identify the internal urethral orifice and insert a probe. Use the probe as a guide and continue the midline cut inferior to the urinary bladder, dividing the urethra. Divide the prostate gland.

4. Extend the midline cut in the posterior direction. Cut through the anterior and posterior walls of the rectum and the distal part of the sigmoid colon. Sponge them clean.

5. In the perineum, insert the scalpel blade inferior to the pubic symphysis with the cutting edge directed inferiorly. Cut between the halves of the bulb of the penis (sectioned earlier). Make a cut in the midline from the pubic symphysis to the coccyx passing through the perineal membrane, perineal body, and anal canal.

6. Use a saw to make two cuts in the midline:
   • Pubic symphysis – Cut through the pubic symphysis from anterior to posterior.
   • Sacrum – Turn the cadaver to the prone position. Cut through the sacrum from posterior to anterior. Do not allow the saw to pass between the soft tissue structures that were cut with the scalpel. Spread the opening and extend the midline cut as far superiorly as the body of the third lumbar vertebra.

7. Return the cadaver to the supine position. To mobilize the right lower limb, use a scalpel to cut the right common iliac vein, right common iliac artery, and right testicular vessels. Cut the right ureter and the branches of the right lumbar plexus.

8. In the transverse plane, cut the psoas major muscle and the quadratus lumborum muscle at vertebral level L3. Use the saw to cut horizontally through the right half of the intervertebral disc between L3 and L4. Now, the right lower limb can be removed.

9. Clean the rectum and anal canal.

MALE INTERNAL GENITALIA [G 209; L 270; N 361; R 336; C 305]

1. Study the cut surface of the sectioned specimen. Use an illustration to guide you.

2. Identify the **perineal membrane**. It is located deep to the bulb of the penis and can be identified as a thin line at the deep edge of the bulb (Fig. 5.15). Superior (deep) to the perineal membrane, the **external urethral sphincter muscle** surrounds the **membranous urethra**. The external urethral sphincter muscle may be difficult to see in the sectioned specimen.

3. On the sectioned pelvis, identify the three parts of the urethra: **prostatic urethra**, **membranous urethra**, and **spongy urethra** (Fig. 5.15).

4. Examine the **interior of the prostatic urethra**. The prostatic urethra is about 3 cm in length and is the part that passes through the prostate. On the posterior wall of the prostatic urethra, identify (Fig. 5.18): [G 221; L 267; N 385; R 338; C 305]
   • **Urethral crest** – a longitudinal ridge
   • **Seminal colliculus** – an enlargement of the urethral crest
   • **Prostatic sinus** – the groove on either side of the seminal colliculus
   • **Prostatic utricle** – a small opening on the midline of the seminal colliculus
   • **Opening of the ejaculatory duct** – one on either side of the prostatic utricle

5. Find the **ductus deferens** where it enters the **deep inguinal ring** lateral to the inferior epigastric vessels. Use a probe to break through the peritoneum at the deep inguinal ring. Use blunt dissection to peel the peritoneum off the lateral wall of the pelvis. Strip the peritoneum from lateral to medial, stopping where it comes in contact with the rectum and urinary bladder. Detach the peritoneum and place it in the tissue container.

6. Use blunt dissection to trace the ductus deferens from the deep inguinal ring toward the midline. Observe that the ductus deferens passes superior and then medial to the branches of the internal iliac artery. Note that the ductus deferens crosses superior to the ureter. [G 216; L 270; N 363; R 337; C 303]

7. Trace the ductus deferens into the **rectovesical septum**, which is the endopelvic fascia between the rectum and the urinary bladder. Observe that the ductus deferens is in contact with the fundus (posterior surface) of the urinary bladder.

8. Identify the **ampulla of the ductus deferens**, which is the enlarged portion just before its termination (Fig. 5.19). [G 220; L 270; N 384; R 339; C 304]

9. Identify the **seminal vesicle**. The seminal vesicle is located lateral to the ampulla of the ductus deferens in the rectovesical septum. Use blunt dissection to release the seminal vesicle from the rectovesical septum.

10. Close to the prostate, the duct of the seminal vesicle joins the ductus deferens to form the **ejaculatory duct**. The ejaculatory duct is delicate and easily torn where it enters the prostate. The ejaculatory duct empties into the prostatic urethra on the seminal colliculus.

11. Observe the **prostate**. The **apex** of the prostate is directed inferiorly and the **base** of the prostate is located superiorly against the neck of the urinary bladder. Use a textbook to study the **lobes of the prostate**.

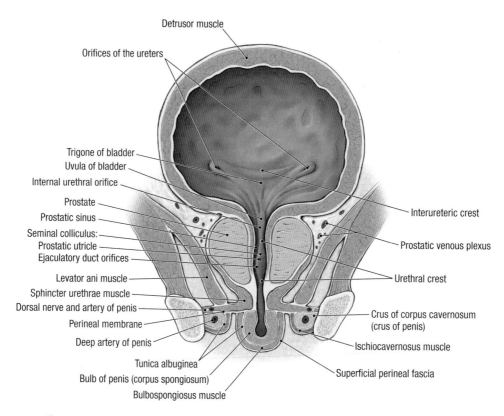

Figure 5.18. Urinary bladder and proximal portion of the male urethra seen in frontal section.

Dissection Review

1. Review the position of the male pelvic viscera within the lesser pelvis. Visit a dissection table with a female cadaver and observe the position of the female pelvic viscera.

2. Review the peritoneum in the male pelvic cavity. Visit a dissection table with a female cadaver and compare differences in the male and female peritoneum (Figs. 5.17 and 5.30).

3. Trace the ductus deferens from the epididymis to the ejaculatory duct, recalling its relationships to vessels, nerves, the ureter, and the seminal vesicle.

4. Visit a dissection table with a female cadaver and trace the round ligament of the uterus from the labium majus to the uterus.

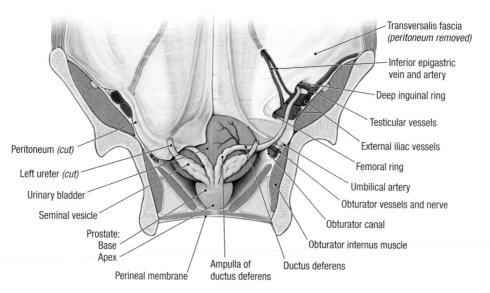

Figure 5.19. Posterior view of the urinary bladder and the male internal genitalia.

5. Compare the pelvic course of the ductus deferens with the pelvic course of the round ligament of the uterus.

URINARY BLADDER, RECTUM, AND ANAL CANAL

Dissection Overview

The urinary bladder is a reservoir for urine. When empty, it is located within the pelvic cavity. When filled, it extends into the abdominal cavity. The urinary bladder is a subperitoneal organ that is surrounded by **endopelvic fascia**. Between the pubic symphysis and the urinary bladder there is a potential space called the **retropubic space (prevesical space)** (Fig. 5.17). The retropubic space is filled with fat and loose connective tissue that accommodates the expansion of the urinary bladder. The **puboprostatic ligament** is a condensation of fascia that ties the prostate to the inner surface of the pubis. The puboprostatic ligament defines the inferior limit of the retropubic space (Fig. 5.17). The lower one-third of the rectum is surrounded by endopelvic fascia. The middle and upper thirds of the rectum are partially covered by peritoneum (Fig. 5.17).

The order of dissection will be as follows: The parts of the urinary bladder will be studied. The interior of the urinary bladder will be studied. The interior of the rectum and anal canal will be studied.

Dissection Instructions

URINARY BLADDER [G 221; L 266, 267; N 366; R 336; C 305]

1. Identify the **parts of the urinary bladder** (Fig. 5.20):
    - **Apex** – the pointed part directed toward the anterior abdominal wall. The apex of the urinary bladder can be identified by the attachment of the urachus.
    - **Body** – between the apex and fundus.
    - **Fundus** – the inferior part of the posterior wall, also called the **base of the urinary bladder**. In the male the fundus is related to the ductus deferens, seminal vesicles, and rectum.
    - **Neck** – where the urethra exits the urinary bladder. In the neck of the urinary bladder, the wall thickens to form the **internal urethral sphincter**, which is an involuntary muscle.
2. Identify the four **surfaces of the urinary bladder** (Fig. 5.20):
    - **Superior** – covered by peritoneum
    - **Posterior** – covered by peritoneum on its superior part and by the endopelvic fascia of the rectovesical septum on its inferior part
    - **Inferolateral (2)** – covered by endopelvic fascia

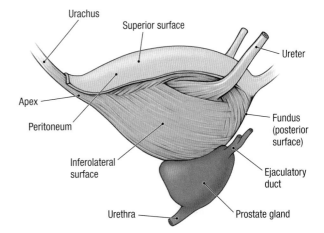

Figure 5.20. Parts of the urinary bladder in the male.

3. Examine the **wall of the urinary bladder** and note its thickness. The wall of the urinary bladder consists of bundles of smooth muscle called the **detrusor muscle** (L. *detrudere*, to thrust out).
4. Identify the **trigone** on the inner surface of the fundus (Fig. 5.18). The angles of the trigone are the **internal urethral orifice** and the two **orifices of the ureters**. The internal urethral orifice is located at the most inferior point in the urinary bladder. [G 221; L 267; N 366; R 338; C 304]
5. Observe that the mucous membrane over the trigone is smooth. The mucous membrane lining the other parts of the urinary bladder lies in folds when the bladder is empty but will accommodate expansion.
6. Insert the tip of a probe into the orifice of the ureter and observe that the ureter passes through the muscular wall of the urinary bladder in an oblique direction. When the urinary bladder is full (distended), the pressure of the accumulated urine flattens the part of the ureter that is within the wall of the bladder and prevents reflux of urine into the ureter.

CLINICAL CORRELATION

Kidney Stones

Kidney stones pass through the ureter to the urinary bladder and they may become lodged in the ureter. The point where the ureter passes through the wall of the urinary bladder is a relatively narrow passage. If a kidney stone becomes lodged, severe colicky pain results. The pain stops suddenly once the stone passes into the bladder.

7. Find the ureter where it crosses the external iliac artery or the bifurcation of the common iliac artery. Use blunt dissection to follow the ureter to the fundus of the urinary bladder.

RECTUM AND ANAL CANAL [G 209, 211; L 272, 273; N 361, 393; R 337; C 305, 309]

1. The rectum begins at the level of the third sacral vertebra. Observe the sectioned pelvis and note that the rectum follows the curvature of the sacrum.
2. Identify the **ampulla of the rectum** (Fig. 5.21). At the ampulla, the rectum bends approximately 80° posteriorly (**anorectal flexure**) and is continuous with the anal canal. Observe that the prostate and seminal vesicles are located close to the anterior wall of the rectum (Fig. 5.17).

CLINICAL CORRELATION

Rectal Examination

Digital rectal examination is part of the physical examination. The size and consistency of the prostate gland can be assessed by palpation through the anterior wall of the rectum.

---

3. Examine the inner surface of the rectum. Note that the mucous membrane is smooth except for the presence of **transverse rectal folds**. There is usually one transverse rectal fold on the right side and two on the left side. The transverse rectal folds may be difficult to identify in some cadavers.

4. Observe that the **anal canal** is only 2.5 to 3.5 cm in length. The anal canal passes out of the pelvic cavity and enters the anal triangle of the perineum.
5. Examine the inner surface of the anal canal (Fig. 5.21). The mucosal features of the anal canal may be difficult to identify in older individuals, but attempt to identify the following:
   • **Anal columns** – 5 to 10 longitudinal ridges of mucosa in the proximal part of the anal canal. The anal columns contain branches of the **superior rectal artery** and **vein**.
   • **Anal valves** – semilunar folds of mucosa that unite the distal ends of the anal columns. Between the anal valve and the wall of the anal canal is a small pocket called an **anal sinus**.
   • **Pectinate line** – the irregular line formed by all of the anal valves.

CLINICAL CORRELATION

Hemorrhoids

In the anal columns, the superior rectal veins of the hepatic portal system anastomose with middle and inferior rectal veins of the inferior vena caval system. An abnormal increase in blood pressure in the hepatic portal system causes engorgement of the veins contained in the anal columns, resulting in **internal hemorrhoids**. Internal hemorrhoids are covered by mucous membrane and are relatively insensitive to painful stimuli because the mucous membrane is innervated by autonomic nerves.

External hemorrhoids are enlargements of the tributaries of the inferior rectal veins. External hemorrhoids are covered by skin and are very sensitive to painful stimuli because they are innervated by somatic nerves (inferior rectal nerves).

---

6. The anal sphincter muscles surround the anal canal. Identify the **external anal sphincter muscle** and the **internal anal sphincter muscle** in the sectioned specimen (Fig. 5.21). The longitudinal muscle of the anal canal separates the two sphincter muscles. If you have difficulty identifying them, use a new scalpel blade to cut another section through the wall of the anal canal to improve the clarity of the dissection.

Dissection Review

1. Use the dissected specimen to review the features of the urinary bladder, rectum, and anal canal.

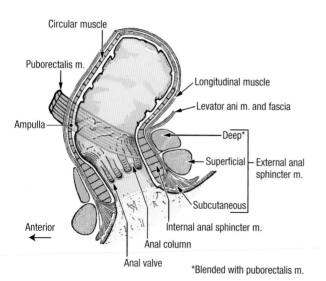

Figure 5.21. Rectum, anal canal, and anal sphincter muscles.

2. Review the relationships of the seminal vesicles, ampulla of the ductus deferens, and ureters to the rectum and fundus of the urinary bladder.

3. Visit a dissection table with a female cadaver and review the relationships of the uterus, vagina, and ureters to the rectum and fundus of the urinary bladder.

4. Review the kidney, the abdominal course of the ureter, the pelvic course of the ureter, and the function of the urinary bladder as a storage organ.

5. Review the parts of the male urethra. Visit a dissection table with a female cadaver and review the female urethra.

6. Review all parts of the large intestine and recall its function in absorption of water and in compaction and elimination of fecal material.

7. Recall that the external anal sphincter muscle is composed of skeletal muscle and is under voluntary control, whereas the internal anal sphincter muscle is composed of smooth muscle and is involuntary.

INTERNAL ILIAC ARTERY AND SACRAL PLEXUS

Dissection Overview

Anterior to the sacroiliac articulation, the **common iliac artery** divides to form the **external** and **internal iliac arteries** (Fig. 5.22). The external iliac artery distributes to the lower limb and the internal iliac artery distributes to the pelvis. *The internal iliac artery has the most variable branching pattern of any artery, and it is worth noting at the outset of this dissection that you must use the distribution of the branches to identify them, not their pattern of branching.*

The internal iliac artery commonly divides into an anterior division and a posterior division. Branches arising from the anterior division are mainly visceral (branches to the urinary bladder, internal genitalia, external genitalia, rectum, and gluteal region). Branches arising from the posterior division are parietal (branches to the pelvic walls and gluteal region).

The order of dissection will be as follows: The branches of the anterior division of the internal iliac artery will be identified. The branches of the posterior division of the internal iliac artery will be identified. The nerves of the sacral plexus will be dissected. Subsequently, the pelvic portion of the sympathetic trunk will be dissected.

Dissection Instructions

BLOOD VESSELS [G 224; L 274; N 402, 403; R 345; C 282]

1. The internal iliac vein is typically plexiform. To clear the dissection field, remove all tributaries to the internal iliac vein.

2. Identify the **common iliac artery** and follow it distally until it bifurcates.

3. Identify the **internal iliac artery**. Use blunt dissection to follow the internal iliac artery into the pelvis.

4. Identify the branches of the anterior division of the internal iliac artery (Fig. 5.22):
   • **Umbilical artery** – in the medial umbilical fold, find the **medial umbilical ligament** (the obliterated portion of the umbilical artery) and use blunt dissection to trace it posteriorly to the umbilical artery. Note that several **superior vesical arteries** arise from the inferior surface of the umbilical artery and descend to the superolateral part of the urinary bladder.

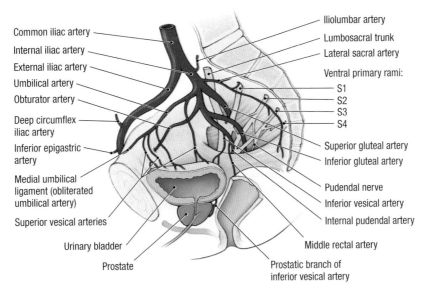

Figure 5.22. Branches of the internal iliac artery in the male.

- **Obturator artery** – passes through the obturator canal. Find the obturator artery where it enters the obturator canal in the lateral wall of the pelvis and follow the artery posteriorly to its origin. In about 20% of cases an **aberrant obturator artery** (a branch of the external iliac artery) crosses the pelvic brim and is at risk of injury during surgical repair of a femoral hernia.
- **Inferior vesical artery** – courses toward the fundus of the urinary bladder to supply the bladder, seminal vesicle, and prostate. The inferior vesical artery is a named branch only in the male; in the female it is an unnamed branch of the vaginal artery.
- **Middle rectal artery** – courses medially toward the rectum. It often arises in common with the inferior vesical artery, making positive identification difficult. Identify the middle rectal artery by tracing it to the rectum. The middle rectal artery, like the inferior vesical artery, sends branches to the seminal vesicle and prostate.
- **Internal pudendal artery** – exits the pelvic cavity by passing through the greater sciatic foramen inferior to the piriformis muscle. The internal pudendal artery often arises from a common trunk with the inferior gluteal artery.
- **Inferior gluteal artery** – usually passes out of the pelvic cavity between ventral rami S2 and S3. The inferior gluteal artery exits the pelvis by passing through the greater sciatic foramen inferior to the piriformis muscle. The inferior gluteal artery may share a common trunk with the internal pudendal artery, or less commonly, with the superior gluteal artery.

5. Identify the branches of the posterior division of the internal iliac artery (Fig. 5.22):
- **Iliolumbar artery** – passes posteriorly, then ascends between the lumbosacral trunk and the obturator nerve. It may arise from a common trunk with the lateral sacral artery.
- **Lateral sacral artery** – gives rise to a superior branch and an inferior branch. Observe the inferior branch that passes anterior to the sacral ventral rami.
- **Superior gluteal artery** – usually exits the pelvic cavity by passing between the lumbosacral trunk and the ventral ramus of S1.

6. Use an illustration to study the **prostatic venous plexus**, **vesical venous plexus**, and **rectal venous plexus**. All of these plexuses drain into the internal iliac vein.

7. On the dissected specimen, observe the **deep dorsal vein of the penis** just inferior to the pubic symphysis. Verify that the deep dorsal vein of the penis empties into the prostatic venous plexus.

NERVES [G 206, 230; L 275, 276; N 410, 499; R 470; C 313]

The somatic plexuses of the pelvic cavity are the **sacral plexus** and **coccygeal plexus**. These plexuses are located between the pelvic viscera and the lateral pelvic wall within the endopelvic fascia. These somatic nerve plexuses are formed by contributions from ventral rami of spinal nerves L4 to S4. The primary visceral nerve plexus of the pelvic cavity is the **inferior hypogastric plexus**. It is formed by contributions from the hypogastric nerves, sympathetic trunks, and pelvic splanchnic nerves.

1. Use your fingers to dissect the rectum from the anterior surface of the sacrum and coccyx.
2. Retract the rectum medially and identify the **sacral plexus** of nerves. The sacral plexus is closely related to the anterior surface of the piriformis muscle. Verify the following (Fig. 5.23):
- The **lumbosacral trunk** (ventral rami of L4 and L5) joins the sacral plexus.
- The ventral rami of S2 and S3 emerge between the proximal attachments of the piriformis muscle.
- The **sciatic nerve** is formed by the ventral rami of spinal nerves L4 through S3. The sciatic nerve exits the pelvis by passing through the greater sciatic foramen, usually inferior to the piriformis muscle.
- The **superior gluteal artery** usually passes between the **lumbosacral trunk** and the **ventral ramus of spinal nerve S1**, and exits the pelvis by passing superior to the piriformis muscle.
- The **inferior gluteal artery** usually passes between the **ventral rami of spinal nerves S2 and S3**. The inferior gluteal artery exits the pelvis by passing inferior to the piriformis muscle.
- The **pudendal nerve** receives a contribution from the ventral rami of spinal nerves S2, S3,

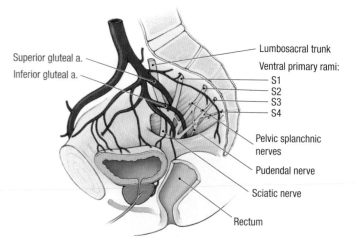

Superior gluteal a.
Inferior gluteal a.

Lumbosacral trunk
Ventral primary rami:
S1
S2
S3
S4
Pelvic splanchnic nerves
Pudendal nerve
Sciatic nerve
Rectum

Figure 5.23. Sacral plexus of nerves in the male.

and S4. The pudendal nerve exits the pelvis by passing inferior to the piriformis muscle.

3. Identify the **pelvic splanchnic nerves (nervi erigentes)**. Pelvic splanchnic nerves are branches of the ventral rami of spinal nerves S2 through S4 (Fig. 5.23). Pelvic splanchnic nerves carry preganglionic parasympathetic axons for the innervation of pelvic organs and the distal gastrointestinal tract (from the left colic flexure through the anal canal). [G 206; L 276; N 410; R 346; C 313]

4. The **sacral portion of the sympathetic trunk** is located on the anterior surface of the sacrum, medial to the ventral sacral foramina. Identify the following:
   - **Sympathetic trunk** – continues from the abdominal region into the pelvis. The sympathetic trunks of the two sides join in the midline near the level of the coccyx to form the **ganglion impar**.
   - **Gray rami communicantes** – connect the sympathetic ganglia to the sacral ventral rami. Each gray ramus communicans carries postganglionic sympathetic fibers to a ventral ramus for distribution to the lower extremity and perineum.
   - **Sacral splanchnic nerves** – arise from two or three of the sacral sympathetic ganglia and pass directly to the **inferior hypogastric plexus**. Sacral splanchnic nerves carry sympathetic fibers that distribute to the pelvic viscera.

CLINICAL CORRELATION

Pelvic Nerve Plexuses

The pelvic splanchnic nerves (parasympathetic outflow of S2, S3, and S4) are closely related to the lateral aspects of the rectum. The inferior hypogastric plexus is located in the connective tissue lateral to the prostate. These autonomic nerve plexuses can be injured during surgery, causing loss of bladder control and erectile dysfunction.

Dissection Review

1. Review the abdominal aorta and its terminal branches.
2. Use the dissected specimen to review the branches of the internal iliac artery. Review the region supplied by each branch.
3. Visit a dissection table with a female cadaver and review the arteries that are unique to the female: uterine artery and vaginal artery. Note their relationship to the ureter.

4. Review the formation of the sacral plexus and the branches that were dissected in the pelvis.
5. Use the dissected specimen and an illustration to review the course of the pudendal nerve from the pelvic cavity to the urogenital triangle.

PELVIC DIAPHRAGM

Dissection Overview

The **pelvic diaphragm** is the muscular floor of the pelvic cavity. The pelvic diaphragm is formed by the levator ani muscle and coccygeus muscle plus the fasciae covering their superior and inferior surfaces (Fig. 5.24A, B). The pelvic diaphragm extends from the pubic symphysis to the coccyx. Laterally, the pelvic diaphragm is attached to the fascia covering the obturator internus muscle. The urethra and anal canal pass through midline openings in the pelvic diaphragm called the **urogenital hiatus** and **anal hiatus**, respectively.

Dissection Instructions

1. Perform the dissection of the pelvic diaphragm on one side of the cadaver. Save the side with the best dissection of arteries and nerves for review. [G 202–204; L 278–279; N 356–358; C 308]
2. Retract the rectum, urinary bladder, prostate, and seminal vesicles medially.
3. Use blunt dissection to remove any remaining fat and connective tissue from the superior surface of the pelvic diaphragm.
4. To find the **tendinous arch of the levator ani muscle** (Fig. 5.24A), palpate the medial surface of the ischial spine and then locate the obturator canal. The tendinous arch lies just inferior to a line connecting these two structures. Note that the tendinous arch is the superior edge of the pelvic diaphragm.
5. Identify the three muscles that form the **levator ani muscle**. The muscles are identified by their proximal attachments. Learn, but do not dissect, their distal attachments. Identify the following:
   - **Puborectalis muscle** – its proximal attachment is the body of the pubis. Its distal attachment is the puborectalis muscle of the opposite side (in a midline raphe). The puborectalis muscle forms the lateral boundary of the urogenital hiatus. The two puborectalis muscles form a "puborectal sling," which causes the **anorectal flexure** at the ampulla of the rectum (Fig. 5.21). During defecation, the puborectalis muscles relax, the anorectal flexure straightens, and the elimination of fecal matter is facilitated.

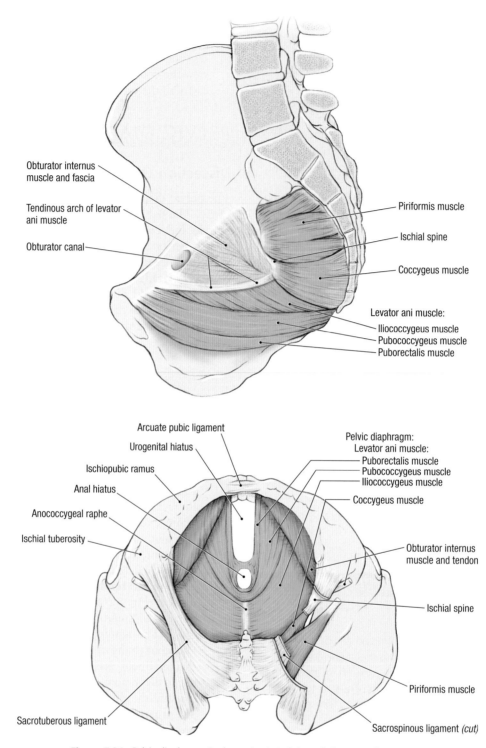

Figure 5.24. Pelvic diaphragm in the male. **A.** Left lateral view. **B.** Inferior view.

- **Pubococcygeus muscle** — its proximal attachment is the body of the pubis. Its distal attachment is the coccyx and the **anococcygeal raphe**.
- **Iliococcygeus muscle** — its proximal attachment is the tendinous arch. Its distal attachment is the coccyx and the anococcygeal raphe.

6. The levator ani muscle supports the pelvic viscera and resists increases in intra-abdominal pressure.
7. Identify the **coccygeus muscle**. The coccygeus muscle completes the pelvic diaphragm posteriorly. The proximal attachment of the coccygeus muscle is the ischial spine and its distal attachment

is the lateral border of the coccyx and the lowest part of the sacrum.

8. Place the fingers of one hand in the ischioanal fossa and the fingers of the other hand on the superior surface of the pelvic diaphragm. Palpate the thinness of the pelvic diaphragm.

9. Observe that the **obturator internus muscle** forms the lateral wall of the ischioanal fossa. The proximal attachment of the obturator internus muscle is the margin of the obturator foramen and inner surface of the obturator membrane. The distal attachment of the obturator internus muscle will be studied when the gluteal region is dissected. Superior to the tendinous arch of the levator ani muscle, the obturator internus muscle forms the lateral wall of the pelvic cavity. Inferior to the tendinous arch, the obturator internus muscle forms the lateral wall of the perineum.

10. Use your textbook to learn the general pattern of lymphatic drainage of the pelvis and the location of each of the following groups of lymph nodes: [G 213, 228, 230; L 291; N 408]

    • **Internal iliac nodes**
    • **External iliac nodes**
    • **Common iliac nodes**
    • **Sacral nodes**
    • **Lumbar nodes**

Dissection Review

1. Use the dissected specimen to review the proximal attachment and action of each muscle of the pelvic diaphragm.

2. Review the relationship of the branches of the internal iliac artery to the pelvic diaphragm.

3. Review the relationship of the sacral plexus to the pelvic diaphragm.

4. Use an illustration to review the role played by the pelvic diaphragm in forming the boundary between the pelvic cavity and the perineum. Review the function of the pelvic diaphragm and perineal body in supporting the pelvic and abdominal viscera.

5. Use an illustration to review the lymphatic drainage from the pelvis and perineum. Realize that structures in the perineum (including the scrotum and the lower part of the anal canal) drain into superficial inguinal lymph nodes. The lymphatic drainage of the testis follows the testicular vessels to the lumbar chain of nodes, bypassing the perineal and pelvic drainage systems.

6. Review the formation of the thoracic duct to complete your understanding of the lymph drainage from this region.

7. Visit a dissection table with a female cadaver and perform a complete review of the dissected female pelvis.

FEMALE EXTERNAL GENITALIA AND PERINEUM

Labium Majus

Dissection Overview

In the female, the round ligament of the uterus passes through the superficial inguinal ring and descends into the fat that forms the labium majus. The layers of the scrotum that are identified in the male are not found in the labium majus.

The order of dissection will be as follows: The anterior surface of the labium majus will be opened by a vertical incision. The round ligament of the uterus will be followed from the superficial inguinal ring for a short distance into the superior part of the labium majus.

Dissection Instructions [G 110; L 221; R220; C188]

1. At the superficial inguinal ring, use blunt dissection to demonstrate that the round ligament of the uterus emerges from the superficial inguinal ring and spreads out into the fatty tissue of the labium majus. The round ligament is a delicate structure that can be demonstrated for only 1 to 2 cm distal to the superficial inguinal ring. [G 111; R 363]

CLINICAL CORRELATION

Lymphatic Drainage of the Labium Majus

Lymphatics from the labium majus drain to the superficial inguinal lymph nodes. Inflammation of the labium majus may cause tender, enlarged superficial inguinal lymph nodes.

Dissection Review

1. Review the course of the round ligament from the abdominal wall to the labium majus.

2. Review the embryology of the ovary and testis and compare the role of the gubernaculum in each case. Review the adult structures that are formed from the gubernaculum in both sexes.

3. Complete the dissection review that follows the dissection of the spermatic cord and testis.

FEMALE UROGENITAL TRIANGLE

Dissection Overview

The order of dissection of the female urogenital triangle will be as follows: The external genitalia will be examined. The skin will be removed from the labia majora. The superficial perineal fascia will be removed and the contents of the superficial perineal pouch will be identified. The contents of the deep perineal pouch will be described, but not dissected.

Dissection Instructions

EXTERNAL GENITALIA [G 253; L 282; N 377; R 362; C 290]

1. Partner with a dissection team that has a male cadaver for the following dissection. You are expected to know the anatomical details for both sexes.
2. Place the cadaver in the supine position. Stretch the thighs widely apart and brace them. Usually, only one student can work on the urogenital triangle at a time. The dissector should be positioned between the thighs with the cadaver pulled to the end of the dissection table.
3. Examine the **vulva** (female external genitalia) (Fig. 5.25). Identify the following structures:
   - **Mons pubis**
   - **Anterior labial commissure**
   - **Labium majus**
   - **Clitoris**
     - **Prepuce**
     - **Glans**
     - **Frenulum of clitoris**
   - **Labium minus**
   - **Vestibule of the vagina** – the area between the labia minora

- **External urethral orifice**
- **Vaginal orifice**
- **Openings of the paraurethral ducts** – on each side of the external urethral orifice
- **Frenulum of labia minora**
- **Posterior labial commissure**

SKIN REMOVAL

1. Refer to Figure 5.26.
2. Make a skin incision in the midline from the anterior margin of the anus to the posterior labial commissure (Fig. 5.26, red dashed lines).
3. Make a skin incision that follows the medial surface of the labium majus on each side. Each incision should begin at the posterior labial commissure, pass lateral to the labium minus, and end at the anterior labial commissure. Extend the incision in the midline to the mons pubis.
4. Make a transverse incision across the mons pubis that extends from the right thigh to the left thigh (Fig. 5.26, blue dashed lines).
5. Remove the skin from the labium majus (lateral to the incisions). Detach each skin flap along the medial surface of the thigh (Fig. 5.26, blue dashed lines) and place the skin in the tissue container.
6. If the cadaver has a large amount of fat in the superficial fascia of the medial thighs, remove a portion of the superficial fascia that corresponds to the skin that was removed.
7. Note that the **posterior labial nerve and vessels** enter the urogenital triangle by passing lateral to the external anal sphincter muscle. The posterior labial nerve and vessels supply the posterior part of the labium majus.

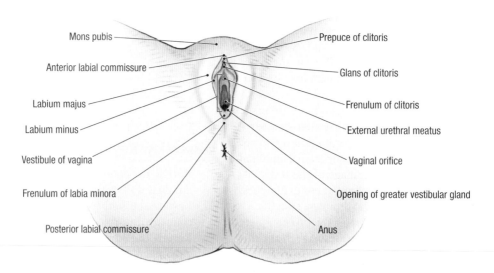

Figure 5.25. Female external genitalia.

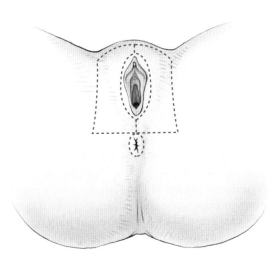

Figure 5.26. Skin incisions.

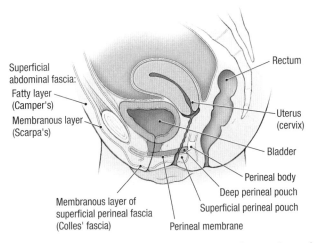

Figure 5.27. Perineal fasciae in the female. The membranous layer of superficial perineal fascia (Colles' fascia) is continuous with the membranous layer of superficial fascia of the lower abdominal wall (Scarpa's fascia). The membranous layer of the superficial perineal fascia is attached along the posterior border of the perineal membrane.

SUPERFICIAL PERINEAL POUCH AND CLITORIS
[G 253, 269–272; L 283, 284; N 378, 379; R 364, 365; C 294, 295]

The superficial perineal fascia has a superficial fatty layer and a deep membranous layer. In the female, the superficial fatty layer provides the shape of the labium majus and is continuous with the fat of the lower abdominal wall, ischioanal fossa, and thigh. The **membranous layer of the superficial perineal fascia (Colles' fascia)** is attached to the ischiopubic ramus as far posteriorly as the ischial tuberosity, and to the posterior edge of the **perineal membrane** (Fig. 5.27). The membranous layer of the superficial perineal fascia forms the superficial boundary of the **superficial perineal pouch (space)**.

1. The **contents of the superficial perineal pouch in the female** include **three muscles (ischiocavernosus, bulbospongiosus, and superficial transverse perineal)**, the **crus of the clitoris**, the **bulb of the vestibule**, and the **greater vestibular gland** (Fig. 5.28). These structures are paired. The superficial perineal pouch also contains the blood vessels and nerves for these structures.

2. It is not necessary to identify the membranous layer of the superficial perineal fascia to complete the dissection. Use a probe to dissect through the superficial perineal fascia about 2 cm lateral to the labium minus. Remove the fat that forms the labium majus and place it in the tissue container.

3. Identify the **bulbospongiosus muscle**, which is lateral to the labium minus (Fig. 5.28A). The bulbospongiosus muscle covers the superficial surface of the bulb of the vestibule. The posterior attachment of the bulbospongiosus muscle is the perineal body. The anterior attachment of the bulbospongiosus muscle is the corpus cavernosum clitoris. The bulbospongiosus muscle in the female does not join the

bulbospongiosus muscle of the opposite side across the midline as it does in the male.

4. Lateral to the bulbospongiosus muscle, use blunt dissection to clean the surface of the **ischiocavernosus muscle** (Fig. 5.28A). The ischiocavernosus muscle covers the superficial surface of the crus of the clitoris. The proximal attachments of the ischiocavernosus muscle are the ischial tuberosity and the ischiopubic ramus. The distal attachment of the ischiocavernosus muscle is the crus of the clitoris. The ischiocavernosus muscle forces blood from the crus of the clitoris into the distal part of the corpus cavernosum clitoris.

5. The **superficial transverse perineal muscle** is difficult to find. Using blunt dissection, attempt to find the superficial transverse perineal muscle at the posterior border of the urogenital triangle (Fig. 5.28A). Limit the time spent looking for it. The lateral attachment of the superficial transverse perineal muscle is the ischial tuberosity and the ischiopubic ramus. The medial attachment of the superficial transverse perineal muscle is the **perineal body**. The perineal body is a fibromuscular mass located between the anal canal and the posterior edge of the perineal membrane that serves as an attachment for several muscles. The superficial transverse perineal muscle helps to support the perineal body.

6. Use a probe to dissect between the three muscles of the superficial perineal pouch until a small triangular opening is created. The membrane that becomes visible through this opening is the **perineal membrane** (Fig. 5.28A). The perineal membrane is the deep boundary of the superficial per-

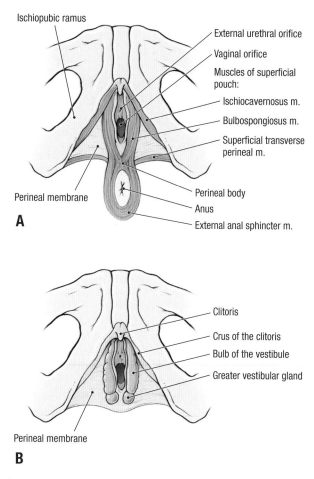

A

B

Figure 5.28. Contents of the superficial perineal pouch in the female. **A.** Muscles. **B.** Erectile bodies.

ineal pouch, and the bulb of the vestibule and crura are attached to it.

7. On the right side of the cadaver, use blunt dissection to remove the bulbospongiosus muscle and identify the **bulb of the vestibule** (Fig. 5.28B). The bulb of the vestibule is an elongated mass of erectile tissue that lies lateral to the vaginal orifice. Note that the **greater vestibular gland** is found in the superficial perineal pouch immediately posterior to the bulb of the vestibule.

8. Anteriorly, the bulbs of the two sides are joined at the **commissure of the bulbs** and the commissure is continuous with the **glans of the clitoris**. Do not attempt to find the commissure of the bulbs.

9. On the right side of the cadaver, use blunt dissection to remove the ischiocavernosus muscle from the **crus of the clitoris** (L. *crus*, a leg-like part; pl. *crura*) (Fig. 5.28B). The crus of the clitoris is the proximal part of the corpus cavernosum clitoris. The two corpora cavernosa form the **body of the clitoris.**

10. Use an illustration to study the erectile bodies of the clitoris. Note that the glans of the clitoris caps the two corpora cavernosa. [G 272; L 284; N 379; R 363]

DEEP PERINEAL POUCH

The deep perineal pouch (space) will not be dissected. The deep perineal pouch lies superior (deep) to the perineal membrane (Fig. 5.27). The **contents of the deep perineal pouch in the female** are the **urethra**, a portion of the **vagina**, the **external urethral sphincter muscle**, **branches of the internal pudendal vessels**, and **branches of the pudendal nerve** (Fig. 5.29).

1. Use an illustration to study the following: [G 254; L 285; N 379; C 296]
   - **Urethra** – extends from the internal urethral orifice in the urinary bladder to the external urethral orifice in the vestibule of the vagina (about 4 cm).
   - **External urethral sphincter (sphincter urethrae) muscle** – a voluntary muscle that surrounds the urethra. When the external urethral sphincter muscle contracts, it compresses the urethra and stops the flow of urine.
   - **Deep transverse perineal muscle** – has a lateral attachment to the ischial tuberosity and the ischiopubic ramus and a medial attachment to the perineal body. Its fiber direction and function are identical to those of the superficial transverse perineal muscle (which is a content of the superficial perineal pouch).

2. Other contents of the deep perineal pouch include **branches of the internal pudendal artery** and **branches of the pudendal nerve** that supply the external urethral sphincter muscle, the deep transverse perineal muscle, and the clitoris (Fig. 5.29).

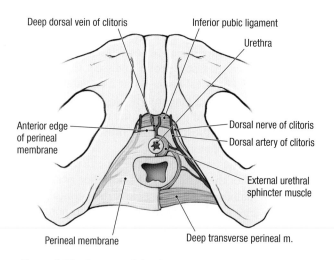

Figure 5.29. Contents of the deep perineal pouch in the female.

3. Collectively, the muscles within the deep perineal pouch plus the perineal membrane are known as the **urogenital diaphragm**. This older anatomical nomenclature is still in clinical use.

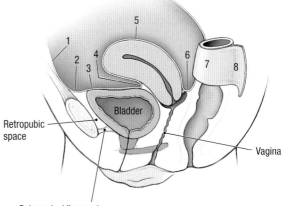

Figure 5.30. Peritoneum in the female pelvis. The numbered features of the peritoneum are explained in the text.

Obstetric Considerations

As the head of the baby passes through the vagina during childbirth, the anus and the levator ani muscle are forced posteriorly toward the sacrum and coccyx. The urethra is forced anteriorly toward the pubic symphysis. Perineal lacerations during childbirth are common, and it may be necessary to surgically widen the vaginal orifice (episiotomy). If the perineal body is lacerated, it must be repaired to prevent weakness of the pelvic floor, which could result in prolapse of the urinary bladder, uterus, or rectum.

To alleviate the pain of childbirth, a **pudendal nerve block** is performed by injecting a local anesthetic around the pudendal nerve near the ischial spine. To perform the injection, the ischial spine is palpated through the vagina, and the needle is directed toward the ischial spine.

The order of dissection will be as follows: The peritoneum will be studied in the female pelvic cavity. The pelvis will be sectioned in the midline and the cut surface of the sectioned pelvis will be studied. The uterus and vagina will be studied. The uterine tube will be traced from the uterus to the ovary. The ovary will be studied.

Dissection Review

1. Replace the muscles of the urogenital triangle in their correct anatomical positions.
2. Review the contents of the female superficial perineal pouch. Visit a dissection table with a male cadaver and view the contents of the superficial perineal pouch.
3. Use an illustration to review the course of the internal pudendal artery from its origin in the pelvis.
4. Use an illustration to review the course and branches of the pudendal nerve.
5. Review an illustration showing the urethra and note its course from the urinary bladder to the perineum.

FEMALE PELVIC CAVITY

Dissection Overview

The female pelvic cavity contains the urinary bladder anteriorly, the female internal genitalia, and the rectum posteriorly (Fig. 5.30). The term **adnexa** (L. *adnexa*, adjacent parts) refers to the ovaries, uterine tubes, and ligaments of the uterus. Removal of the uterus (hysterectomy), with or without the ovaries, is a common surgical procedure. If the uterus has been surgically removed from your cadaver, examine it in other cadavers.

Dissection Instructions

PERITONEUM [G 232, 233; L 265; N 360; R 357; C 274]

1. Using Figure 5.30 as a reference, examine the **peritoneum** in the female pelvis. Note that the peritoneum:
   (1, 2) Passes from the anterior abdominal wall superior to the pubis
   (3) Covers the superior surface of the urinary bladder
   (4) Passes from the superior surface of the urinary bladder to the uterus where it forms the **vesicouterine pouch**
   (5) Covers the fundus and body of the uterus and contacts the wall of the posterior part of the vaginal fornix
   (6) Forms the **rectouterine pouch** between the uterus and the rectum
   (7) Covers the anterior surface and sides of the rectum
   (8) Forms the sigmoid mesocolon beginning at the level of the third sacral vertebra
2. Laterally, a **paravesical fossa** is apparent on each side of the urinary bladder. Further posteriorly, a **pararectal fossa** is apparent on each side of the rectum.

Pelvic Peritoneum

As the urinary bladder fills, the peritoneal reflection from the anterior abdominal wall to the bladder is elevated above the level of the pubis. A filled urinary bladder can be approached with a needle superior to the pubis without entering the peritoneal cavity.

3. Identify the **broad ligament of the uterus**. The broad ligament of the uterus is formed by two layers of peritoneum that extend from the lateral side of the uterus to the lateral pelvic wall. The **uterine tube** is contained within the superior margin of the broad ligament. The broad ligament has three parts (Fig. 5.31): [G 236; L 269; N 370; R 359; C 278]
    - **Mesosalpinx** (Gr. *salpinx*, tube) – supports the uterine tube
    - **Mesovarium** – attaches the ovary to the posterior aspect of the broad ligament
    - **Mesometrium** – the part of the broad ligament that is below the attachment of the mesovarium
4. The tissue enclosed between the two layers of the broad ligament is called **parametrium** (Gr. *para*, beside; *metra*, womb, uterus).
5. Identify the **round ligament of the uterus**, which is visible through the anterior layer of the broad ligament (Fig. 5.31). Observe that the round ligament of the uterus passes over the pelvic brim and exits the abdominal cavity by passing through the deep inguinal ring, lateral to the inferior epigastric vessels. The round ligament of the uterus passes through the inguinal canal and ends in the labium majus.

6. Identify the **ovarian ligament**, which is a fibrous cord within the broad ligament that connects the ovary to the uterus.
7. Identify the **suspensory ligament of the ovary**, which is a peritoneal fold that covers the ovarian vessels. The suspensory ligament of the ovary extends into the greater pelvis from the superior aspect of the ovary.
8. The **endopelvic fascia** (extraperitoneal fascia) contains condensations of connective tissue that passively support the uterus. Study an illustration and note the following: [G 251; L 270; N 364; C 305]
    - **Uterosacral (sacrogenital) ligament** – extends from the cervix to the sacrum. The uterosacral ligament underlies the **uterosacral fold**.
    - **Transverse cervical ligament (cardinal ligament)** – extends from the cervix to the lateral wall of the pelvis.
    - **Pubocervical (pubovesical) ligament** – extends from the pubis to the cervix.

SECTION OF THE PELVIS

The pelvis will be divided in the midline. First, the pelvic viscera and the soft tissues of the perineum will be cut in the midline with a scalpel. The pubic symphysis and vertebral column (up to vertebral level L3) will be cut in the midline with a saw. Subsequently, the right side of the body will be transected at vertebral level L3. The left lower limb and left side of the pelvis will remain attached to the trunk.

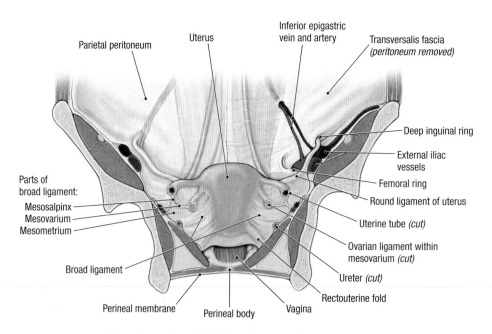

Figure 5.31. Parts of the broad ligament of the uterus.

Both halves of the pelvis will be used to dissect the pelvic viscera, pelvic vasculature, and nerves of the pelvis. One half of the pelvis will be used to demonstrate the muscles of the pelvic diaphragm.

1. Begin this dissection with a new scalpel blade.
2. Use your hand to position the uterus in the midline. Use a scalpel to divide the uterus in *its* median plane. Extend the cut through the cervix and into the fornix of the vagina.
3. Beginning posterior to the pubic symphysis, make a midline cut through the superior surface of the urinary bladder. Open the bladder and sponge the interior, if necessary.
4. Identify the internal urethral orifice and insert a probe. Using the probe as a guide, cut through the inferior part of the bladder, dividing the urethra.
5. Extend the midline cut in the posterior direction. Cut through the anterior and posterior walls of the rectum and the distal part of sigmoid colon. Sponge them clean.
6. In the perineum, insert the tip of a probe into the external urethral orifice. Use the probe as a guide to make a midline cut through the clitoris, dividing it into right and left sides. Extend this cut posteriorly, dividing the urethra and vagina into right and left sides.
7. In the midline, cut through the perineal membrane, perineal body, and anal canal. Extend the cut to the tip of the coccyx.
8. Use a saw to make two cuts in the midline:
   - **Pubic symphysis** – cut through the pubic symphysis from anterior to posterior.
   - **Sacrum** – turn the cadaver to the prone position. Cut through the sacrum from posterior to anterior. Do not allow the saw to pass between

the soft tissue structures that were cut with the scalpel. Spread the opening and extend the midline cut as far superiorly as the body of the third lumbar vertebra.

9. Return the cadaver to the supine position. To mobilize the right lower limb, use a scalpel to cut the right common iliac vein, right common iliac artery, and right ovarian vessels. Cut the right ureter and the branches of the right lumbar plexus.
10. In the transverse plane, cut the psoas major muscle and the quadratus lumborum muscle at vertebral level L3. Use the saw to cut horizontally through the right half of the intervertebral disc between L3 and L4. Now, the right lower limb can be removed.
11. Clean the rectum and anal canal.

FEMALE INTERNAL GENITALIA [G 232; L 268, 269; N 360, 365; R 357; C 274]

1. Study the cut surface of the sectioned specimen. Use an illustration to guide you.
2. Trace the sectioned urethra anteroinferiorly from the urinary bladder to the **external urethral orifice**. Attempt to identify the **external urethral sphincter muscle** that surrounds the urethra. The external urethral sphincter muscle may be difficult to see.
3. In the sectioned specimen, observe the **vagina**. Identify the **vaginal fornix**. The vaginal fornix has four parts: **anterior**, **lateral (2)**, and **posterior** (Fig. 5.32). Observe that the anterior vaginal wall is shorter than the posterior vaginal wall.
4. Observe that the posterior wall of the vagina (near the posterior part of the vaginal fornix) is in contact with the peritoneum that lines the rectouterine pouch.

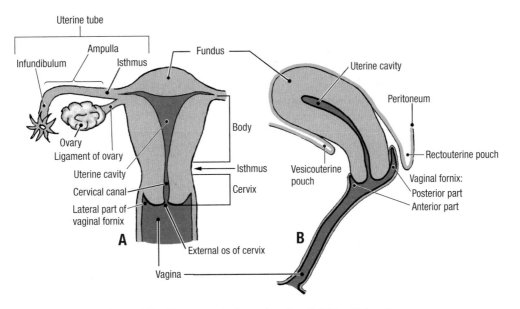

Figure 5.32. The uterus. **A.** Coronal section. **B.** Midsagittal section.

5. Study the **uterus** (Fig. 5.32). Observe that the uterus is tilted approximately 90° anterior to the axis of the vagina (anteverted). The position of the uterus changes as the bladder fills, and during pregnancy. [G 237, 283; L 270; N 371; R 358, 359; C 278, 279]

6. Identify the following features of the uterus (Fig. 5.32A):
   - **Fundus** – the rounded part of the body that lies superior to the attachments of the uterine tubes
   - **Body** – the part of the uterus between the fundus and the cervix. The **vesical surface** of the body of the uterus faces the vesicouterine pouch and the **intestinal surface** faces the rectouterine pouch. Note that the broad ligament is attached to the lateral surface of the body of the uterus.
   - **Isthmus** – the narrowed portion of the body that is superior to the cervix.
   - **Cervix** – the thick-walled portion of the uterus that protrudes into the vaginal canal.

7. Identify the **uterine cavity**. In a coronal section, it is triangular (Fig. 5.32A). In a sagittal section, it is a slit (Fig. 5.32B).

8. Note that the uterine mucosa is called **endometrium**. The thick muscular wall of the uterus is called **myometrium**. The peritoneal covering on the surface of the uterus is called **perimetrium** (Gr. *pari*, around). The tissues within the broad ligament are called **parametrium** (Gr. *para*, beyond).

9. Identify the **uterine tube** (Fig. 5.32A). Use your fingers to follow the uterine tube as it passes laterally within the mesosalpinx. Observe:
   - **Isthmus** – the narrow, medial one-third of the uterine tube
   - **Ampulla** – the widest and longest part of the uterine tube
   - **Infundibulum** – the funnel-like end of the uterine tube
   - **Fimbriae** – multiple processes that surround the distal margin of the infundibulum

10. Observe the **ovary**. The ovary is ovoid, with a **tubal (distal) extremity** and a **uterine (proximal) extremity**. The ovarian vessels enter the tubal extremity of the ovary, and the ligament of the ovary is attached to the uterine extremity.

11. The ovary sits in the **ovarian fossa**. The ovarian fossa is a shallow depression in the lateral pelvic wall bounded by the ureter, external iliac vein, and uterine tube.

12. Review the abdominal origin and course of the ovarian vessels. Note that they pass through the **suspensory ligament of the ovary**.

Dissection Review

1. Review the position of the female pelvic viscera within the lesser pelvis. Visit a dissection table with a male cadaver and observe the position of the male pelvic viscera.

2. Review the peritoneum in the female pelvic cavity. Visit a dissection table with a male cadaver and compare differences in the female and male peritoneum (Figs. 5.17 and 5.30).

3. Trace the round ligament of the uterus from the superficial inguinal ring to the uterus.

4. Visit a table with a male cadaver and trace the ductus deferens from the epididymis to the ejaculatory duct, noting its relationships to vessels, nerves, the ureter, and the seminal vesicle.

5. Compare the pelvic course of the ductus deferens with the pelvic course of the round ligament of the uterus.

6. Review the parts of the broad ligament and review the function of the endopelvic fascia in passive support of the uterus.

URINARY BLADDER, RECTUM, AND ANAL CANAL

Dissection Overview

The urinary bladder is a reservoir for urine. When empty, it is located within the pelvic cavity. When filled, it extends into the abdominal cavity. The urinary bladder is a retroperitoneal organ that is surrounded by **endopelvic fascia**. Between the pubic symphysis and the urinary bladder there is a potential space called the **retropubic space (prevesical space)** (Fig. 5.30). The retropubic space is filled with fat and loose connective tissue that accommodates the expansion of the urinary bladder. The **pubovesical ligament** is a condensation of fascia that ties the neck of the urinary bladder to the pubis across the retropubic space. The pubovesical ligament defines the inferior limit of the retropubic space (Fig. 5.30). The lower one-third of the rectum is surrounded by endopelvic fascia. The middle and upper thirds of the rectum are partially covered by peritoneum (Fig. 5.30).

The order of dissection will be as follows: The parts of the urinary bladder will be studied. The interior of the urinary bladder will be studied. The interior of the rectum and anal canal will be studied.

Dissection Instructions

URINARY BLADDER [L 266, 267; N 366]

1. Identify the **parts of the urinary bladder** (Fig. 5.33):
   - **Apex** – the pointed part directed toward the anterior abdominal wall. The apex of the uri-

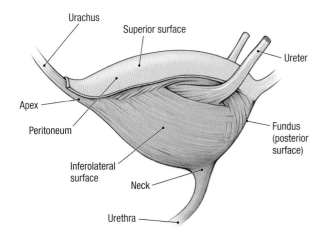

Figure 5.33. Parts of the urinary bladder in the female.

2. Identify the four **surfaces of the urinary bladder** (Fig. 5.33):
   - **Superior** – covered by peritoneum
   - **Posterior** – covered by peritoneum on its superior part and by the endopelvic fascia on its inferior part
   - **Inferolateral (2)** – covered by endopelvic fascia
3. Examine the **wall of the urinary bladder** and note its thickness. The wall of the urinary bladder consists of bundles of smooth muscle called the **detrusor muscle** (L. *detrudere*, to thrust out).
4. Identify the **trigone** on the inner surface of the fundus (Fig. 5.34). The angles of the trigone are the **internal urethral orifice** and the two **orifices of the ureters**. The internal urethral orifice is located at the most inferior point in the urinary bladder. [L 267; N 366]
5. Observe that the mucous membrane over the trigone is smooth. The mucous membrane lining the other parts of the urinary bladder lies in folds when the bladder is empty but will accommodate expansion.
6. Insert the tip of a probe into the orifice of the ureter and observe that the ureter passes through the wall of the urinary bladder in an oblique direction. When the urinary bladder is full (distended), the pressure of the accumulated urine flattens the part of the ureter that is within the wall of the bladder and prevents reflux of urine into the ureter.

nary bladder can be identified by the attachment of the urachus.
- **Body** – between the apex and fundus.
- **Fundus** – the inferior part of the posterior wall, also called the **base of the bladder**. In the female the fundus is related to the vagina and cervix.
- **Neck** – where the urethra exits the urinary bladder. In the neck of the urinary bladder, the wall thickens to form the **internal urethral sphincter**, which is an involuntary muscle.

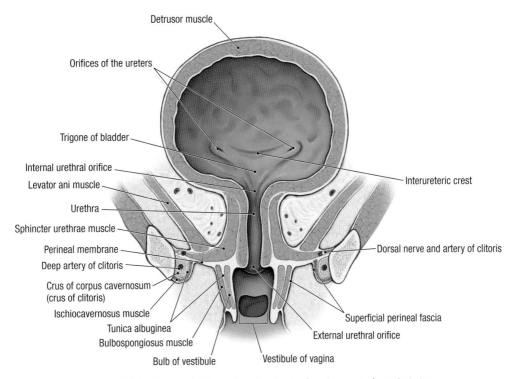

Figure 5.34. Urinary bladder and urethra in the female seen in frontal section.

Kidney Stones

Kidney stones pass through the ureter to the urinary bladder and they may become lodged in the ureter. The point where the ureter passes through the wall of the urinary bladder is a relatively narrow passage. If a kidney stone becomes lodged, severe colicky pain results. The pain stops suddenly once the stone passes into the bladder.

7. Find the ureter where it crosses the external iliac artery or the bifurcation of the common iliac artery. Use a probe to follow the ureter to the fundus of the urinary bladder. Observe that the ureter crosses inferior to the **uterine artery** and superior to the **vaginal artery**. [G 234; L 268; N 400; R 356; C 285]

RECTUM AND ANAL CANAL [G 211, 232; L 272; N 360, 393; R 357; C 274, 309]

1. Recall that the rectum begins at the level of the third sacral vertebra. Observe the sectioned pelvis and note that the rectum follows the curvature of the sacrum.
2. Identify the **ampulla of the rectum** (Fig. 5.35). At the ampulla, the rectum bends approximately 80° posteriorly (**anorectal flexure**) and is continuous with the anal canal.
3. Examine the inner surface of the rectum. Note that the mucous membrane is smooth except for the presence of **transverse rectal folds**. There is usually one transverse rectal fold on the right side and two on the left side. The transverse rectal folds may be difficult to identify in some cadavers.

4. Observe that the **anal canal** is only 2.5 to 3.5 cm in length. The anal canal passes out of the pelvic cavity and enters the anal triangle of the perineum.
5. Examine the inner surface of the anal canal (Fig. 5.35). Note that the mucosal features of the anal canal may be difficult to identify in older individuals, but attempt to identify the following:
   • **Anal columns** – 5 to 10 longitudinal ridges of mucosa in the proximal part of the anal canal. The anal columns contain branches of the **superior rectal artery** and **vein**.
   • **Anal valves** – semilunar folds of mucosa that unite the distal ends of the anal columns. External to each anal valve is a small pocket called an **anal sinus**.
   • **Pectinate line** – the irregular line formed by all of the anal valves.

Hemorrhoids

In the anal columns, the superior rectal veins of the hepatic portal system anastomose with middle and inferior rectal veins of the inferior vena caval system. An abnormal increase in blood pressure in the hepatic portal system causes engorgement of the veins contained in the anal columns, resulting in **internal hemorrhoids**. Internal hemorrhoids are covered by mucous membrane and are relatively insensitive to painful stimuli because the mucous membrane is innervated by autonomic nerves.

External hemorrhoids are enlargements of the tributaries of the inferior rectal veins. External hemorrhoids are covered by skin and are very sensitive to painful stimuli because they are innervated by somatic nerves (inferior rectal nerves).

6. The anal sphincter muscles surround the anal canal. Identify the **external anal sphincter muscle** and the **internal anal sphincter muscle** in the sectioned specimen (Fig. 5.35). The longitudinal muscle of the anal canal separates the two sphincter muscles. If you have difficulty identifying them, use a new scalpel blade to cut another section through the wall of the anal canal to improve the clarity of the dissection.

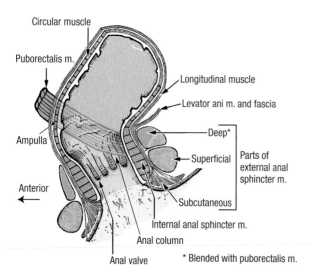

Figure 5.35. Rectum, anal canal, and anal sphincter muscles.

Dissection Review

1. Use the dissected specimen to review the features of the urinary bladder, rectum, and anal canal.
2. Review the relationships of the uterus, vagina, and ureters to the rectum and fundus of the urinary bladder.
3. Visit a dissection table with a male cadaver and review the relationships of the seminal vesicles, ampulla of the ductus deferens, and ureters to the rectum and fundus of the urinary bladder.
4. Review the kidney, the abdominal course of the ureter, the pelvic course of the ureter, and the function of the urinary bladder as a storage organ.
5. Review the female urethra. Visit a table with a male cadaver and review the parts of the male urethra.
6. Review all parts of the large intestine and recall its function in absorption of water and in compaction and elimination of fecal material.
7. Recall that the external anal sphincter muscle is composed of skeletal muscle and is under voluntary control, whereas the internal anal sphincter muscle is composed of smooth muscle and is involuntary.

INTERNAL ILIAC ARTERY AND SACRAL PLEXUS

Dissection Overview

Anterior to the sacroiliac articulation, the **common iliac artery** divides to form the **external** and **internal iliac arteries** (Fig. 5.36). The external iliac artery distributes to the lower limb and the internal iliac artery distributes to the pelvis. *The internal iliac artery has the most variable branching pattern of any artery, and it is worth noting at the outset of this dissection that you must use the distribution of the branches to identify them, not their pattern of branching.*

The internal iliac artery commonly divides into an anterior division and a posterior division. Branches arising from the anterior division are mainly visceral (branches to the urinary bladder, internal genitalia, external genitalia, rectum, and gluteal region). Branches arising from the posterior division are parietal (branches to the pelvic walls and gluteal region).

The order of dissection will be as follows: The branches of the anterior division of the internal iliac artery will be identified. The branches of the posterior division of the internal iliac artery will be identified. The nerves of the sacral plexus will be dissected. Finally, the pelvic portion of the sympathetic trunk will be dissected.

Dissection Instructions

BLOOD VESSELS [G 242; L 274; N 400, 402; C 285]

1. The internal iliac vein is typically plexiform. To clear the dissection field, remove all tributaries to the internal iliac vein.
2. Identify the **common iliac artery** and follow it distally until it bifurcates.
3. Identify the **internal iliac artery**. Use blunt dissection to follow the internal iliac artery into the pelvis.
4. Identify the branches of the anterior division of the internal iliac artery (Fig. 5.36):
   - **Umbilical artery** – in the medial umbilical fold, find the **medial umbilical ligament** (the obliterated portion of the umbilical artery) and use blunt dissection to trace it posteriorly to the

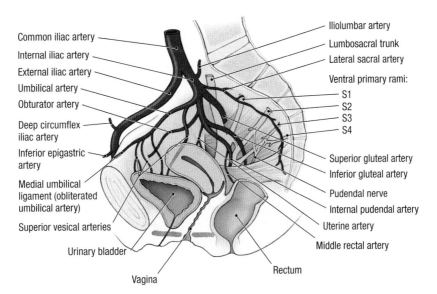

Figure 5.36. Branches of the internal iliac artery in the female.

umbilical artery. Note that several **superior vesical arteries** arise from the inferior surface of the umbilical artery and descend to the superolateral aspect of the urinary bladder.

- **Obturator artery** – passes through the obturator canal. Find the obturator artery where it enters the obturator canal in the lateral wall of the pelvis, and follow the artery posteriorly to its origin. In about 20% of cases, an **aberrant obturator artery** (a branch of the external iliac artery) crosses the pelvic brim and is at risk of injury during surgical repair of a femoral hernia.
- **Uterine artery** – courses along the inferior attachment of the broad ligament. Use blunt dissection to trace it to the lateral aspect of the uterus and note that it passes superior to the ureter. The uterine artery divides into a large superior branch to the body and fundus of the uterus and a smaller branch to the cervix and vagina. Observe the close relationship of the lateral part of the vaginal fornix to the uterine artery. In a living person, the pulsations of the uterine artery may be felt through the lateral part of the vaginal fornix.

CLINICAL CORRELATION

UTERINE ARTERY

The close proximity of the ureter and the uterine artery near the lateral fornix of the vagina is of clinical importance. During hysterectomy, the uterine artery is tied off and cut. The ureter may be unintentionally clamped, tied off, and cut where it crosses the uterine artery. This would have serious consequences for the corresponding kidney. To recall this relationship, use the mnemonic device "water under the bridge." The "water" is urine; the "bridge" is the uterine artery.

- **Vaginal artery** – passes across the floor of the pelvis, inferior to the ureter. The vaginal artery supplies the vagina and the urinary bladder. Note that the ureter passes between the vaginal artery and the uterine artery.
- **Middle rectal artery** – courses medially toward the rectum. To confirm the identity of the middle rectal artery, follow it to the rectum.
- **Internal pudendal artery** – exits the pelvic cavity by passing through the greater sciatic foramen inferior to the piriformis muscle. The internal pudendal artery often arises from a common trunk with the inferior gluteal artery.
- **Inferior gluteal artery** – usually passes out of the pelvic cavity between ventral rami S2 and

S3. The inferior gluteal artery exits the pelvis by passing through the greater sciatic foramen inferior to the piriformis muscle. The inferior gluteal artery may share a common trunk with the internal pudendal artery, or less commonly, with the superior gluteal artery.

5. Identify the branches of the posterior division of the internal iliac artery (Fig. 5.36):
   - **Iliolumbar artery** – passes posteriorly, then ascends between the lumbosacral trunk and the obturator nerve. It may arise from a common trunk with the lateral sacral artery.
   - **Lateral sacral artery** – gives rise to a superior branch and an inferior branch. Observe the inferior branch that passes anterior to the sacral ventral rami.
   - **Superior gluteal artery** – usually exits the pelvic cavity by passing between the lumbosacral trunk and the ventral ramus of spinal nerve S1.
6. Use an illustration to study the **vesical venous plexus, uterine venous plexus, vaginal venous plexus**, and **rectal venous plexus**. All of these plexuses drain into the internal iliac vein.

NERVES [G 206, 242; L 275; N 412, 499; R 470; C 313]

The somatic plexuses of the pelvic cavity are the **sacral plexus** and **coccygeal plexus**. These plexuses are located between the pelvic viscera and the lateral pelvic wall, within the endopelvic fascia. These somatic nerve plexuses are formed by contributions from ventral rami of spinal nerves L4 to S4. The primary visceral nerve plexus of the pelvic cavity is the **inferior hypogastric plexus**. It is formed by contributions from the hypogastric nerves, sympathetic trunks, and pelvic splanchnic nerves.

1. Use your fingers to dissect the rectum from the anterior surface of the sacrum and coccyx.
2. Retract the rectum medially and identify the **sacral plexus** of nerves. The sacral plexus is closely related to the anterior surface of the piriformis muscle. Verify the following (Fig. 5.37):
   - The **lumbosacral trunk** (ventral rami of L4 and L5) joins the sacral plexus.
   - The ventral rami of S2 and S3 emerge between the proximal attachments of the piriformis muscle.
   - The **sciatic nerve** is formed by the ventral rami of spinal nerves L4 through S3. The sciatic nerve exits the pelvis by passing through the greater sciatic foramen, usually inferior to the piriformis muscle.
   - The **superior gluteal artery** usually passes between the **lumbosacral trunk** and the **ventral**

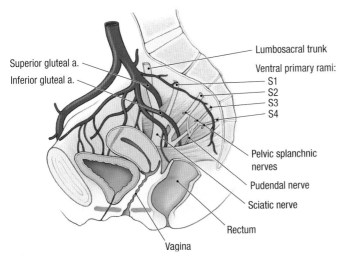

Superior gluteal a.
Inferior gluteal a.
Lumbosacral trunk
Ventral primary rami:
S1
S2
S3
S4
Pelvic splanchnic nerves
Pudendal nerve
Sciatic nerve
Rectum
Vagina

Figure 5.37. Sacral plexus of nerves in the female.

ramus of spinal nerve **S1**, and exits the pelvis by passing superior to the piriformis muscle.

- The **inferior gluteal artery** usually passes between the **ventral rami of spinal nerves S2 and S3**. The inferior gluteal artery exits the pelvis by passing inferior to the piriformis muscle.
- The **pudendal nerve** receives a contribution from the ventral rami of spinal nerves S2, S3, and S4. The pudendal nerve exits the pelvis by passing inferior to the piriformis muscle.

3. Identify the **pelvic splanchnic nerves (nervi erigentes)**. Pelvic splanchnic nerves are branches of the ventral rami of spinal nerves S2 through S4 (Fig. 5.37). Pelvic splanchnic nerves carry preganglionic parasympathetic axons for the innervation of pelvic organs and the distal gastrointestinal tract (from the left colic flexure through the anal canal). [G 247; L 275, 276; N 412; C 313]

4. The **sacral portion of the sympathetic trunk** is located on the anterior surface of the sacrum, medial to the ventral sacral foramina. Identify the following:
   - **Sympathetic trunk** – continues from the abdominal region into the pelvis. The sympathetic trunks of the two sides join in the midline near the level of the coccyx to form the **ganglion impar**.
   - **Gray rami communicantes** – connect the sympathetic ganglia to the sacral ventral rami. Each gray ramus communicans carries postganglionic sympathetic fibers to a ventral ramus for distribution to the lower extremity and the perineum.
   - **Sacral splanchnic nerves** – arise from two or three of the sacral sympathetic ganglia and pass directly to the **inferior hypogastric plexus**. Sacral splanchnic nerves carry sympathetic fibers that distribute to the pelvic viscera.

Pelvic Nerve Plexuses

The pelvic splanchnic nerves (parasympathetic outflow of S2, S3, and S4) are closely related to the lateral aspects of the rectum. The inferior hypogastric plexus is located in the connective tissue lateral to the uterus. These autonomic nerve plexuses can be injured during surgery, causing loss of bladder control.

Dissection Review

1. Review the abdominal aorta and its terminal branches.
2. Use the dissected specimen to review the branches of the internal iliac artery. Review the region supplied by each branch.
3. Review the relationship of the uterine and vaginal arteries to the ureter.
4. Review the formation of the sacral plexus and the branches that were dissected in the pelvis.
5. Use the dissected specimen and an illustration to review the course of the pudendal nerve from the pelvic cavity to the urogenital triangle.

PELVIC DIAPHRAGM

Dissection Overview

The **pelvic diaphragm** is the muscular floor of the pelvic cavity. The pelvic diaphragm is formed by the levator ani muscle and coccygeus muscle plus the fasciae covering their superior and inferior surfaces (Fig. 5.38A, B). The pelvic diaphragm extends from the pubic symphysis to the coccyx. Laterally, the pelvic diaphragm is attached to the fascia covering the obturator internus muscle. The urethra and vagina and the anal canal pass through midline openings in the pelvic diaphragm called the **urogenital hiatus** and **anal hiatus**, respectively.

Dissection Instructions

1. Perform the dissection of the pelvic diaphragm on one side of the cadaver. Save the side with the best dissection of arteries and nerves for review. [G 202, 205; L 278, 279; N 356, 357; C 287, 289]
2. Retract the urinary bladder, uterus, and rectum toward the midline.
3. Use blunt dissection to remove any remaining fat and connective tissue from the superior surface of the pelvic diaphragm.
4. To find the **tendinous arch of the levator ani muscle** (Fig. 5.38A), palpate the medial surface of the ischial spine and then locate the obturator

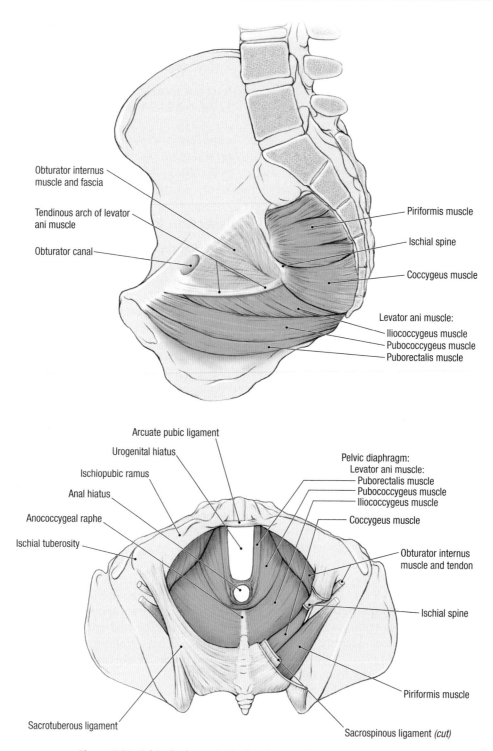

Figure 5.38. Pelvic diaphragm in the female. **A.** Left lateral view. **B.** Inferior view.

canal. The tendinous arch lies just inferior to a line connecting these two structures. Note that the tendinous arch is the superior edge of the pelvic diaphragm.

5. Identify the three muscles that form the **levator ani muscle**. The muscles are identified by their proximal attachments. Learn, but do not dissect, their distal attachments. Identify the following:

- **Puborectalis muscle** – its proximal attachment is the body of the pubis. Its distal attachment is the puborectalis muscle of the opposite side (in a midline raphe). The puborectalis muscle forms the lateral boundary of the urogenital hiatus. The two puborectalis muscles form a "puborectal sling," which causes the **anorectal flexure** at the ampulla of the rectum

(Fig. 5.35). During defecation, the puborectalis muscles relax, the anorectal flexure straightens, and the elimination of fecal matter is facilitated.

- **Pubococcygeus muscle** – its proximal attachment is the body of the pubis. Its distal attachment is the coccyx and the **anococcygeal raphe**.
- **Iliococcygeus muscle** – its proximal attachment is the tendinous arch. Its distal attachment is the coccyx and the anococcygeal raphe.

6. The levator ani muscle supports the pelvic viscera and resists increases in intra-abdominal pressure.
7. Identify the **coccygeus muscle**. The coccygeus muscle completes the pelvic diaphragm posteriorly. The proximal attachment of the coccygeus muscle is the ischial spine and its distal attachment is the lateral border of the coccyx and the lowest part of the sacrum.
8. Place the fingers of one hand in the ischioanal fossa and the fingers of the other hand on the superior surface of the pelvic diaphragm. Palpate the thinness of the pelvic diaphragm.
9. Observe that the **obturator internus muscle** forms the lateral wall of the ischioanal fossa. The proximal attachment of the obturator internus muscle is the margin of the obturator foramen and inner surface of the obturator membrane. The distal attachment of the obturator internus muscle will be studied when the gluteal region is dissected. Superior to the tendinous arch of the levator ani muscle, the obturator internus muscle forms the lateral wall of the pelvic cavity. Inferior to the tendinous arch, the obturator internus muscle forms the lateral wall of the perineum.
10. Use your textbook to learn the general pattern of lymphatic drainage of the pelvis and the location of each of the following groups of lymph nodes: [G 213, 244, 245; L 290; N 406; R 361; C 285]

- **Internal iliac nodes**
- **External iliac nodes**
- **Common iliac nodes**
- **Sacral nodes**
- **Lumbar nodes**

Dissection Review

1. Use the dissected specimen to review the proximal attachment and action of each muscle of the pelvic diaphragm.
2. Review the relationship of the branches of the internal iliac artery to the pelvic diaphragm.
3. Review the relationship of the sacral plexus to the pelvic diaphragm.
4. Use an illustration to review the role played by the pelvic diaphragm in forming the boundary between the pelvic cavity and the perineum. Review the function of the pelvic diaphragm and perineal body in supporting the pelvic and abdominal viscera.
5. Use an illustration to review the lymphatic drainage from the pelvis and perineum. Realize that structures in the perineum (including the labia majora and the lower part of the anal canal) drain into superficial inguinal lymph nodes. The lymphatic drainage of the ovary follows the ovarian vessels to the lumbar chain of nodes, bypassing the pelvic drainage systems.
6. Review the formation of the thoracic duct to complete your understanding of the lymph drainage from this region.
7. Visit a dissection table with a male cadaver and perform a complete review of the dissected male pelvis.

THE LOWER LIMB

The functional requirements of the lower limb are weight bearing, locomotion, and maintenance of equilibrium. As such, it is constructed for strength at the cost of mobility. The lower limb is divided into four parts: **hip**, **thigh**, **leg**, and **foot** (Fig. 6.1). It is worth noting that the term *leg* refers only to the portion of the lower limb between the knee and ankle, not to the entire lower limb.

SURFACE ANATOMY [G 365; L 87; N 485; C 364]

The surface anatomy of the lower limb can be studied on a living subject or the cadaver. Place the cadaver in the supine position and palpate the following structures (Fig. 6.1):

- **Iliac crest**
- **Anterior superior iliac spine**
- **Pubic tubercle**
- **Patella**
- **Medial femoral epicondyle**
- **Lateral femoral epicondyle**
- **Medial malleolus**
- **Lateral malleolus**

SUPERFICIAL VEINS AND CUTANEOUS NERVES

Dissection Overview

The order of dissection will be as follows: The entire lower limb will be skinned. The superficial veins and cutaneous nerves will be dissected. The subcutaneous connective tissue and fat will be removed leaving selected superficial veins and cutaneous nerves intact. The deep fascia of the thigh will be studied.

Dissection Instructions

SKIN INCISIONS

1. The objective is to remove the skin from the lower limb, leaving the superficial fascia, superficial veins, and cutaneous nerves undisturbed. Refer to Figure 6.2A.
2. Make a cut from the anterior superior iliac spine (D) along the inguinal ligament to the pubic tubercle. Extend this cut around the medial side of the thigh to the posterior surface of the thigh (E). If the abdomen and perineum have been dissected, this cut has been made previously.
3. Make a vertical cut from the midpoint of the inguinal ligament (F) passing over the patella to the dorsum of the foot (G).

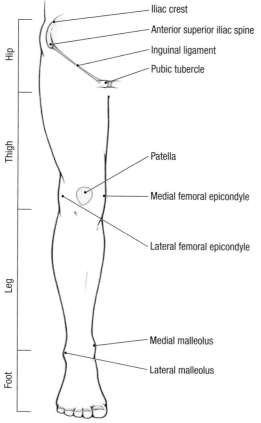

Iliac crest
Anterior superior iliac spine
Inguinal ligament
Pubic tubercle

Patella

Medial femoral epicondyle

Lateral femoral epicondyle

Medial malleolus

Lateral malleolus

Hip

Thigh

Leg

Foot

Figure 6.1. Surface anatomy of the lower limb.

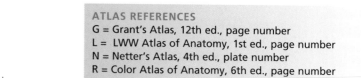

ATLAS REFERENCES
G = Grant's Atlas, 12th ed., page number
L = LWW Atlas of Anatomy, 1st ed., page number
N = Netter's Atlas, 4th ed., plate number
R = Color Atlas of Anatomy, 6th ed., page number

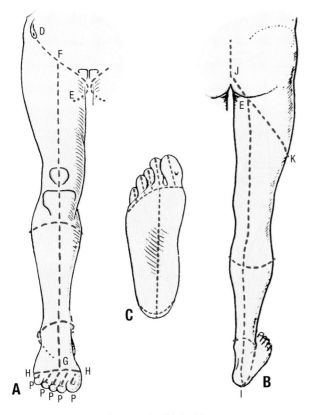

Figure 6.2. Skin incisions.

4. Make a cut across the dorsum of the foot at the webs of the toes (H to H). The skin is very thin on the dorsum of the foot. Do not cut too deep.

5. Make one cut along the dorsal midline of each toe to the proximal end of the nail (H to P).

6. Remove the skin from the thigh, leg, and dorsum of the foot as far laterally and medially as possible. Make as many transverse skin incisions as are needed to speed up the skinning process.

7. Turn the cadaver into the prone position and refer to Figure 6.2B.

8. If not already done during the dissection of the pelvis, remove the skin from the gluteal region. Make a midline incision and work from medial to lateral. Detach the skin along line J–K and the lateral side of the hip and place it in the tissue container.

9. Make a cut along the midline of the thigh and leg from the gluteal fold to the heel (E to I).

10. Extend the previous transverse skin incisions around the limb to join incision E–I. Begin at line E–I and work both medially and laterally. Remove the skin completely from the lower limb and place it in the tissue container.

11. Remove the skin from the sole of the foot using the cuts indicated in Figure 6.2C. The skin is thick

over the heel and over the heads of the metatarsal bones, but it is thinner on the toes and the instep.

SUPERFICIAL FASCIA OF THE POSTERIOR LOWER LIMB
[G 359, 364; L 89; N 545; R 474, 489; C 382, 412]

1. With the cadaver still in the prone position, examine the structures contained in the superficial fascia of the posterior aspect of the lower limb (Fig. 6.3B).

2. Find the **small saphenous vein** where it passes posterior to the lateral malleolus at the ankle (Fig. 6.3B). The small saphenous vein arises from the lateral end of the **dorsal venous arch**. Clean the small saphenous vein and follow it superiorly until it pierces the deep fascia in the popliteal fossa where it drains into the popliteal vein.

3. Identify the **sural nerve** (L. *sura*, calf of the leg). The sural nerve pierces the deep fascia halfway down the posterior aspect of the leg and courses parallel to the small saphenous vein. The sural nerve innervates the skin of the lateral aspect of the ankle and foot.

4. Use an illustration to study the cutaneous innervation of the posterior surface of the lower limb and note the following:
   - **Cluneal nerves** innervate the skin of the gluteal region (L. *clunis*, buttock) (Fig. 6.3B):
     - **Superior cluneal nerves** – branches of the dorsal rami of L1 to L3 innervate the upper buttock.
     - **Middle cluneal nerves** – branches of the dorsal rami of S1 to S3 innervate the middle part of the buttock.
     - **Inferior cluneal nerves** – branches of the posterior cutaneous nerve of the thigh wrap around the inferior border of the gluteus maximus muscle and innervate the skin over the lower part of the buttock.
   - **Posterior cutaneous nerve of the thigh** – lies deep to the deep fascia (Fig. 6.3B, *ghosted*). Branches of the posterior cutaneous nerve pierce the deep fascia to supply the skin on the posterior surface of the thigh and popliteal fossa.

5. Remove all remnants of **superficial fascia** from the posterior aspect of the gluteal region, thigh, and leg. Preserve the deep fascia, cutaneous nerves, and superficial veins that you have dissected.

SUPERFICIAL FASCIA OF THE ANTERIOR LOWER LIMB
[G 359, 364; L 88; N 544; R 478, 492; C 368, 398, 406]

1. Turn the cadaver to the supine position and refer to Figure 6.3A.

2. Find the **great saphenous vein** (Gr. *saphenous*, manifest; obvious) where it arises from the medial

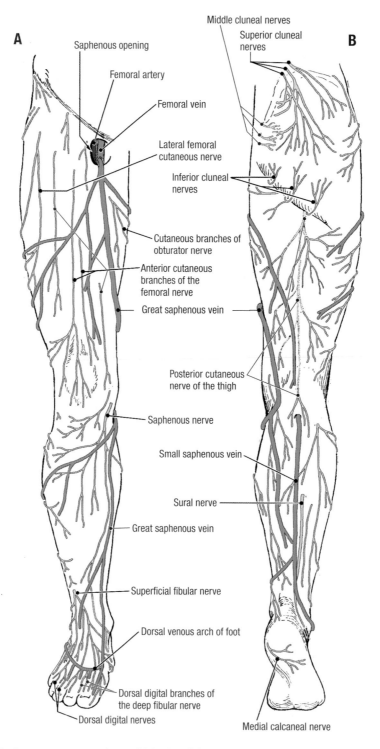

Figure 6.3. Cutaneous nerves and superficial veins of the lower limb. **A.** Anterior view. **B.** Posterior view.

end of the **dorsal venous arch of the foot** (Fig. 6.3A). Use blunt dissection to follow it proximally. Note the following:

- At the ankle, the great saphenous vein passes anterior to the medial malleolus.
- At the knee, it passes over the posterior border of the medial epicondyle of the femur.
- Beginning at the level of the knee, the great

saphenous vein courses anterolaterally to eventually lie on the anterior surface of the proximal thigh.

- **Perforating veins** connect the great saphenous vein to the deep venous system.
- Many superficial veins join the great saphenous vein, and some of these are quite large. Most of these are not named.

- The **accessory saphenous vein** drains the superficial fascia and skin of the medial side of the thigh (Fig. 6.3A).
- Three small superficial veins (**superficial external pudendal**, **superficial epigastric**, and **superficial circumflex iliac**) join the great saphenous vein near its proximal end.

3. About 4 cm inferior to the inguinal ligament, the great saphenous vein passes deeply through the **saphenous opening** and drains into the femoral vein. The saphenous opening is an opening in the deep fascia that will be dissected later.

CLINICAL CORRELATION

Great Saphenous Vein

Superficial veins and perforating veins have valves that prevent the backflow of blood. If these valves become incompetent, then the veins become distended, a condition known as varicose veins.

Portions of the great saphenous vein may be removed and used as graft vessels in coronary bypass surgery. The distal end of the vein is attached to the aorta, reversing the direction of blood flow through the vessel so that the valves do not impede the flow of blood.

---

4. Use an illustration to study the cutaneous innervation of the anterior surface of the lower limb and note the following (Fig. 6.3A):
   - **Lateral femoral cutaneous nerve** – passes deep to the lateral end of the inguinal ligament and innervates the skin of the lateral thigh.
   - **Anterior cutaneous branches of the femoral nerve** – innervate the skin of the anterior thigh. These branches enter the superficial fascia lateral to the great saphenous vein.
   - **Cutaneous branches of the obturator nerve** – innervate the skin of the medial thigh.
   - **Saphenous nerve** – a branch of the femoral nerve that pierces the deep fascia on the medial aspect of the knee and accompanies the great saphenous vein into the leg. The saphenous nerve innervates the skin on the anterior and medial aspects of the leg and the medial side of the ankle and foot.
5. In the distal third of the leg, identify the **superficial fibular nerve**. The superficial fibular nerve pierces the deep fascia proximal to the lateral malleolus. Follow the superficial fibular nerve distally and note that it innervates the dorsum of the foot and sends **dorsal digital nerves** to the skin of the toes.

6. The skin between the first toe and the second toe is innervated by the **dorsal digital branches of the deep fibular nerve**. This innervation pattern is used for the assessment of deep fibular nerve function.
7. Identify the **superficial inguinal lymph nodes**. Two subgroups can be identified (Fig. 6.4):
   - **Horizontal group** – about 2 cm below the inguinal ligament
   - **Vertical group** – around the proximal end of the great saphenous vein
8. Note that the superficial inguinal lymph nodes collect lymph from the lower limb, inferior part of the anterior abdominal wall, gluteal region, perineum, and external genitalia. The superficial inguinal lymph nodes drain into the **deep inguinal lymph nodes**. Do not attempt to dissect the deep inguinal lymph nodes at this time.
9. Remove the remnants of superficial fascia from the anterior thigh, leg, and foot. Preserve the superficial veins, cutaneous nerves, and deep fascia.
10. Examine the deep fascia of the lower limb. It is named regionally: **fascia lata** (L. *latus*, broad) in the thigh, **crural fascia** in the leg, and **pedal fascia** in the foot. The lateral portion of the fascia lata is particularly strong and is called the **iliotibial tract**.

Dissection Review

1. Review the superficial fascia of the lower limb.
2. Trace the course of the superficial veins from distal to proximal.

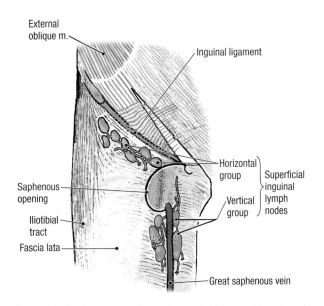

Figure 6.4. Saphenous opening and superficial inguinal lymph nodes.

3. Review the location and pattern of distribution of each cutaneous nerve that you have dissected in the lower limb.
4. Review the extent and bony attachments of the deep fascia and name its parts.

ANTERIOR COMPARTMENT OF THE THIGH

Dissection Overview

The fascia lata is connected to the femur by intermuscular septa (Fig. 6.5) to form the three fascial compartments of the thigh: **anterior (extensor)**, **medial (adductor)**, and **posterior (flexor)**. The anterior compartment of the thigh contains five muscles: **sartorius**, **rectus femoris**, **vastus lateralis**, **vastus intermedius**, and **vastus medialis**. The rectus femoris, vastus lateralis, vastus intermedius, and vastus medialis collectively are called the **quadriceps femoris muscle**. The shared action of the anterior thigh muscles is extension of the leg. The major blood supply to the lower limb (femoral artery and deep femoral artery) passes through the anterior compartment of the thigh. [G 368, 369; L 101; N 505; R 455]

The order of dissection will be as follows: The fascia lata of the thigh will be reviewed and its saphenous opening will be studied. The anterior surface of the superior part of the fascia lata will be opened to expose the femoral triangle. The femoral triangle will be dissected and its contents traced distally. The adductor canal will be dissected and the sartorius muscle identified. The anterior surface of the inferior part of the fascia lata will be incised and the remaining anterior thigh muscles will be studied.

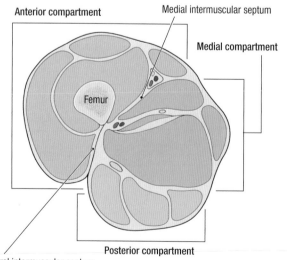

Figure 6.5. Compartments of the right thigh from an inferior view

SKELETON OF THE THIGH

Refer to a skeleton and Figure 6.6.
On the pelvis, identify: [G 380; L 92; N 486; R 436; C 266]

- **Anterior superior iliac spine**
- **Anterior inferior iliac spine**
- **Pecten pubis**
- **Pubic tubercle**

On the femur, identify: [G 380; L 92; N 489; R 439; C 430, 431]

- **Greater trochanter**
- **Lesser trochanter**
- **Lateral condyle** and **lateral epicondyle**
- **Medial condyle** and **medial epicondyle**
- **Medial supracondylar line**
- **Adductor tubercle**
- **Linea aspera**
- **Pectineal line**

On the tibia, identify: [G 380; L 94; N 513; R 440; C 446]

- **Tuberosity**

On the patella, identify:

- **Anterior surface**
- **Articular surface**

Dissection Instructions

SAPHENOUS OPENING [G 370, 371; L 88; N 544; R 468; C 368]

1. Remove any remnants of superficial fascia that remain on the anterior surface of the fascia lata from the level of the inguinal ligament to the knee. The superficial inguinal lymph nodes must be removed during this step of the dissection. Preserve the great saphenous vein.
2. Follow the great saphenous vein superiorly and observe that it turns posteriorly to disappear approximately 4 cm inferior to the inguinal ligament. Use a probe to dissect the connective tissue around the great saphenous vein where it passes deeply. Insert your finger beside the great saphenous vein and move your finger around the vein to define the margins of the **saphenous opening** (Fig. 6.7). The saphenous opening is a natural opening in the fascia lata that is filled with a rather weak layer of fascia. Observe that the great saphenous vein passes through the saphenous opening to enter the deeper part of the anterior thigh. Trace the great saphenous vein through the saphenous opening and observe that it drains into the anterior surface of the **femoral vein**.
3. Again insert your finger into the saphenous opening inferior to the great saphenous vein. Push your

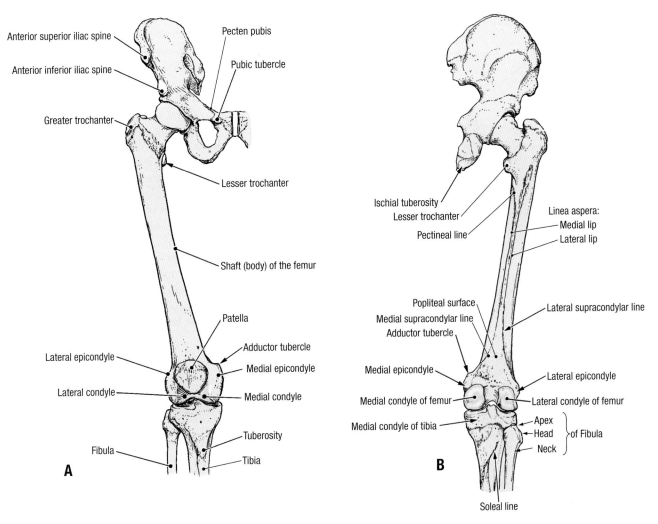

Figure 6.6. Bones of the thigh. **A.** Anterior view. **B.** Posterior view.

finger inferiorly deep to the fascia lata until your fingertip reaches the level of the sartorius muscle. Use scissors to make an incision through the fascia lata from the saphenous opening to the sartorius muscle (Fig. 6.7, incision 1).

4. Use scissors to make a second incision through the fascia lata that extends laterally from the superior margin of the saphenous opening, parallel to the inguinal ligament (Fig. 6.7, incision 2). This incision should extend laterally to a point that is directly inferior to the anterior superior iliac spine.

5. Use scissors to make a third incision through the fascia lata that extends medially from the superior margin of the saphenous opening, parallel to the inguinal ligament (Fig. 6.7, incision 3). This incision should extend medially to a point that is directly inferior to the pubic tubercle.

6. Use blunt dissection to separate the fascia lata from deeper structures. Reflect the flaps of fascia

lata medially and laterally. You have opened the superficial boundary (roof) of the femoral triangle.

FEMORAL TRIANGLE [G 372, 373; L 103; 104, N 500; R 479–481; C 372, 377]

1. Identify the **femoral triangle** (Fig. 6.8). The femoral triangle is bounded superiorly by the **inguinal ligament,** laterally by the **sartorius muscle,** and medially by the **adductor longus muscle.** The base of the femoral triangle is the inguinal ligament and the apex is located inferiorly.

2. The **contents of the femoral triangle** are:
   • **Femoral nerve** and its branches
   • **Femoral artery** and some of its branches
   • **Femoral vein** and some of its tributaries (notably, the great saphenous vein)
   • **Femoral sheath**

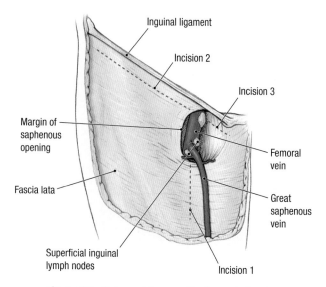

Figure 6.7. Cuts used to open the femoral triangle.

Femoral Triangle

The pulse of the femoral artery can be palpated about 3 cm inferior to the midpoint of the inguinal ligament. Within the femoral triangle, the femoral vessels are accessed for diagnostic purposes. A catheter introduced into the femoral artery can be advanced proximally into the aorta and its branches. A catheter introduced into the femoral vein can be advanced through the inferior vena cava into the right atrium of the heart.

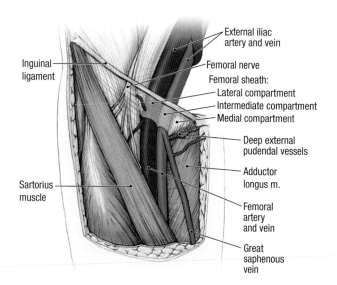

Figure 6.8. Boundaries and contents of the femoral triangle.

3. Identify the **femoral sheath** (Fig. 6.8). The femoral sheath is an extension of transversalis fascia into the thigh that envelops the proximal end of the femoral artery and femoral vein, and some deep inguinal lymph nodes. The femoral sheath is subdivided into **three compartments** (Fig. 6.8):
   • **Lateral** – containing the femoral artery
   • **Intermediate** – containing the femoral vein
   • **Medial** – containing lymphatics
4. Note that the lateral to medial arrangement of structures that pass under the inguinal ligament (including the contents of the femoral sheath) can be arranged by use of the mnemonic device **NAVL** (pronounced navel): femoral **N**erve, femoral **A**rtery, femoral **V**ein, **L**ymphatics.
5. The medial compartment of the femoral sheath is also called the **femoral canal** and its proximal opening into the abdominal cavity is called the **femoral ring**. The femoral canal and femoral ring are seen from the abdominal side of the inguinal ligament.

Femoral Hernia

The femoral ring is a site of potential herniation. A femoral hernia is a protrusion of abdominal viscera through the femoral ring into the femoral canal. A femoral hernia may become strangulated due to the inflexibility of the inguinal ligament.

6. Use blunt dissection to clean the **femoral artery** and **femoral vein** within the femoral triangle. Three small arteries arise from the femoral artery just distal to the inguinal ligament (Fig. 6.9B): **superficial external pudendal artery**, **superficial epigastric artery**, and **superficial circumflex iliac artery**. Respectively, these arteries pass medially, superiorly, and laterally from their origin and they supply the superficial fascia of the abdominal wall, proximal thigh, and part of the perineum. Do not attempt to follow these vessels.
7. Three large arteries arise within the femoral triangle (Fig. 6.9B): **deep artery of the thigh (deep femoral artery, profunda femoris artery)**, **lateral circumflex femoral artery**, and **medial circumflex femoral artery**. The medial and lateral circumflex femoral arteries usually arise from the deep artery of the thigh, but each may arise from the femoral artery very close to the origin of the deep artery of the thigh.

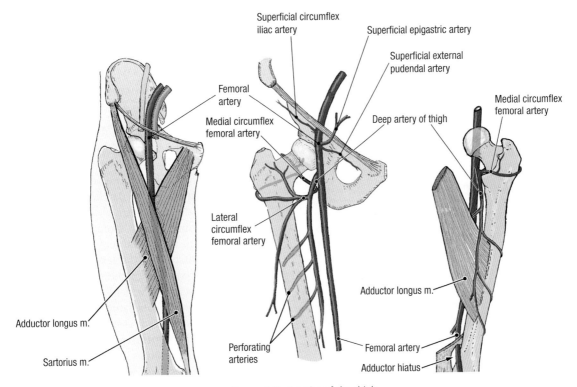

Figure 6.9. Arteries of the thigh.

8. Preserve the major veins (femoral vein, deep vein of the thigh, great saphenous vein), but remove their tributaries to clear the dissection field.

9. Inferior to the apex of the femoral triangle, note that the **femoral artery** courses distally between the sartorius muscle and the adductor longus muscle (Fig. 6.9A).

10. Retract the femoral artery medially and identify the **deep artery of the thigh**. The deep artery of the thigh courses parallel to the femoral artery but posterior to the adductor longus muscle (Fig. 6.9C). The deep artery of the thigh supplies the medial and posterior compartments of the thigh.

11. Identify the **lateral circumflex femoral artery**. The lateral circumflex femoral artery usually arises from the deep artery of the thigh very close to the femoral artery. The lateral circumflex femoral artery passes laterally, deep to the proximal end of the rectus femoris muscle, and supplies the muscles and soft tissues of the lateral part of the thigh. It has three branches, each of which participates in an anastomosis:
   - **Ascending branch** – anastomoses with the superior gluteal artery
   - **Transverse branch** – anastomoses with the medial circumflex femoral artery
   - **Descending branch** – courses inferiorly on the anterior surface of the vastus intermedius

muscle and anastomoses with the genicular arteries at the knee

12. Identify the **medial circumflex femoral artery**. The medial circumflex femoral artery typically arises from the deep artery of the thigh close to the femoral artery. The medial circumflex femoral artery passes posteriorly, between the pectineus and iliopsoas muscles. In addition to supplying the soft tissues of the region, the medial circumflex femoral artery is an important blood supply to the head and neck of the femur.

13. The floor of the femoral triangle is formed by the iliopsoas muscle and the pectineus muscle.

14. The iliacus and psoas major muscles collectively are named the **iliopsoas muscle**. The proximal attachment of the iliacus muscle is the iliac fossa and the proximal attachments of the psoas major muscle are the transverse processes and bodies of vertebrae T12 to L5. The distal attachment of the iliopsoas tendon is the lesser trochanter of the femur. The iliopsoas muscle is a strong flexor of the thigh.

15. The proximal attachment of the **pectineus muscle** is the pecten pubis and the superior ramus of the pubis, and its distal attachment is the pectineal line of the femur. The pectineus muscle adducts and flexes the thigh.

16. Use blunt dissection to clean the floor of the femoral triangle.

17. Expose the **femoral nerve**, which lies on the floor of the femoral triangle on the lateral side of the femoral artery (Fig. 6.8). Follow the femoral nerve inferiorly and observe that it divides into numerous branches. The femoral nerve innervates the anterior thigh muscles and the skin of the anterior thigh. Its motor branches will be identified later.

18. Verify that the **anterior cutaneous branches of the femoral nerve** enter the superficial fascia by penetrating the fascia lata along the anterior surface of the sartorius muscle (Fig. 6.3).

ADDUCTOR CANAL AND SARTORIUS MUSCLE [G 382; L 102, 103; N 500; R 480; C 377]

1. The **adductor canal** is a fascial compartment located deep to the sartorius muscle that conducts the femoral artery and vein through the inferior part of the thigh. The adductor canal begins at the **apex of the femoral triangle** and ends at the **adductor hiatus**, which is located just above the knee (Fig. 6.9C). The femoral vessels pass through the adductor hiatus to reach the popliteal fossa.

2. Use scissors to cut the fascia lata along the superficial surface of the sartorius muscle. The cut should extend from the anterior superior iliac spine to the medial epicondyle of the femur.

3. Use a probe and your fingers to separate the **sartorius muscle** from the deep fascia that is both anterior and posterior to it. Retract the sartorius muscle laterally so that its superior and inferior attachments can be defined and its blood and nerve supplies can be identified. The proximal attachment of the sartorius muscle is the anterior superior iliac spine and its distal attachment is the medial surface of the proximal tibia. Observe that the sartorius muscle crosses both the hip joint and the knee joint. It flexes and laterally rotates the thigh and flexes the leg.

4. Transect the sartorius muscle near the apex of the femoral triangle. Reflect the distal part of the sartorius muscle inferiorly. Posterior to the sartorius muscle observe a sheath of connective tissue that encloses the femoral vessels. This connective tissue sheath is the adductor canal.

5. Use scissors to open the adductor canal and examine the femoral vessels. Observe that the **femoral vein** lies posterior to the **femoral artery**. Use blunt dissection to follow the femoral artery distally through the adductor hiatus, where its name changes to **popliteal artery** (Fig. 6.9C).

6. The **nerve to vastus medialis** and the **saphenous nerve** accompany the femoral vessels in the adductor canal. The nerve to vastus medialis is the motor nerve to the vastus medialis muscle, and the

saphenous nerve is a cutaneous nerve that innervates the skin of the medial side of the leg, ankle, and foot.

QUADRICEPS FEMORIS MUSCLE [G 377, 382; L 103; N 501; R 481; C 375]

1. Insert your finger deep to the fascial lata near the apex of the femoral triangle and direct it inferiorly toward the knee. Use scissors to make a vertical cut through the fascia lata from the apex of the femoral triangle to the patella. Make a transverse incision in the fascia lata above the patella. This incision should extend from the medial femoral epicondyle to the lateral femoral epicondyle.

2. Use blunt dissection to release the fascia lata from the anterior surface of the deeper structures and open the fascia lata widely. Follow the inner surface of the fascia lata laterally with your fingers. Here, the fascia lata is continuous with the **lateral intermuscular septum** (Fig. 6.10). The lateral intermuscular septum is attached to the **linea aspera** on the posterior aspect of the femur.

3. The **quadriceps femoris muscle** occupies most of the anterior compartment of the thigh (Fig. 6.10). The four parts of the quadriceps femoris muscle are the rectus femoris, vastus lateralis, vas-

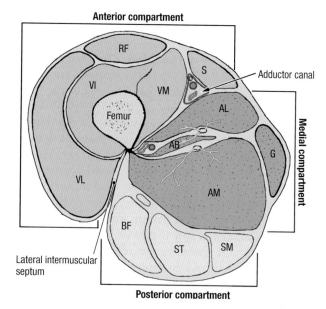

Figure 6.10. Transverse section through the right thigh, inferior view. Anterior compartment: VI, vastus intermedius; VL, vastus lateralis; VM, vastus medialis; RF, rectus femoris; S, sartorius. Medial compartment: AB, adductor brevis; AL, adductor longus; AM, adductor magnus; G, gracilis. Posterior compartment: BF, biceps femoris; ST, semitendinosus; SM, semimembranosus.

tus intermedius, and vastus medialis. The tendons of all four muscles unite to form the **quadriceps femoris tendon**. The quadriceps femoris tendon is attached to the patella. The **patellar ligament** attaches the patella to the tibial tuberosity, so the ultimate attachment of the quadriceps femoris muscle is the tibial tuberosity (Fig. 6.11).

4. Identify the **rectus femoris muscle** in the midline of the anterior thigh. The proximal attachment of the rectus femoris muscle is the anterior inferior iliac spine and its distal attachment is the tibial tuberosity. The rectus femoris muscle crosses both the hip joint and the knee joint. It flexes the thigh and extends the leg.

5. Transect the rectus femoris muscle near its midlength and reflect its halves superiorly and inferiorly as shown in Figure 6.11.

6. Identify the **vastus lateralis muscle** on the lateral side of the anterior thigh (Fig. 6.11). The proximal attachments of the vastus lateralis muscle are the lateral lip of the linea aspera and the greater trochanter of the femur. The distal attachment of the vastus lateralis muscle is the tibial tuberosity and it extends the leg.

7. Identify the **vastus medialis muscle** on the medial side of the anterior thigh. The proximal attachments of the vastus medialis muscle are the medial lip of the linea aspera of the femur and the intertrochanteric line. The distal attachment of the vastus medialis muscle is the tibial tuberosity and it extends the leg.

8. Identify the **vastus intermedius muscle,** which is between the vastus lateralis and vastus intermedius muscles. The proximal attachments of the vastus intermedius muscle are the anterior and lateral surfaces of the femur (Fig. 6.10). The distal attachment of the vastus intermedius muscle is the tibial tuberosity and it extends the leg.

9. Observe the **descending branch of the lateral circumflex femoral artery,** which can be seen on the anterior surface of the vastus intermedius muscle, deep to the rectus femoris muscle.

10. Identify the **motor branches of the femoral nerve** to the anterior thigh muscles (Fig. 6.11). The motor branches of the femoral nerve are located between the rectus femoris muscle and the three vastus muscles. Note that the femoral nerve innervates the sartorius muscle and the pectineus muscle in addition to innervating the quadriceps femoris muscle.

Dissection Review

1. Replace the anterior thigh muscles in their correct anatomical positions.
2. Use the dissected specimen to review the boundaries and contents of the femoral triangle.
3. Review the origin and course of the femoral artery and its branches in the thigh.
4. Use the dissected specimen to review the attachments and actions of the muscles of the anterior compartment of the thigh.

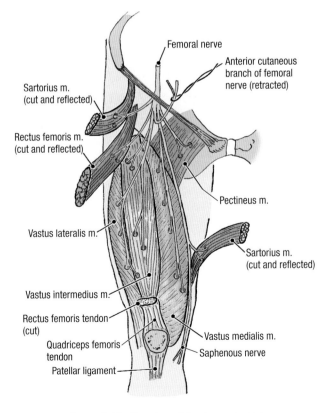

Sartorius m. (cut and reflected)

Rectus femoris m. (cut and reflected)

Vastus lateralis m.

Vastus intermedius m.

Rectus femoris tendon (cut)

Quadriceps femoris tendon

Patellar ligament

Femoral nerve

Anterior cutaneous branch of femoral nerve (retracted)

Pectineus m.

Sartorius m. (cut and reflected)

Vastus medialis m.

Saphenous nerve

Figure 6.11. Branches of the femoral nerve.

5. Recall the rule of innervation of the anterior compartment of the thigh: [L 149]
   - **All muscles in the anterior compartment of the thigh are innervated by the femoral nerve.**

MEDIAL COMPARTMENT OF THE THIGH [G 378; L 105–107; N 501; R 481; C 379]

Dissection Overview

The medial compartment of the thigh contains six muscles: **gracilis**, **adductor longus**, **adductor brevis**, **pectineus**, **adductor magnus**, and **obturator externus**. The shared function of this group of muscles is to adduct the thigh. Therefore, they are also known as the adductor group of thigh muscles.

The order of dissection will be as follows: The fascia lata will be removed from the medial thigh. The gracilis muscle will be studied. The adductor muscles will be dissected by following the medial circumflex femoral artery, the deep artery of the thigh, and the branches of the obturator nerve. Note: The anterior and posterior branches of the obturator nerve pass anterior and posterior, respectively, to the adductor brevis muscle. *The branches of the deep artery of the thigh and the obturator nerve are excellent aids to help you define the plane of separation between the muscles of the medial compartment of the thigh.*

Dissection Instructions

1. On the medial aspect of the thigh, use your hands to separate the fascia lata from the muscles of the medial compartment. Begin at the medial border of the femoral triangle and work medially. Be careful not to remove the gracilis muscle. Use scissors to cut the fascia lata and remove it and any remnants of superficial fascia that may adhere to it.
2. Identify the **gracilis muscle**. The proximal attachment of the gracilis muscle is the pubic bone and its distal attachment is the medial condyle of the tibia. With your fingers, define the gracilis muscle from its proximal attachment to its distal attachment. Using scissors, trim away any remaining superficial fascia or fascia lata so that the gracilis muscle is clearly visible and separated from deeper structures. The gracilis muscle crosses both the hip and knee joints. It adducts the thigh and assists in flexion of the leg.
3. Use an illustration to observe the proximal attachments of the **gracilis muscle**, **pectineus muscle**, and **adductor longus muscle** along a curved line on the pubic bone. [G 380; L 98; N 490; R 453; C 430]
4. Observe the anterior surface of the **pectineus** and **adductor longus muscles**. They fan out to their distal attachments on the pectineal line or the linea aspera of the femur. Both muscles are adductors of the thigh.
5. Note that the **deep artery of the thigh** passes between the pectineus and adductor longus muscles, then courses inferiorly between the adductor longus muscle and the adductor brevis muscle. Follow the deep artery of the thigh distally between the pectineus and adductor longus muscles and use blunt dissection to define the muscle borders.
6. Continue to follow the deep artery of the thigh posterior to the adductor longus muscle to separate the adductor longus muscle from the adductor brevis muscle. Transect the adductor longus muscle 5 cm inferior to its proximal attachment and reflect it as shown in Figure 6.12.
7. The **adductor brevis muscle** can now be seen at a deeper plane. The proximal attachments of the adductor brevis muscle are the body and inferior ramus of the pubis and its distal attachments are the pectineal line and linea aspera of the femur. The adductor brevis muscle adducts the thigh.

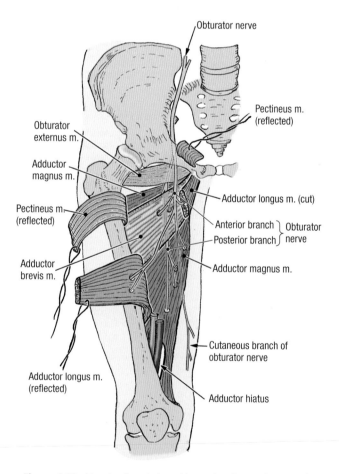

Figure 6.12. How to dissect the adductor brevis muscle using the branches of the obturator nerve.

8. Clean the deep artery of the thigh and identify one or two **perforating arteries**. Perforating arteries penetrate the adductor brevis and adductor magnus muscles. They encircle the femur and supply the muscles of the posterior compartment of the thigh.

9. Refer to Figure 6.12 and note that the **anterior branch of the obturator nerve** crosses the anterior surface of the adductor brevis muscle and that the **posterior branch of the obturator nerve** crosses its posterior surface.

10. Superiorly, the anterior branch of the obturator nerve passes deep to the pectineus muscle but is superficial to the adductor brevis muscle (Fig. 6.12). Follow the anterior branch of the obturator nerve superiorly to separate the pectineus muscle from the adductor brevis muscle. Note that the superior border of the adductor brevis muscle is deep to the pectineus muscle. Use blunt dissection to clean the adductor brevis. Do not damage the anterior branches of the obturator nerve.

11. The posterior branch of the obturator nerve lies between the adductor brevis muscle and the **adductor magnus muscle**. Use blunt dissection to follow the posterior branch of the obturator nerve superiorly to separate the adductor brevis muscle from the adductor magnus muscle.

12. Raise the adductor brevis muscle and observe the **adductor magnus muscle**. The proximal attachments of the adductor magnus muscle are the ischiopubic ramus and the ischial tuberosity, and its distal attachments are the gluteal tuberosity, linea aspera, medial supracondylar line, and adductor tubercle of the femur. The most medial part of the adductor magnus muscle (the part that attaches to the adductor tubercle) is the **ischiocondylar portion** and it is innervated by the tibial division of the sciatic nerve rather than by the obturator nerve. The adductor magnus muscle adducts and extends the thigh.

13. Trace the tendon of the ischiocondylar portion of the adductor magnus muscle inferiorly to its attachment on the **adductor tubercle**. On the lateral side of this tendon, observe the **adductor hiatus**, which is an opening in the adductor magnus tendon (Fig. 6.12). Note that the femoral artery and vein pass from the anterior compartment of the thigh into the posterior compartment of the thigh by passing through the adductor hiatus.

14. Study an illustration of the **obturator externus muscle**. Do not attempt to dissect this muscle, as it lies deep to the pectineus muscle and iliopsoas tendon. The proximal attachment of the obturator externus muscle is the superior pubic ramus, the ischiopubic ramus, and the external surface of the obturator membrane. Its distal attachment is into the trochanteric fossa on the medial side of the greater trochanter of the femur. The obturator externus muscle is a lateral rotator of the thigh. [G 394; L 107; N 501; C 378]

Dissection Review

1. Replace the medial thigh muscles in their correct anatomical positions.

2. Use the dissected specimen to review the attachments and action of each muscle dissected.

3. Trace the deep artery of the thigh from its origin to its termination as the fourth perforating artery.

4. Trace the medial circumflex femoral artery from its origin to where it passes between the iliopsoas and pectineus muscles.

5. Trace the course of the anterior and posterior branches of the obturator nerve superiorly as far as the superior border of the adductor brevis muscle.

6. Recall the rule for innervation of the medial thigh muscles: [L 150]
   - **The obturator nerve innervates the muscles of the medial compartment of the thigh** with the following exceptions:
     ○ The pectineus muscle receives motor innervation from both the femoral nerve and the obturator nerve.
     ○ The ischiocondylar portion of the adductor magnus muscle is innervated by the tibial division of the sciatic nerve.

GLUTEAL REGION

Dissection Overview

The gluteal region (Gr. *gloutos*, buttock) lies on the posterior aspect of the pelvis. It is the most superior part of the lower limb. It contains muscles that adduct and laterally rotate the thigh.

The order of dissection will be as follows: The fat and superficial fascia will be removed from the gluteal region. The borders of the gluteus maximus muscle will be defined and it will be reflected laterally to expose the muscles that lie deep to it. Muscles that lie deep to the gluteus maximus muscle will be studied. Arteries and nerves in the region will be studied. Note that the piriformis muscle will be a key landmark in understanding the relationships of this region.

SKELETON OF THE GLUTEAL REGION

Refer to a skeleton and an illustration of an articulated pelvis with intact ligaments. On the pelvis, identify (Fig. 6.13): [G 381; L 93; N 486; R 437; C 265]

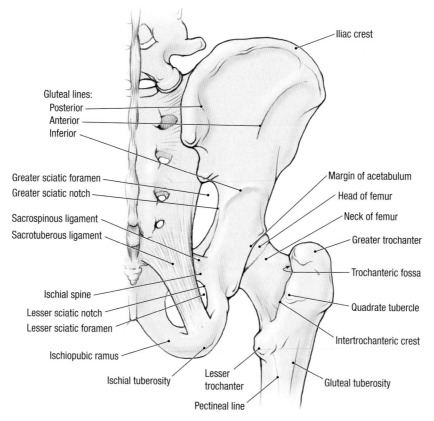

Figure 6.13. Skeleton of the gluteal region.

- **Gluteal lines (posterior, anterior, inferior)**
- **Greater sciatic foramen**
- **Greater sciatic notch**
- **Ischial spine**
- **Lesser sciatic notch**
- **Lesser sciatic foramen**
- **Ischial tuberosity**
- **Sacrotuberous ligament**
- **Sacrospinous ligament**

On the femur, identify (Fig. 6.13): [G 381; L 93; N 489; R 439; C 431]

- **Greater trochanter**
- **Intertrochanteric crest**
- **Trochanteric fossa**
- **Quadrate tubercle**
- **Gluteal tuberosity**

Dissection Instructions

1. Place the cadaver in the prone position.
2. Remove the superficial fascia from the surface of the fascia lata in the gluteal region. You should be able to see the gluteal aponeurosis (Fig. 6.14) before you proceed to step 3.
3. Identify the **gluteus maximus muscle** (Fig. 6.14). The proximal attachment of the gluteus maximus muscle is the part of the ilium that lies posterior to the posterior gluteal line, the posterior surface of the sacrum and coccyx, and the sacrotuberous ligament. The distal attachment of the gluteus maximus muscle is the iliotibial tract, and through it, the lateral condyle of the tibia. The deeper part of the inferior half of the gluteus maximus muscle attaches to the gluteal tuberosity of the femur. The gluteus maximus muscle is a powerful extensor of the thigh. [G 384; L 112; N 495; R 426; C 385]
4. Clean the superficial fascia from the inferior border of the gluteus maximus muscle. The inferior border should be visible from its proximal attachment on the sacrum and coccyx to its distal attachment on the iliotibial tract (Fig. 6.14).
5. Remove the fascia lata from the surface of the gluteus maximus muscle and use your fingers or a probe to define the superior border of the muscle. The superior border of the muscle should be visible from its proximal attachment on the iliac crest to its distal attachment on the iliotibial tract (Fig. 6.14)
6. The fascia lata is relatively thin over the superficial surface of the gluteus maximus muscle, but superior to the muscle it becomes thicker and forms the **gluteal aponeurosis.** The gluteal aponeurosis spans from the superior border of the gluteus maximus muscle to the iliac crest.

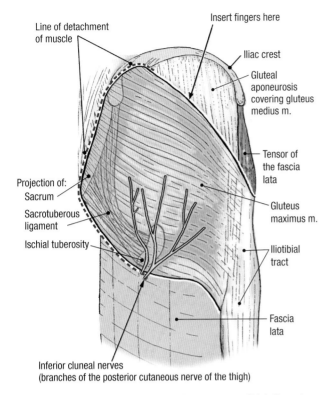

Line of detachment of muscle

Insert fingers here

Iliac crest

Gluteal aponeurosis covering gluteus medius m.

Tensor of the fascia lata

Projection of: Sacrum

Gluteus maximus m.

Sacrotuberous ligament

Ischial tuberosity

Iliotibial tract

Fascia lata

Inferior cluneal nerves (branches of the posterior cutaneous nerve of the thigh)

Figure 6.14. Muscles of the gluteal region, superficial dissection.

7. Insert your fingers between the gluteus maximus muscle and the gluteal aponeurosis (Fig. 6.14, arrow) and separate the gluteus maximus muscle from the aponeurosis.

8. Use scissors to detach the gluteus maximus from its proximal attachment. Start at the superior border of the muscle and cut the gluteus maximus muscle close to the ilium, sacrum, and sacrotuberous ligament (Fig. 6.14, dashed line).

9. Push your fingers deep to the gluteus maximus muscle and palpate the **inferior gluteal artery, vein,** and **nerve,** which are located near the center of the muscle. The inferior gluteal nerve is the only nerve supply to the gluteus maximus muscle, but the muscle receives blood from both the superior gluteal artery and the inferior gluteal artery.

10. Use scissors to cut the inferior gluteal vessels and nerve. Use your fingers to loosen the gluteus maximus muscle from deeper structures and reflect it laterally. The gluteus maximus muscle should remain attached only along its distal attachment, widely exposing the deeper structures of the gluteal region (Fig. 6.15). [G 386, 389; L 112; N 495; R 426; C 386]

11. Use a scalpel to incise the gluteal aponeurosis along the iliac crest. Use skinning motions to remove the gluteal aponeurosis from the superficial surface of the gluteus medius muscle. Note that the aponeurosis is firmly attached to the underly-

ing gluteus medius muscle and that it serves as an origin for that muscle.

12. Identify the **gluteus medius muscle.** To define its inferior border, insert your finger or a probe lateral to the superior gluteal vessels (Fig. 6.15) and open the interval between the gluteus medius muscle and the piriformis muscle.

13. The proximal attachment of the **gluteus medius muscle** is the deep surface of the gluteal aponeurosis and the lateral surface of the ilium between the **posterior gluteal line** and the **anterior gluteal line.** The distal attachment of the gluteus medius muscle is the greater trochanter of the femur and it is an abductor of the thigh.

14. The **piriformis muscle** is located inferior to the gluteus medius muscle. Note that its superior border lies adjacent to the inferior border of the gluteus medius muscle. To define its inferior border, insert your finger or a probe lateral to the inferior gluteal vessels (Fig. 6.15) and open the interval between the piriformis muscle and the superior gemellus muscle.

15. The proximal attachment of the piriformis muscle is the anterior surface of the sacrum and its distal attachment is the greater trochanter of the femur. The piriformis muscle is a lateral rotator of the thigh. Verify that the piriformis muscle passes through the greater sciatic foramen and nearly fills it.

16. Note that the **superior gluteal artery, vein,** and **nerve** exit the pelvic cavity and enter the gluteal region by passing over the superior border of the piriformis muscle (i.e., they pass between the piriformis muscle and the gluteus medius muscle).

17. Use blunt dissection to clean the inferior border of the piriformis muscle. Note that the **sciatic nerve, posterior cutaneous nerve of the thigh, inferior gluteal vessels, inferior gluteal nerve, nerve to obturator internus, internal pudendal vessels,** and **pudendal nerve** exit the pelvic cavity and enter the gluteal region by passing under the inferior border of the piriformis muscle.

18. Identify the **sciatic nerve** (Fig. 6.15). The sciatic nerve is the largest nerve in the body and it has a **tibial division** and a **common fibular division.** In about 12% of specimens the divisions may emerge separately with the common fibular division passing over the superior border of the piriformis muscle or through the center of the piriformis muscle.

19. Use your fingers to tear the fascia lata posterior to the sciatic nerve and follow the sciatic nerve for 6 or 7 cm into the thigh.

20. Identify the **posterior cutaneous nerve of the thigh,** which lies on the medial side of the sciatic nerve (Fig. 6.15).

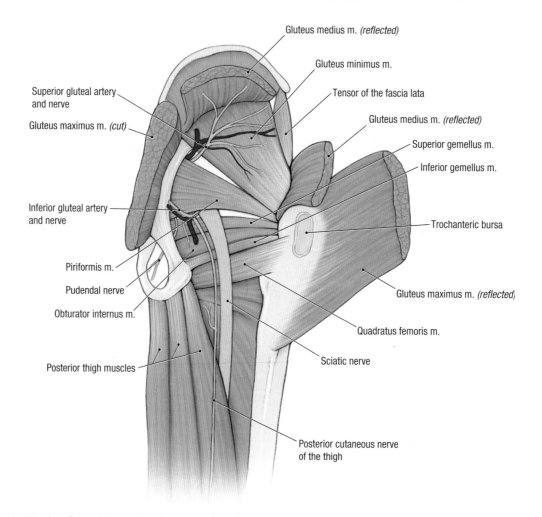

Gluteus medius m. *(reflected)*

Gluteus minimus m.

Tensor of the fascia lata

Superior gluteal artery and nerve

Gluteus maximus m. *(cut)*

Gluteus medius m. *(reflected)*

Superior gemellus m.

Inferior gemellus m.

Trochanteric bursa

Inferior gluteal artery and nerve

Piriformis m.

Pudendal nerve

Obturator internus m.

Gluteus maximus m. *(reflected)*

Quadratus femoris m.

Sciatic nerve

Posterior thigh muscles

Posterior cutaneous nerve of the thigh

Figure 6.15. Muscles of the gluteal region, deep dissection. The gluteus maximus and gluteus medius muscles have been reflected.

21. At the inferior border of the piriformis muscle, identify the cut ends of the **inferior gluteal vessels** and **nerve,** which lie on the medial side of the posterior cutaneous nerve of the thigh (Fig. 6.15).

22. Identify the **nerve to obturator internus, internal pudendal artery** and **vein,** and **pudendal nerve** near the medial end of the inferior border of the piriformis muscle (Fig. 6.15). The pudendal nerve and internal pudendal vessels enter the gluteal region by passing through the greater sciatic foramen and enter the perineum by passing through the lesser sciatic foramen. The pudendal nerve and internal pudendal vessels supply the anal and urogenital triangles.

23. Identify the tendon of the **obturator internus muscle** (Fig. 6.15). The obturator internus tendon is inferior to the superior gemellus muscle. The proximal attachment of the obturator inter-

nus muscle is the margin of the obturator foramen and the inner surface of the obturator membrane. The distal attachment of the obturator internus muscle is on the medial side of the greater trochanter of the femur, superior to the trochanteric fossa. The obturator internus muscle is a lateral rotator of the thigh. The obturator internus muscle exits the lesser pelvis by passing through the lesser sciatic foramen.

24. Identify the two **gemellus muscles** (L. *gemellus,* twin) (Fig. 6.15). The proximal attachment of the **superior gemellus muscle** is the ischial spine superior to the obturator internus muscle. The proximal attachment of the **inferior gemellus muscle** is the ischial tuberosity inferior to the obturator internus muscle. Both gemellus muscles attach with the obturator internus tendon on the greater trochanter of the femur and both are lateral rota-

tors of the thigh. Note: The two gemellus muscles may be large enough to hide the obturator internus tendon.

25. Identify the **quadratus femoris muscle** (Fig. 6.15), which is inferior to the inferior gemellus muscle. The proximal attachment of the quadratus femoris muscle is the ischial tuberosity and its distal attachment is onto the quadrate tubercle on the intertrochanteric crest of the femur. The quadratus femoris muscle is a lateral rotator of the thigh.

26. To expose the gluteus minimus muscle, first locate the branches of the **superior gluteal vessels** superior to the piriformis muscle (Fig. 6.15). Insert your finger superior to the superior gluteal vessels and deep to the gluteus medius muscle. Push your finger superiorly along the course of these vessels to open the plane of separation between the gluteus medius muscle and the gluteus minimus muscle.

27. Use scissors to transect the gluteus medius muscle, following the course of the superior gluteal vessels. Gently reflect the proximal portion of the muscle superiorly and observe the **superior gluteal nerve**.

28. Reflect the distal part of the gluteus medius muscle and identify the **gluteus minimus muscle** (Fig. 6.15). The proximal attachment of the gluteus minimus muscle is the lateral surface of the ilium between the **anterior gluteal line** and the **inferior gluteal line**. The distal attachment of the gluteus minimus muscle is on the greater trochanter of the femur and it abducts the thigh.

29. Identify the **tensor of the fascia lata (tensor fasciae latae muscle)**. It is within the fascia lata inferior to the anterior superior iliac spine (Fig. 6.15). The proximal attachment of the tensor of the fascia lata is the anterior superior iliac spine and its distal attachment is the **iliotibial tract**. The tensor of the fascia lata is an abductor and medial rotator of the thigh.

CLINICAL CORRELATION

Intragluteal Injections

The gluteal region is commonly used for intramuscular injections. These injections are made in the **superior lateral quadrant of the gluteal region**. Injections into the two inferior quadrants of the gluteal region would endanger the sciatic nerve, or the nerves and vessels that pass inferior to the piriformis muscle. Injections into the superior medial quadrant may injure the superior gluteal nerve and vessels. Intragluteal injections into the superior lateral quadrant are relatively safe since the superior gluteal nerve and vessels are well branched in this region.

Dissection Review

1. Replace the muscles of the gluteal region in their correct anatomical positions.
2. Review the attachments, action, and innervation of each muscle.
3. Study the functions of muscles in the gluteal region:
   - Extend your thigh. This movement is accomplished by the gluteus maximus muscle.
   - Abduct your thigh. This movement is accomplished by the gluteus medius muscle, gluteus minimus muscle, and tensor of the fascia lata.
   - Laterally rotate your thigh. This motion is accomplished by the piriformis muscle, obturator internus muscle, superior gemellus muscle, inferior gemellus muscle, and quadratus femoris muscle.
4. Review the anatomy of the safe intragluteal injection site.
5. If you have completed the dissection of the pelvis and perineum prior to dissection of the lower limb, study the continuity of muscles, vessels, and nerves observed in the gluteal and pelvic regions:
   - Within the pelvis identify the obturator internus muscle and follow the muscle posteriorly into the gluteal region.
   - Within the pelvis identify the piriformis muscle and then follow this muscle laterally to its attachment on the greater trochanter of the femur.
   - Within the pelvis study the gluteal vessels and their relationship to the piriformis muscle and the sacral plexus.
6. Review the sacral plexus and its contribution to the sciatic nerve. Note that the muscles of the gluteal region are innervated by branches of the sacral plexus. [L 111]

POSTERIOR COMPARTMENT OF THE THIGH

Dissection Overview

The posterior compartment of the thigh contains the posterior thigh muscles: **biceps femoris**, **semimembranosus**, and **semitendinosus**. The muscles of the posterior group extend the thigh and flex the leg. The posterior thigh muscles are commonly known as the "hamstring" muscles.

The order of dissection will be as follows: The muscles of the posterior compartment of the thigh will be studied. The course and branches of the sciatic nerve will be studied. The dissection will be extended inferiorly to include the popliteal fossa. The muscular boundaries of the popliteal fossa will be identified and the contents of the popliteal fossa will be studied.

SKELETON OF THE POSTERIOR THIGH

Refer to a skeleton. On the pelvis, identify (Fig. 6.6B): [G 381; L 93; N 486; R 438; C 265]

- **Ischial tuberosity**

  On the femur, identify: [G 381; L 93; N 489; R 439; C 431]

- **Lateral lip of linea aspera**
- **Lateral supracondylar line**
- **Medial condyle**
- **Lateral condyle**
- **Popliteal surface**

  On the fibula, identify: [G 381; L 95; N 513; R 440; C 447]

- **Apex**
- **Head**
- **Neck**

  On the tibia, identify:

- **Medial condyle**
- **Soleal line**

Dissection Instructions

POSTERIOR THIGH [G 385, 387; L 115; N 495; R 485; C 384, 390–393]

1. Place the cadaver in the prone position. Use scissors to incise the fascia lata from the level of the gluteus maximus muscle to the knee and open it widely.
2. Use blunt dissection to clean the **sciatic nerve** and follow it inferiorly. Note that the sciatic nerve passes deep to the long head of the biceps femoris muscle (Fig. 6.16).
3. Identify the **long head of the biceps femoris muscle**. The proximal attachment of the long head of the biceps femoris muscle is the ischial

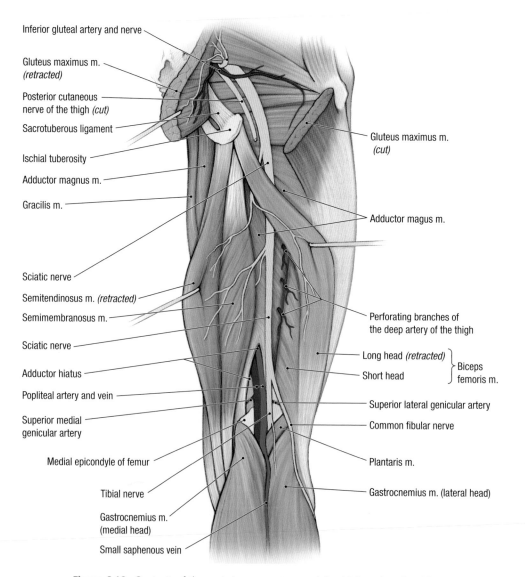

Figure 6.16. Contents of the posterior compartment of the thigh and popliteal fossa.

tuberosity and its distal attachment is the head of the fibula. The long head of the biceps femoris muscle is innervated by the tibial division of the sciatic nerve.

4. Retract the long head of the biceps femoris muscle laterally to observe the **short head of the biceps femoris muscle** (Fig. 6.16). The proximal attachment of the short head of the biceps femoris muscle is the lateral lip of the linea aspera of the femur. The tendon of the short head of the biceps femoris muscle joins the tendon of the long head. The biceps femoris muscle extends the thigh and flexes the leg. The short head of the biceps femoris muscle is innervated by the common fibular division of the sciatic nerve.

5. On the medial side of the thigh, identify the **semitendinosus muscle** (Fig. 6.16). The semitendinosus ("half tendon") muscle is named for the long, cord-like tendon at its distal end. The proximal attachment of the semitendinosus muscle is the ischial tuberosity and its distal attachment is the medial surface of the superior part of the tibia. The semitendinosus muscle extends the thigh and flexes the leg. The semimembranosus muscle is innervated by the tibial division of the sciatic nerve.

6. Use your fingers to separate the semitendinosus muscle from the **semimembranosus muscle**. The semimembranosus ("half membrane") muscle is named for the broad, membrane-like tendon at its proximal end. The proximal attachment of the semimembranosus muscle is the ischial tuberosity and its distal attachment is the posterior part of the medial condyle of the tibia. The semimembranosus muscle extends the thigh and flexes the leg. The semimembranosus muscle is innervated by the tibial division of the sciatic nerve.

7. Verify that the **hamstring part of the adductor magnus muscle** arises from the ischial tuberosity deep to the proximal attachment of the posterior thigh muscles. Confirm that the adductor magnus muscle forms the deep boundary of the posterior compartment of the thigh (Fig. 6.16). The hamstring part of the adductor magnus muscle is innervated by the tibial division of the sciatic nerve.

8. Follow the sciatic nerve through the posterior compartment of the thigh to the area behind the knee (Fig. 6.16). Note that the sciatic nerve gives off unnamed muscular branches to the posterior thigh muscles. The sciatic nerve typically divides at the level of the knee but this division may occur more superiorly, in the thigh or in the gluteal region.

CLINICAL CORRELATION

Sciatic Nerve

The sciatic nerve and its branches innervate the posterior muscles of the thigh and the muscles of the leg (which act on the foot). The cutaneous branches of the sciatic nerve innervate a large area of the lower limb. Thus, when the sciatic nerve is injured, significant peripheral neurologic deficits may occur: paralysis of the flexors of the knee and all muscles below the knee, and widespread numbness of the skin on the posterior aspect of the lower limb.

POPLITEAL FOSSA [G 402–404; L 117; N 502; R 487, 488; C 394–396]

1. Define the **borders of the popliteal fossa** (L. *poples*, ham):
   • **Superolateral** – biceps femoris muscle
   • **Superomedial** – semitendinosus and semimembranosus muscles
   • **Inferolateral and inferomedial** – the two heads of the gastrocnemius muscle
   • **Posterior** – skin and deep (popliteal) fascia
   • **Anterior** – popliteal surface of the femur, the posterior surface of the capsule of the knee joint, and the popliteus muscle

2. At the superior border of the popliteal fossa, the sciatic nerve divides into the **tibial** and **common fibular nerves** (Fig. 6.16).

3. Use blunt dissection to follow the **common fibular nerve** laterally along the superolateral border of the popliteal fossa. Note that the common fibular nerve parallels the biceps femoris tendon and passes superficial to the lateral head of the gastrocnemius muscle.

4. Remove the remnants of the deep fascia (popliteal fascia) to expose the medial and lateral heads of the gastrocnemius muscle. Use your fingers to separate the **tibial nerve** from the loose connective tissue that surrounds it and follow the nerve inferiorly. The tibial nerve passes deep to the plantaris and gastrocnemius muscles at the inferior border of the popliteal fossa (Fig. 6.16).

5. At the inferior border of the popliteal fossa, insert your index fingers between the two bellies of the gastrocnemius muscle. Pull the muscle bellies apart for a distance of 5 to 10 cm. This will expose the structures that pass from the popliteal fossa into the leg.

6. The **popliteal artery** and **vein** are located deep to the tibial nerve. Note that the popliteal artery and vein are enclosed by a connective tissue sheath. Use scissors to open the sheath. Extend the incision superiorly and inferiorly.

7. Use a probe to separate the popliteal artery from the popliteal vein. Preserve the popliteal vein but remove its tributaries to clear the dissection field.

8. Use an illustration to study the branches of the popliteal artery that participate in the formation of the arterial anastomoses around the knee joint (**genicular anastomosis**) (Fig. 6.17). Identify the **superior lateral genicular artery** and the **superior medial genicular artery**. These arteries are located deep in the popliteal fossa, proximal to the attachments of the gastrocnemius muscle. [G 416; L 117, 124; N 518; R 467; C 396]

9. Distally, the popliteal artery passes deep to the plantaris and gastrocnemius muscles (Fig. 6.16). Retract the popliteal artery posteriorly and identify the **inferior lateral genicular artery** and the **inferior medial genicular artery**. The inferior genicular arteries pass deep (distal) to the proximal attachments of the gastrocnemius muscle.

10. Use an illustration [G 416; L 148; N 530; R 482; C 396] to observe that the genicular anastomosis receives contributions from the femoral artery, lateral circumflex femoral artery, and anterior tibial artery.

11. Part of the floor of the popliteal fossa is formed by the **popliteus muscle** (Fig. 6.17). Retract the inferior end of the popliteal artery and vein and identify the popliteus muscle. It will be seen better when the posterior muscles of the leg are dissected.

12. At the medial side of the knee, observe that the **sartorius, gracilis**, and **semitendinosus tendons** converge on the proximal end of the tibia in an arrangement that is named the **pes anserinus** (L., goose's foot).

Dissection Review

1. Replace the muscles of the posterior compartment of the thigh into their correct anatomical positions.

2. Using the dissected specimen, review the attachments and actions of the posterior thigh muscles.

3. Trace the course of the sciatic nerve from the pelvis to the knee. Review its terminal branches.

4. Trace the femoral artery and vein from the level of the inguinal ligament to the popliteal fossa, naming its branches.

5. Review the course of the deep artery of the thigh through the medial compartment of the thigh, and then review the course of its perforating vessels through the adductor magnus and brevis muscles into the posterior compartment of the thigh.

6. Review the genicular anastomosis around the knee, naming the branches of the popliteal artery and lateral circumflex femoral artery that participate.

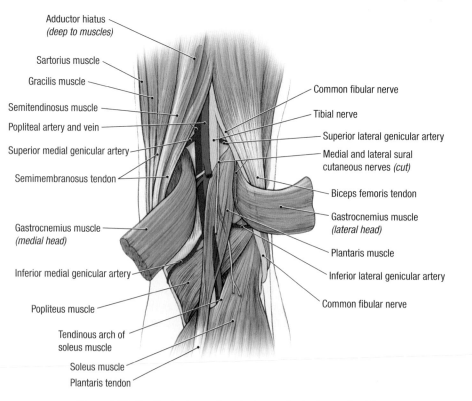

Figure 6.17. Popliteal artery and genicular arteries in the popliteal fossa.

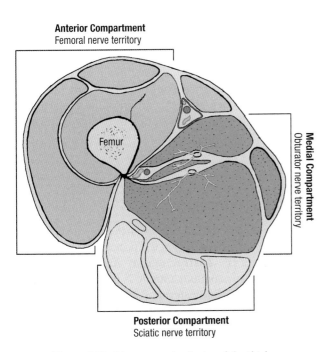

Figure 6.18. Motor nerve territories of the thigh.

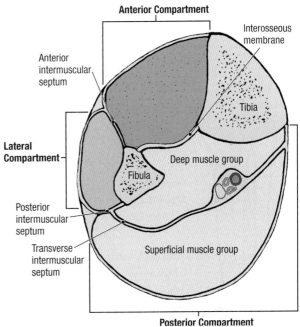

Figure 6.19. Compartments of the right leg, inferior view.

7. Review the principal muscle groups of the thigh, the group functions, and the innervation of each muscle group (Fig. 6.18):
   • **The anterior thigh muscles are innervated by the femoral nerve.**
   • **The medial thigh muscles are innervated by the obturator nerve.**
   • **The posterior thigh muscles are innervated by the tibial and common fibular divisions of the sciatic nerve.** [L 152]
8. Recall the exceptions to the rules of innervation stated above:
   • The pectineus muscle receives motor innervation from both the femoral nerve and the obturator nerve.
   • The ischiocondylar portion of the adductor magnus muscle is innervated by the tibial division of the sciatic nerve.

LEG AND DORSUM OF THE FOOT

The two bones of the leg are unequal in size. The larger **tibia** is the weight-bearing bone of the leg. The **fibula** is surrounded by muscles except at its proximal and distal ends. The tibia and fibula are joined by an **interosseous membrane** (Fig. 6.19). The **crural fascia** is attached to the fibula by two **intermuscular septa: anterior** and **posterior**. The tibia, fibula, interosseous membrane, and intermuscular septa divide the leg into **three compartments: posterior, lateral (fibular),** and **anterior** (Fig. 6.19). [G 369; L 118; N 522; C 400]

Skeleton of the Leg

Refer to a skeleton. On the tibia, identify (Fig. 6.20): [G 423; L 94, 95; N 513; R 440; C 447]

• **Medial condyle**
• **Lateral condyle**
• **Shaft (body)**
• **Anterior border**
• **Medial malleolus**
• **Soleal line**

On the fibula, identify (Fig. 6.20):

• **Head**
• **Neck**
• **Shaft (body)**
• **Lateral malleolus**

In the articulated foot, identify the seven tarsal bones (Fig. 6.21): [G 431, 444; L 94; N 523; R 442; C 450, 451]

• **Talus**
• **Calcaneus**
• **Navicular**
• **Cuboid**
• **Three cuneiform bones** – first (medial), second (intermediate, middle), and third (lateral)

On the **calcaneus**, identify (Fig. 6.21):

• **Calcaneal tuberosity**
• **Sustentaculum tali**

Identify the **five metatarsal bones** and the **tuberosity of the fifth metatarsal bone**.

Identify **14 phalanges**. Note that the first toe has only two phalanges, whereas the other toes each have three phalanges.

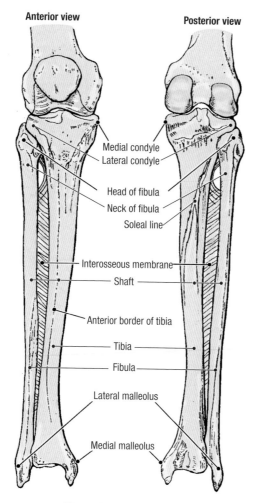

Anterior view

Posterior view

Medial condyle
Lateral condyle

Head of fibula
Neck of fibula
Soleal line

Interosseous membrane
Shaft

Anterior border of tibia

Tibia

Fibula

Lateral malleolus

Medial malleolus

Figure 6.20. Skeleton of the leg.

POSTERIOR COMPARTMENT OF THE LEG

Dissection Overview

The **posterior compartment of the leg** lies posterior to the interosseous membrane, tibia, and fibula (Fig. 6.19). A **transverse intermuscular septum** divides the muscles of the posterior compartment into superficial and deep groups. The superficial posterior group contains three muscles: **gastrocnemius**, **soleus**, and **plantaris**. The group action of the superficial posterior muscle group is plantar flexion of the foot. The deep posterior group contains four muscles: **popliteus**, **tibialis posterior**, **flexor digitorum longus**, and **flexor hallucis longus**. The shared actions of the deep posterior muscle group are inversion of the foot, plantar flexion of the foot, and flexion of the toes. The tibial nerve innervates both the superficial and deep posterior muscle groups.

The order of dissection will be as follows: The superficial veins and cutaneous nerves of the posterior aspect of the leg will be reviewed. The crural fascia of the posterior aspect of the leg will be incised and the superficial poste-

rior group of leg muscles will be examined. The muscles in the superficial posterior group will be reflected to expose the muscles of the deep posterior group. The vessels and nerves of the posterior compartment will be dissected. The muscles of the deep posterior group will be identified. The tendons of the deep posterior group of muscles will be organized where they pass posterior to the medial malleolus by use of a mnemonic device.

Dissection Instructions

1. Incise the crural fascia from the popliteal fossa to the calcaneus and open the posterior compartment.
2. Identify the **gastrocnemius muscle** (Fig. 6.22). The gastrocnemius muscle is the most superficial muscle in the posterior compartment of the leg. The proximal attachments of the **two heads of the gastrocnemius muscle** are the femoral condyles. The distal attachment of the gastrocnemius muscle is on the calcaneal tuberosity by way of the **calcaneal tendon (Achilles' tendon)**. The gastrocnemius muscle plantar flexes the foot. [G 434; L 119; N 516; R 457; C 413]
3. Use scissors to transect the two heads of the gastrocnemius muscle at the point where they join (Fig. 6.22). Reflect the proximal and distal portions of the muscle.
4. Identify the **soleus muscle**, which is located deep to the gastrocnemius muscle. The proximal attachments of the soleus muscle are the soleal line of the tibia and the head of the fibula. The distal attachment of the soleus muscle is the calcaneal tendon. The soleus muscle plantar flexes the foot. [G 435; L 120; N 517; R 457; C 415]
5. Identify the tendon of the **plantaris muscle** (Fig. 6.22). The belly of the plantaris muscle lies in the popliteal fossa and its proximal attachment is the lateral supracondylar line of the femur. In the proximal part of the leg the plantaris tendon courses between the gastrocnemius and soleus muscles. In the distal part of the leg the plantaris tendon may be seen on the medial side of the tendon of the gastrocnemius muscle. The plantaris tendon joins the calcaneal tendon and ultimately attaches to the calcaneus. The plantaris muscle is a plantar flexor of the foot and a weak flexor of the knee. The plantaris muscle and tendon may be absent.
6. The **tibial nerve** and **posterior tibial vessels** exit the popliteal fossa by passing deep to the tendinous arch of the soleus muscle (Fig. 6.22). They course distally in the **transverse intermuscular septum** that separates the superficial posterior muscle group from the deep posterior muscle group (Fig. 6.19).

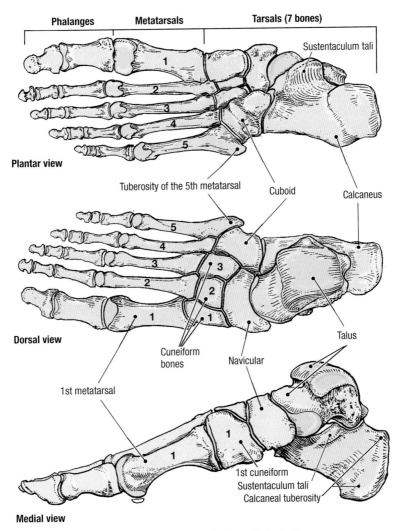

Phalanges   Metatarsals   Tarsals (7 bones)

Sustentaculum tali

Plantar view

Tuberosity of the 5th metatarsal   Cuboid   Calcaneus

Dorsal view

Cuneiform bones   Navicular   Talus

1st metatarsal

1st cuneiform
Sustentaculum tali
Calcaneal tuberosity

Medial view

Figure 6.21. Skeleton of the foot.

7. Use scissors to transect the calcaneal tendon about 5 cm superior to the tuberosity of the calcaneus (Fig. 6.22, dashed line). Use your fingers to separate the calcaneal tendon from the muscles that lie deep to it.

8. Use scissors to cut the soleus muscle beginning at its tibial (medial) attachment and extending across the leg to its fibular attachment (Fig. 6.22, dashed line), but leave the muscle attached to the fibula. This cut should pass 2.5 cm inferior to the tendinous arch of the soleus muscle (Fig. 6.23). Retract the soleus muscle and the distal part of the gastrocnemius muscle laterally to expose the transverse intermuscular septum.

9. Identify the **posterior tibial vessels** and the **tibial nerve** in the transverse intermuscular septum (Fig. 6.23). The posterior tibial artery is usually accompanied by two veins. Remove the veins to clear the dissection field. [G 436; L 121; N 518; R 490; C 417]

10. Use a probe to follow the posterior tibial artery and the tibial nerve proximally. Observe that the

popliteal artery bifurcates at the inferior border of the popliteus muscle to form the **posterior tibial artery** and the **anterior tibial artery**.

11. Retract the contents of the popliteal fossa laterally and identify the **popliteus muscle** (Fig. 6.23). The proximal attachment of the popliteus muscle is the lateral condyle of the femur and its distal attachment is the posterior surface of the proximal tibia. The popliteus muscle rotates the femur on the tibia to unlock the extended knee. It is also a weak flexor of the leg. [G 437; L 121; N 518; R 460; C 418]

12. Identify the **tibialis posterior muscle**. The proximal attachments of the tibialis posterior muscle are the tibia, fibula, and interosseous membrane. The distal attachments of the tibialis posterior muscle are the plantar surfaces of several tarsal bones. The tibialis posterior muscle is an inverter and plantar flexor of the foot.

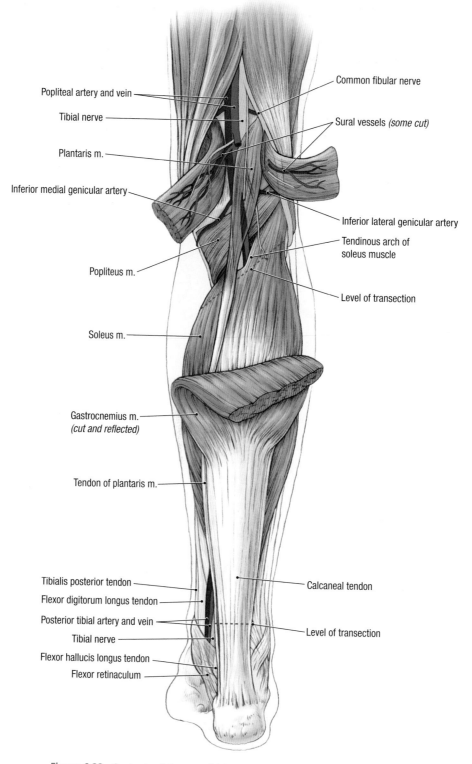

Popliteal artery and vein

Tibial nerve

Plantaris m.

Inferior medial genicular artery

Popliteus m.

Soleus m.

Gastrocnemius m.
(cut and reflected)

Tendon of plantaris m.

Tibialis posterior tendon

Flexor digitorum longus tendon

Posterior tibial artery and vein

Tibial nerve

Flexor hallucis longus tendon

Flexor retinaculum

Common fibular nerve

Sural vessels *(some cut)*

Inferior lateral genicular artery

Tendinous arch of
soleus muscle

Level of transection

Calcaneal tendon

Level of transection

Figure 6.22. Contents of the superficial posterior compartment of the leg.

13. The proximal attachment of the **flexor digitorum longus muscle** is the tibia. Distally, its tendons attach to the bases of the distal phalanges of the lateral four toes. The flexor digitorum longus muscle flexes toes 2 to 5 and plantar flexes the foot.

14. The proximal attachment of the **flexor hallucis longus muscle** (L. *hallux*, great toe; genitive, *hallucis*) is the inferior two-thirds of the fibula and interosseous membrane, and its distal attachment is the base of the distal phalanx of the great toe. The

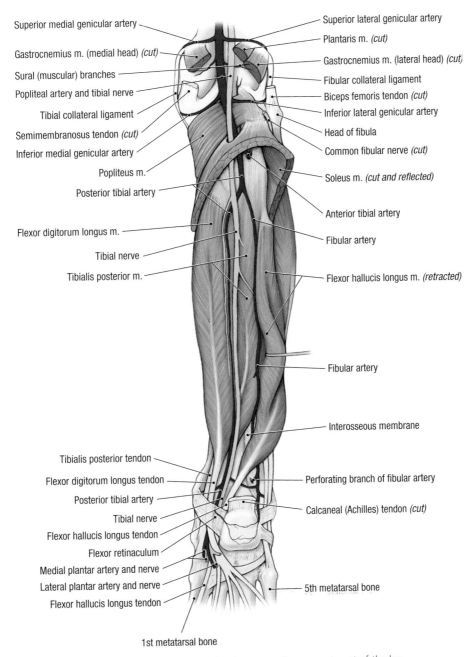

Superior medial genicular artery

Gastrocnemius m. (medial head) *(cut)*

Sural (muscular) branches

Popliteal artery and tibial nerve

Tibial collateral ligament

Semimembranosus tendon *(cut)*

Inferior medial genicular artery

Popliteus m.

Posterior tibial artery

Flexor digitorum longus m.

Tibial nerve

Tibialis posterior m.

Tibialis posterior tendon

Flexor digitorum longus tendon

Posterior tibial artery

Tibial nerve

Flexor hallucis longus tendon

Flexor retinaculum

Medial plantar artery and nerve

Lateral plantar artery and nerve

Flexor hallucis longus tendon

1st metatarsal bone

Superior lateral genicular artery

Plantaris m. *(cut)*

Gastrocnemius m. (lateral head) *(cut)*

Fibular collateral ligament

Biceps femoris tendon *(cut)*

Inferior lateral genicular artery

Head of fibula

Common fibular nerve *(cut)*

Soleus m. *(cut and reflected)*

Anterior tibial artery

Fibular artery

Flexor hallucis longus m. *(retracted)*

Fibular artery

Interosseous membrane

Perforating branch of fibular artery

Calcaneal (Achilles) tendon *(cut)*

5th metatarsal bone

Figure 6.23. Contents of the deep posterior compartment of the leg.

flexor hallucis longus muscle flexes the great toe and plantar flexes the foot.

15. Posterior to the medial malleolus, observe that the **posterior tibial artery** and the **tibial nerve** lie between the tendons of the flexor digitorum longus and flexor hallucis longus muscles, deep to the flexor retinaculum. (Fig. 6.23) Posterior to the medial malleolus, the following mnemonic device may be used to identify the tendons and vessels in anterior to posterior order: **T**om, **D**ick **AN**d **H**arry (**T**ibialis posterior, flexor **D**igitorum longus, posterior tibial **A**rtery, tibial **N**erve, flexor **H**allucis longus). [G 438; L 120, 121; N 516; C 416]

16. Once again, observe the vascular distribution in the posterior compartment of the leg (Fig. 6.23). Identify the **fibular artery**. The fibular artery arises from the posterior tibial artery about 2 or 3 cm distal to the inferior border of the popliteus muscle. The fibular artery courses distally between the tibialis posterior muscle and the flexor hallucis longus muscle. It supplies blood to the muscles of the lateral compartment of the leg and lateral side of the posterior compartment of the leg.

17. The **perforating branch of the fibular artery** usually arises just above the ankle joint (Fig 6.23).

It perforates the interosseous membrane and anastomoses with a branch of the anterior tibial artery. Occasionally, the perforating branch of the fibular artery will give rise to the dorsalis pedis artery.

Dissection Review

1. Replace the muscles of the posterior compartment of the leg into their correct anatomical positions.
2. Use the dissected specimen to review the attachments and action of each muscle dissected.
3. Follow the popliteal artery into the posterior compartment of the leg and identify its branches. Follow the posterior tibial artery distally and identify the origin of the fibular artery. Review the distribution of the arteries of the posterior compartment of the leg.
4. Follow the tibial nerve through the popliteal fossa and posterior compartment of the leg, observing that it gives off numerous muscular branches.
5. Review the relationships of the nerve, tendons, and vessels posterior to the medial malleolus and use this pattern to organize the contents of the deep posterior compartment of the leg.
6. Recall the rule of innervation of the posterior compartment of the leg:
   - **All muscles in the posterior compartment of the leg are innervated by the tibial nerve.**

LATERAL COMPARTMENT OF THE LEG [G 428, 429; L 122; N 521; R 459; C 404]

Dissection Overview

The lateral compartment of the leg contains two muscles: **fibularis brevis** and **fibularis longus**. The nerve of the lateral compartment is the superficial fibular nerve. The group action of the muscles in the lateral compartment of the leg is to evert and plantar flex the foot.

Dissection Instructions

1. Examine the crural fascia on the lateral side of the leg. Identify the **superior fibular retinaculum**, a thickening of the crural fascia. It is found on the lateral side of the ankle posterior to the lateral malleolus.
2. At the midlevel of the leg, identify the **superficial fibular nerve** where it penetrates the crural fascia (Figs. 6.3A and 6.24). Follow the superficial fibular nerve distally. It is the primary cutaneous nerve to the dorsum of the foot and gives rise to several **dorsal digital branches** (Fig. 6.24). The superfi-

cial fibular nerve is a branch of the common fibular nerve.
3. Use scissors to incise the crural fascia overlying the lateral compartment of the leg. Carry the incision as far inferiorly as the superior fibular retinaculum. Open the crural fascia and observe that the fibularis longus muscle is attached to its inner surface.
4. Follow the tendons of the **fibularis brevis** and **fibularis longus muscles** distally and observe that their tendons pass deep to the superior and inferior fibular retinacula. Note that the tendon of the fibularis brevis is anterior to the tendon of the fibularis longus where they pass posterior to the lateral malleolus.
5. Follow the tendon of the fibularis brevis muscle inferiorly to its distal attachment on the tuberosity of the fifth metatarsal bone (Fig. 6.24).
6. Follow the tendon of the fibularis longus muscle inferiorly and observe that it turns around the lateral side of the cuboid bone and enters the sole of the foot. The tendon of the fibularis longus muscle attaches to the plantar surface of the medial cuneiform and first metatarsal bones and it will be dissected with the sole of the foot.

CLINICAL CORRELATION

Common Fibular Nerve

The common fibular nerve is the most frequently injured nerve in the body because of its superficial position and relationship to the head and neck of the fibula. When the common fibular nerve is injured, there is impairment of eversion, dorsiflexion of the foot, and extension of the toes. The result is a condition called "foot drop," resulting in steppage gait (the advancing foot hangs with the toes pointed toward the ground, the knee being lifted high so that the toes may clear the ground). There will also be sensory loss on the dorsum of the foot and toes.

Dissection Review

1. Use the dissected specimen to review the attachments and actions of the muscles in the lateral compartment of the leg.
2. Understand that the fibular artery supplies the muscles of the lateral compartment of the leg by several small perforating branches that penetrate the posterior intermuscular septum.
3. Recall the rule of innervation for the lateral compartment of the leg: [L 151]
   - **Both of the muscles in the lateral compartment of the leg are innervated by the superficial fibular nerve.**

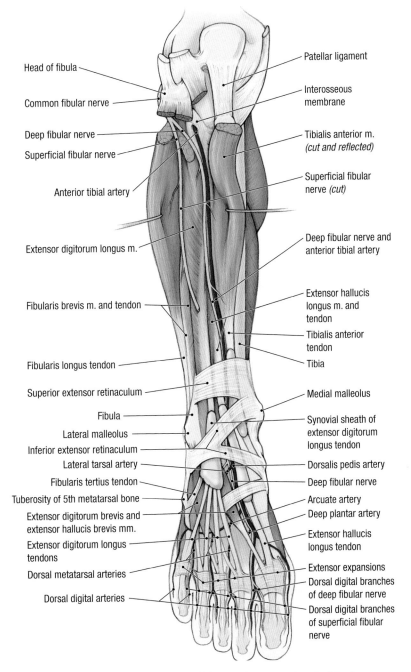

Head of fibula

Common fibular nerve

Deep fibular nerve

Superficial fibular nerve

Anterior tibial artery

Extensor digitorum longus m.

Fibularis brevis m. and tendon

Fibularis longus tendon

Superior extensor retinaculum

Fibula

Lateral malleolus

Inferior extensor retinaculum

Lateral tarsal artery

Fibularis tertius tendon

Tuberosity of 5th metatarsal bone

Extensor digitorum brevis and
extensor hallucis brevis mm.

Extensor digitorum longus
tendons

Dorsal metatarsal arteries

Dorsal digital arteries

Patellar ligament

Interosseous
membrane

Tibialis anterior m.
(cut and reflected)

Superficial fibular
nerve *(cut)*

Deep fibular nerve and
anterior tibial artery

Extensor hallucis
longus m. and
tendon

Tibialis anterior
tendon

Tibia

Medial malleolus

Synovial sheath of
extensor digitorum
longus tendon

Dorsalis pedis artery

Deep fibular nerve

Arcuate artery

Deep plantar artery

Extensor hallucis
longus tendon

Extensor expansions

Dorsal digital branches
of deep fibular nerve

Dorsal digital branches
of superficial fibular
nerve

Figure 6.24. Contents of the anterior compartment of the leg.

ANTERIOR COMPARTMENT OF THE LEG AND DORSUM OF THE FOOT [G 422, 423; L 123, 131; N 519, 520; R 462; C 399, 402]

Dissection Overview

The **anterior compartment** of the leg contains four muscles: **tibialis anterior**, **extensor hallucis longus**, **extensor digitorum longus**, and **fibularis tertius**. The deep fibular nerve innervates the muscles of the anterior compartment.

The group actions of the muscles in the anterior compartment are dorsiflexion of the foot, inversion of the foot, and extension of the toes.

The order of dissection will be as follows: The distribution of cutaneous nerves over the lower anterior surface of the leg and dorsal surface of the foot will be reviewed. The anterior aspect of the deep fascia of the leg and foot will be examined and the extensor retinacula will be identified. The anterior compartment of the leg will be opened and the relationships of tendons, vessels, and nerves will be examined on the anterior surface of the ankle. The tendon of each muscle of the anterior compartment will be followed into the foot. The intrinsic muscles of the dorsum of the foot will be identified. The deep vessels and deep nerve of the leg and dorsum of the foot will be dissected.

Dissection Instructions

1. Place the cadaver in the supine position.
2. Recall that the superficial fibular nerve provides most of the cutaneous innervation to the anterior surface of the ankle and dorsum of the foot (Fig. 6.3A).
3. Remove the remnants of superficial fascia on the anterior surface of the leg and dorsum of the foot. Preserve the branches of the superficial fibular nerve.
4. Observe the crural fascia and note that it is firmly attached to the anterior border of the tibia.
5. Identify the **superior** and **inferior extensor retinacula** on the anterior surface of the ankle. The retinacula are transverse thickenings of the crural fascia that hold tendons in place. The superior extensor retinaculum extends across the tendons superior to the ankle joint. The inferior extensor retinaculum is at the level of the ankle joint and it is Y-shaped. The stem of the "Y" is attached to the calcaneus.
6. Use a scalpel to make a vertical cut through the crural fascia just below the lateral condyle of the tibia. Use forceps to lift the edges of the crural fascia and observe that the muscles of the anterior compartment are attached to its deep surface. Extend the cut through the crural fascia in the distal direction as far as the inferior extensor retinaculum.
7. The proximal attachments of the anterior muscles of the leg are on the proximal tibia, fibula, and interosseous membrane. Do not attempt to dissect the proximal attachments.
8. Observe the vessels and nerves and the tendons of the anterior muscles of the leg where they cross the anterior surface of the ankle joint. From medial to lateral, identify (Fig. 6.24):
   • **Tibialis anterior tendon**
   • **Extensor hallucis longus tendon**
   • **Anterior tibial vessels**
   • **Deep fibular nerve**
   • **Extensor digitorum longus tendon**
   • **Fibularis tertius tendon**
9. Follow the tendon of the **tibialis anterior muscle** into the foot. Observe that the distal attachment of the tibialis anterior tendon is the first cuneiform bone and the base of the first metatarsal bone. The tibialis anterior muscle dorsiflexes and inverts the foot.
10. Follow the tendon of the **extensor hallucis longus muscle** into the foot. Observe that the distal attachment of the extensor hallucis longus tendon is the base of the distal phalanx of the great toe. The extensor hallucis longus muscle extends the great toe and dorsiflexes the foot.
11. Observe that the tendons of the **extensor digitorum longus muscle** attach to the middle and distal phalanges of the lateral four toes. The extensor digitorum longus muscle extends the toes and dorsiflexes the foot. Note that each of these tendons forms an **extensor expansion**.
12. Follow the tendon of the **fibularis tertius muscle** to its distal attachment on the dorsal surface of the shaft of the fifth metatarsal bone (Fig. 6.24). The fibularis tertius muscle dorsiflexes the foot and assists in eversion of the foot. The fibularis tertius muscle is absent in about 5% of specimens.
13. At the level of the superior extensor retinaculum, identify the **anterior tibial artery** (Fig. 6.24). Trace the anterior tibial artery proximally. Use your fingers to forcibly separate the extensor digitorum longus muscle and the tibialis anterior muscle. Follow the anterior tibial artery proximally between these two muscle bellies. [G 424; L 132; N 519; R 462; C 399]
14. Use a probe to clean the anterior tibial artery. Note that it passes over the superior border of the interosseous membrane (Fig. 6.24). Note that the anterior tibial artery lies directly on the anterior surface of the interosseous membrane and that it gives rise to unnamed muscular branches.
15. Observe that the **deep fibular nerve** joins the anterior tibial artery just below the knee (Fig. 6.24). The deep fibular nerve is the motor nerve of the anterior compartment of the leg and the muscles in the dorsum of the foot. Trace the deep fibular nerve proximally and confirm that it is a branch of the **common fibular nerve**.
16. Return to the ankle region and trace the distal end of the anterior tibial artery deep to the inferior extensor retinaculum. As the anterior tibial artery crosses the ankle joint, its name changes to **dorsalis pedis artery** (L. *pes, pedis*, foot). [G 426; L 133; N 520; R 497; C 402]
17. Use scissors to cut the inferior extensor retinaculum over the extensor digitorum longus tendons. Retract the tendons of the extensor digitorum longus muscle in the lateral direction.
18. On the dorsum of the foot deep to the tendons of the extensor digitorum longus muscle, identify the **extensor digitorum brevis muscle** and the **extensor hallucis brevis muscle** (Fig. 6.24). The extensor digitorum brevis and extensor hallucis brevis muscles share a common muscle belly that

attaches to the calcaneus. Four tendons arise from this muscle belly and attach to the extensor expansions of toes 1 to 4. The portion of this muscle that attaches on the great toe is called the extensor hallucis brevis muscle. These muscles extend the toes and they are innervated by the deep fibular nerve.

19. Follow the dorsalis pedis artery onto the dorsum of the foot. In the distal part of the leg, the dorsalis pedis artery passes deep to the extensor hallucis longus tendon to lie on the lateral side of the tendon at the ankle. In the living person, the pulse of the dorsalis pedis artery can be palpated between the tendons of the extensor hallucis longus muscle and the extensor digitorum longus muscle.

20. Identify the **arcuate artery**. The arcuate artery is a branch of the dorsalis pedis artery that crosses the proximal ends of the metatarsal bones. The lateral three **dorsal metatarsal arteries** are branches of the arcuate artery. [G 427; L 133; N 520; R 497; C 411]

21. Identify the **lateral tarsal artery**. The lateral tarsal artery arises from the dorsalis pedis artery near the ankle joint and passes deep to the extensor digitorum brevis and extensor hallucis brevis muscles. The lateral tarsal artery joins the lateral end of the arcuate artery to complete an arterial arch.

22. Identify the **deep plantar artery**. The deep plantar artery arises from the dorsalis pedis artery near the origin of the arcuate artery. The deep plantar artery passes between the first and second metatarsal bones to enter the sole of the foot. In the sole of the foot, the deep plantar artery anastomoses with the plantar arch.

23. At the level of the ankle, identify the **deep fibular nerve** (Fig. 6.24). Use blunt dissection to follow the deep fibular nerve into the dorsum of the foot. Note that the deep fibular nerve innervates the extensor digitorum brevis muscle and the extensor hallucis brevis muscle. The deep fibular nerve then continues toward the great toe to give rise to two **dorsal digital branches**.

24. Use an illustration and your cadaver specimen to trace the cutaneous branch of the deep fibular nerve to the region of skin between the great toe and the second toe (Fig. 6.24). Understand that the skin between the great toe and the second toe is the only skin on the dorsum of the foot that is innervated by the deep fibular nerve.

Dissection Review

1. Use the dissected specimen to review the attachments and actions of the muscles in the anterior compartment of the leg.

2. Trace the anterior tibial artery through the anterior compartment to the foot, where its name changes to dorsalis pedis artery. Review the branches of this arterial system.

3. Recall the rule of innervation for the anterior compartment of the leg and the dorsum of the foot: [L 151]
   • **All muscles in the anterior compartment of the leg and the dorsum of the foot are innervated by the deep fibular nerve.**

4. Review the principal muscle groups of the leg, the group functions, and the innervation of each muscle group (Fig. 6.25):
   • **The posterior leg muscles are innervated by the tibial nerve.**
   • **The lateral leg muscles are innervated by the superficial fibular nerve.**
   • **The anterior leg muscles are innervated by the deep fibular nerve.**

SOLE OF THE FOOT

Dissection Overview

The **foot is arched longitudinally** (Fig. 6.21). The **weight-bearing points** of the foot are the calcaneus posteriorly and the heads of the five metatarsal bones anteriorly. The **plantar aponeurosis** supports the longitudinal arch. Deep to the plantar aponeurosis are four layers of intrinsic foot muscles, tendons, vessels, and nerves.

The order of dissection will be as follows: The plantar aponeurosis will be cleaned of superficial fascia and stud-

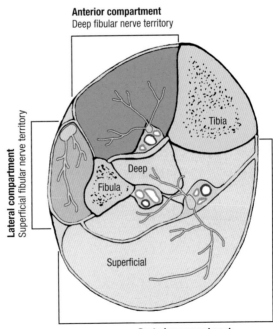

Figure 6.25. Motor nerve territories of the leg.

ied. It will then be reflected to expose the first layer of the sole. The dissection will proceed from superficial (inferior) to deep (superior) and each of the four layers of the sole will be dissected. Note that abduction and adduction movements of the toes are described around an axis of reference that passes through the second digit (second toe). This convention differs from the hand, in which the axis of reference passes through the third digit.

Dissection Instructions

PLANTAR APONEUROSIS AND CUTANEOUS NERVES
[G 443; L 134; N 532; R 463; C 422]

1. Place the cadaver in the prone position.
2. If the skin has not been removed from the sole of the foot, refer to Figure 6.2C and complete the skin removal.

3. Note that the plantar fascia over the medial and lateral portions of the sole is thin. In the median plane of the sole it is thickened to form the **plantar aponeurosis** (Fig. 6.26A).
4. Use a dull scalpel blade to scrape the superficial fascia off the plantar aponeurosis. The plantar aponeurosis is attached to the calcaneus posteriorly and it divides distally into five bands, one to each toe. Note that the five bands are joined by the superficial transverse metatarsal ligaments.
5. Use a scalpel to cut the plantar aponeurosis longitudinally (Fig. 6.26B). The plantar aponeurosis is approximately 4 mm thick. Do not cut too deeply.
6. Make two transverse cuts through the plantar aponeurosis: one cut at the proximal end close to the calcaneus and one cut in the anterior one-third of the foot (Fig. 6.26B).

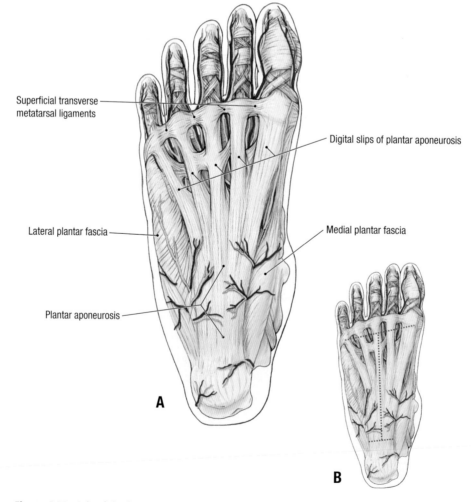

Figure 6.26. Sole of the foot. **A.** Plantar aponeurosis. **B.** Cuts used to open the plantar aponeurosis.

7. Tough bands of connective tissue attach the plantar aponeurosis to the metatarsal bones. Use a scalpel to cut these bands and release the plantar aponeurosis from the underlying structures. Reflect the flaps medially or laterally, respectively, and remove them (Fig. 6.26B).

FIRST LAYER OF THE SOLE [G 444; L 135; N 533; R 463; C 423]

1. Identify the **flexor digitorum brevis muscle** (Fig. 6.27). The proximal attachments of the flexor digitorum brevis muscle are the calcaneal tuberosity and the plantar aponeurosis. The distal attachments of the flexor digitorum brevis muscle are the middle phalanges of the lateral four toes. The flexor digitorum brevis muscle flexes the lateral four toes. Trace the flexor digitorum brevis tendons to their distal attachments. Remove remnants of the plantar aponeurosis as necessary.

2. Identify the **abductor hallucis muscle** (Fig. 6.27). The abductor hallucis muscle is located on the medial side of the flexor digitorum brevis muscle. The proximal attachments of the abductor hallucis muscle are the medial side of the calcaneal tuberosity and the plantar aponeurosis. The distal attachment of the abductor hallucis muscle is the medial side of the base of the proximal phalanx of the great toe and it abducts the great toe. Use blunt dissection to follow the tendon to its distal attachment.

3. Identify the **abductor digiti minimi muscle** (Fig. 6.27). The proximal attachments of the abductor digiti minimi muscle are the lateral side of the calcaneal tuberosity and the plantar aponeurosis and its distal attachment is the lateral side of the base of the proximal phalanx of the fifth (small) toe. The abductor digiti minimi muscle abducts the fifth toe. Follow the tendon to its distal attachment.

4. In the distal one-third of the sole of the foot, look for **common** and **proper plantar digital nerves**, which are branches of the **medial** and **lateral plantar nerves** (Fig. 6.27). The common and proper digital nerves lie between the tendons just identified.

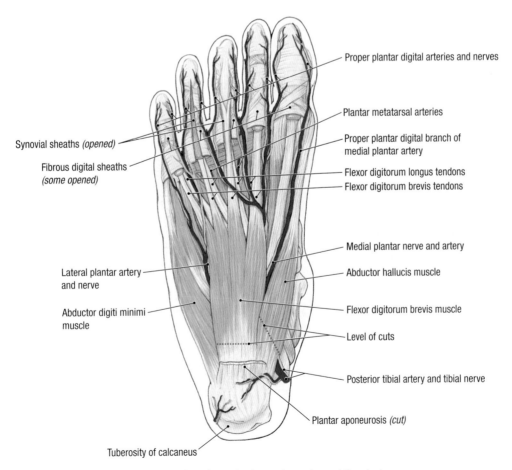

Figure 6.27. Sole of the foot. First layer of muscles and the plantar nerves.

SECOND LAYER OF THE SOLE [G 445; L 136; N 534; R 464; C 424]

1. Use scissors to transect the flexor digitorum brevis muscle close to the calcaneus (Fig. 6.27, dashed line). Reflect the muscle distally.
2. Push a probe deep to the abductor hallucis muscle from superior to inferior along the course of the posterior tibial artery and tibial nerve. Cut the abductor muscle over the probe (Fig. 6.27, dashed line).
3. Use blunt dissection to follow the posterior tibial artery and tibial nerve into the sole. Identify the **medial** and **lateral plantar nerves** and **arteries** (Fig. 6.28).
4. Identify the **quadratus plantae muscle**, which is deep to the flexor digitorum brevis muscle (Fig. 6.28). The proximal attachment of the quadratus plantae muscle is the calcaneus and its distal attachment is the tendon of the flexor digitorum longus muscle. The quadratus plantae muscle assists the flexor digitorum longus muscle in flexing the lateral four toes.

5. Use a probe to dissect the **flexor digitorum longus tendons** in the sole of the foot. Observe that its four tendons pass through the tendons of the flexor digitorum brevis muscle in the toes (Fig. 6.28).
6. Observe that four **lumbrical muscles** arise from the tendons of the flexor digitorum longus muscle. The distal attachments of the lumbrical muscles are the extensor expansions of the lateral four toes.

THIRD LAYER OF THE SOLE [G 446; L 137; N 535; R 465; C 427]

1. Use scissors to transect the flexor digitorum longus tendon where it is joined by the quadratus plantae muscle (Fig. 6.28, dashed line). Reflect the tendons distally, along with the lumbrical muscles.
2. Identify the **flexor hallucis brevis muscle** (Fig. 6.29). The flexor hallucis brevis muscle has a **medial head** and a **lateral head**, and each head has its own tendon. A **sesamoid bone** is found in each of the tendons. The proximal attachments of the flexor hallucis brevis muscle are the first

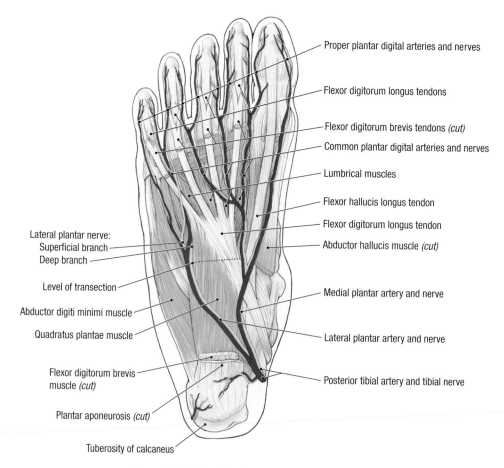

Proper plantar digital arteries and nerves

Flexor digitorum longus tendons

Flexor digitorum brevis tendons *(cut)*

Common plantar digital arteries and nerves

Lumbrical muscles

Flexor hallucis longus tendon

Flexor digitorum longus tendon

Abductor hallucis muscle *(cut)*

Medial plantar artery and nerve

Lateral plantar artery and nerve

Posterior tibial artery and tibial nerve

Lateral plantar nerve:
Superficial branch
Deep branch

Level of transection

Abductor digiti minimi muscle

Quadratus plantae muscle

Flexor digitorum brevis muscle *(cut)*

Plantar aponeurosis *(cut)*

Tuberosity of calcaneus

Figure 6.28. Sole of the foot. Second layer of muscles.

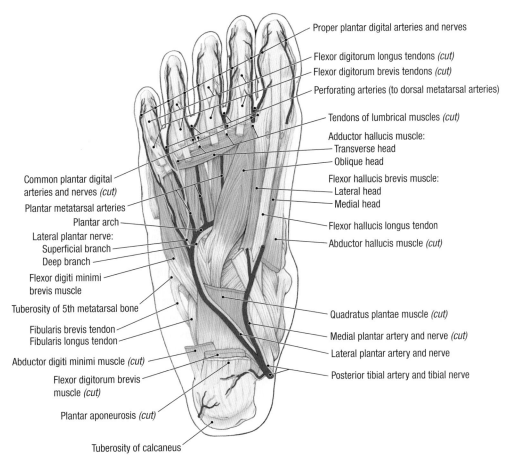

Proper plantar digital arteries and nerves

Flexor digitorum longus tendons *(cut)*
Flexor digitorum brevis tendons *(cut)*
Perforating arteries (to dorsal metatarsal arteries)

Tendons of lumbrical muscles *(cut)*
Adductor hallucis muscle:
Transverse head
Oblique head
Flexor hallucis brevis muscle:
Lateral head
Medial head
Flexor hallucis longus tendon
Abductor hallucis muscle *(cut)*

Quadratus plantae muscle *(cut)*
Medial plantar artery and nerve *(cut)*
Lateral plantar artery and nerve
Posterior tibial artery and tibial nerve

Common plantar digital
arteries and nerves *(cut)*
Plantar metatarsal arteries
Plantar arch
Lateral plantar nerve:
Superficial branch
Deep branch
Flexor digiti minimi
brevis muscle
Tuberosity of 5th metatarsal bone
Fibularis brevis tendon
Fibularis longus tendon
Abductor digiti minimi muscle *(cut)*
Flexor digitorum brevis
muscle *(cut)*
Plantar aponeurosis *(cut)*
Tuberosity of calcaneus

Figure 6.29. Sole of the foot. Third layer of muscles.

metatarsal bone, the cuboid bone, and the third cuneiform bone. The distal attachment of the flexor hallucis brevis muscle is the base of the proximal phalanx of the great toe and it flexes the great toe.

3. Observe that the **tendon of the flexor hallucis longus muscle** lies between the two sesamoid bones of the flexor hallucis brevis muscle. Verify that the tendon of the flexor hallucis longus is attached to the base of the distal phalanx of the great toe (Fig. 6.29).

4. Identify the **adductor hallucis muscle**. The adductor hallucis muscle has a **transverse head** and an **oblique head** (Fig. 6.29). Both heads attach to the lateral side of the base of the proximal phalanx of the great toe. The adductor hallucis muscle adducts the great toe (i.e., moves it toward the second toe).

5. Identify the **flexor digiti minimi muscle**. The proximal attachment of the flexor digiti minimi muscle is the base of the fifth metatarsal bone and its distal attachment is the base of the proximal phalanx of the fifth toe. The flexor digiti minimi muscle flexes the fifth toe.

FOURTH LAYER OF THE SOLE [G 447; L 138; N 536; R 465; C 428]

1. Use blunt dissection to trace the lateral plantar artery distally. At the level of the base of the metatarsal bones, the lateral plantar artery turns deeply to form the **plantar arch** (Fig. 6.29). Follow the plantar arch medially until it passes deep to the oblique head of the adductor hallucis muscle.

2. The medial end of the plantar arch is formed by the **deep plantar branch of the dorsalis pedis artery** (Fig. 6.24). Use an illustration to study the pattern of distribution of the **plantar metatarsal arteries** that arise from the plantar arch. [G 446; L 139; N 536; R 502; C 428]

3. The **interosseous muscles** are located superior (deep) to the plantar arch. Use an illustration to study the **interosseous muscles.** [G 447; L 138; N 537; R497, 502; C 428] The four **D**orsal interosseous muscles are **AB**ductors (**DAB**) and the three **P**lantar interosseous muscles are **AD**ductors (**PAD**) of the toes. Recall that the reference axis for abduction and adduction passes through the second toe.

4. Locate the **fibularis longus tendon** posterior to the lateral malleolus (Fig. 6.29). Insert a probe along its superficial surface, deep to the abductor digiti minimi muscle. Use scissors to transect the abductor digiti minimi muscle over the probe and reflect the muscle. Follow the fibularis longus tendon into the sole of the foot and note that it turns deeply around the lateral surface of the navicular bone.

5. In the sole, insert the probe along the superficial surface of the fibularis longus tendon (into its tendon sheath) and gently push the probe medially across the sole as far as it will go. The tip of the probe will stop near the distal attachment of the fibularis longus tendon. Wiggle the probe so that you can see where the tip is and note that the fibularis longus tendon crosses the sole of the foot at its deepest plane. The distal attachment of the fibularis longus tendon is onto the base of the first metatarsal bone and the first cuneiform bone.

6. Follow the **tibialis posterior tendon** distally and verify that it has a broad distal attachment on the navicular bone, all three cuneiform bones, and the bases of the second, third, and fourth metatarsal bones.

7. Once again, identify the **flexor hallucis longus muscle** in the posterior compartment of the leg. Follow its tendon distally until it disappears into an osseofibrous tunnel at the medial side of the ankle. Push a probe into the tunnel, and then open it with a scalpel. Lift the tendon of the flexor hallucis longus muscle with a probe and verify that it crosses the inferior surface of the **sustentaculum tali**. The sustentaculum tali acts as a pulley to change the direction of force of the flexor hallucis longus muscle.

Dissection Review

1. Replace the structures of the four layers of the sole of the foot into their correct anatomical positions.
2. Using the dissected specimen, review the attachments and action of each muscle. Organize the muscles from superficial (inferior) to deep (superior).
3. Follow the posterior tibial artery from its origin in the leg to its bifurcation in the sole of the foot. Use an illustration and the dissected specimen to review the distribution of the medial and lateral plantar arteries. Review the connection between the deep plantar arch and the deep plantar branch of the dorsalis pedis artery.
4. Trace the course of the tibial nerve from the popliteal fossa to the medial side of the ankle. Follow its two branches in the sole of the foot (medial and lateral plantar nerves). Use a textbook description to help you relate the motor and sensory function of the lateral and medial plantar nerves to your dissected specimen: [L 153]

- The medial plantar nerve innervates the abductor hallucis muscle, flexor digitorum brevis muscle, flexor hallucis brevis muscle, and medial lumbrical muscle. The medial plantar nerve will provide cutaneous innervation to the plantar surfaces of the medial $3\frac{1}{2}$ toes. The motor and cutaneous distribution of the medial plantar nerve is comparable to the distribution of the median nerve in the hand.
- The lateral plantar nerve innervates all other muscles in the sole of the foot and provides cutaneous innervation to the plantar surfaces of the lateral $1\frac{1}{2}$ toes. The motor and cutaneous distribution of the lateral plantar nerve is comparable to the distribution of the ulnar nerve in the hand.
- The proper plantar digital nerves innervate the dorsal surface of the toes as far proximally as the distal interphalangeal joint. The nail bed is included in the area innervated by the proper plantar digital nerves. This pattern of innervation has significance for proper application of local anesthesia prior to removal of damaged toe nails.

JOINTS OF THE LOWER LIMB

Dissection Overview

Dissect the joints of one lower limb. Keep the soft tissue structures of the other limb intact for review purposes.

The order of dissection will be as follows: The hip will be dissected, then the knee joint. The ankle joint will be dissected. The intermetatarsal joints, which are responsible for inversion and eversion, will be studied. During this dissection, the muscles of one limb will be removed. Take advantage of this opportunity to review the attachments, innervation, and action of each muscle as it is removed.

Dissection Instructions

HIP JOINT

1. Review the bony features of the hip joint. Three bones form the acetabulum: **ilium**, **ischium**, and **pubis**. Review the proximal end of the femur and identify the following: **head, fovea for the ligament of the head, neck**, and **intertrochanteric line**.
2. Remove the sartorius muscle, rectus femoris muscle, and pectineus muscle.
3. Identify the **iliopsoas muscle**. Trace its tendon to the lesser trochanter. Sever the tendon of the iliopsoas muscle close to the lesser trochanter and reflect the muscle superiorly.

4. Use an illustration to identify the ligaments that contribute to the formation of the **fibrous joint capsule: iliofemoral ligament, ischiofemoral ligament**, and **pubofemoral ligament** (Figs. 6.30 and 6.31). [G 394, 395; L 140; N 487; R 444, 445; C 432]

5. Examine the **iliofemoral ligament**. Verify that the distal end of the iliofemoral ligament is attached to the intertrochanteric line of the femur. The proximal end is attached to the anterior inferior iliac spine and the margin of the acetabulum.

6. Flex and extend the femur. Observe that the iliofemoral ligament becomes lax in flexion and taut in extension. The iliofemoral ligament prevents overextension of the hip joint.

7. Use a scalpel to open the anterior aspect of the **joint capsule** as illustrated in Figure 6.30.

8. Inside the joint capsule, observe the **cartilage on the articular surface of the head of the femur**. Rotate the femur laterally and note that you can see more of the articular surface of the head. Rotate the femur medially and observe that the articular surface disappears into the acetabulum. [G 394; L 141; N 487; R 445; C 433]

9. Abduct and laterally rotate the femur. Identify the **ligament of the head of the femur** (Fig. 6.30).

10. Identify the **obturator externus muscle**. Note that the obturator externus muscle passes inferior to the neck of the femur.

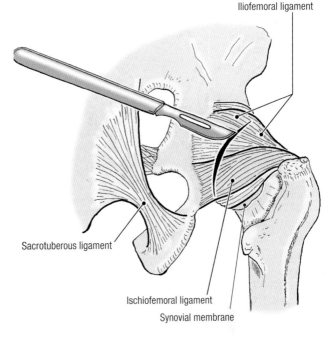

Figure 6.31. How to open the posterior aspect of the hip joint capsule.

11. Remove the obturator externus muscle to expose the **pubofemoral ligament**.

12. Turn the specimen to the prone position.

13. Remove the piriformis, superior gemellus, obturator internus, inferior gemellus, quadratus femoris, gluteus medius, and gluteus minimus muscles.

14. Use a scalpel and scraping motions to clean the posterior surface of the **joint capsule** (Fig. 6.31).

15. Identify the **ischiofemoral ligament**, which runs from the acetabular margin to the neck of the femur. Note that the ischiofemoral ligament does not attach to the intertrochanteric crest but leaves an area where the synovial membrane of the hip joint is exposed.

16. Extend the femur. Observe that the ischiofemoral ligament becomes taut and limits extension of the hip joint.

17. Open the posterior wall of the joint cavity by incising the capsule as shown in Figure 6.31. Observe the thickness of the joint capsule.

18. The next objective is to disarticulate the hip joint. Return the specimen to the supine position. Insert a probe under the ligament of the head of the femur (Fig. 6.30) and cut the ligament with a scalpel. Rotate the femur laterally and the head of the femur will come out of the acetabulum.

19. Examine the head and neck of the femur (Fig. 6.32). Identify the **articular surface** of the head of the femur. Observe the cut end of the **ligament of the head of the femur** and identify the **artery of the ligament of the head of the femur** in the

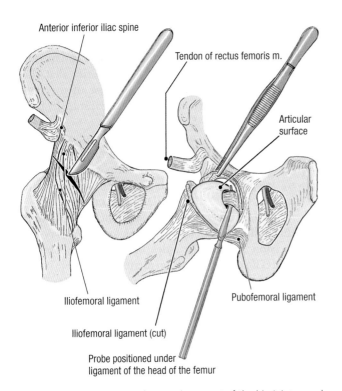

Figure 6.30. How to open the anterior aspect of the hip joint capsule.

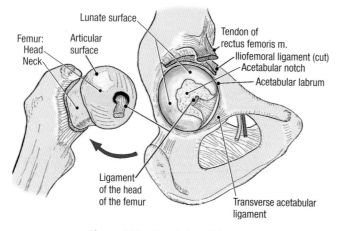

Femur:
Head
Neck
Articular
surface
Lunate surface
Tendon of
rectus femoris m.
Iliofemoral ligament (cut)
Acetabular notch
Acetabular labrum
Ligament
of the head
of the femur
Transverse acetabular
ligament

Figure 6.32. Disarticulated hip joint.

center of the ligament. Use an illustration to review the blood supply to the head and neck of the femur.

20. Identify the **lunate surface** in the acetabulum (Fig. 6.32). Note that the **ligament of the head of the femur** lies in the **acetabular notch**. [G 396; L 141; N 487; R 445; C 433]

21. Identify the **transverse acetabular ligament** that bridges the acetabular notch and the **acetabular labrum** that surrounds the rim of the acetabulum.

CLINICAL CORRELATION

Neck of the Femur

A fracture of the neck of the femur disrupts the blood supply to the head of the femur. If the blood supply (via the artery of the ligament of the head) is insufficient, the head will become necrotic. Necrosis of the femoral head is a common complication in femoral neck fractures in the elderly.

KNEE JOINT

1. Review the skeleton of the knee. On the distal end of the femur, identify the **medial condyle, lateral condyle**, and **intercondylar fossa**. On the proximal end of the tibia, identify the **superior articular surface, medial condyle, lateral condyle**, and **intercondylar eminence**. On the patella, identify the **articular surface** and **anterior surface**.

2. On the medial side of the knee, use a scalpel to detach the tendons of the sartorius, gracilis, and semitendinosus muscles from their distal attachments (pes anserinus). [G 408; L 142, 143; N 506; R 446; C 436]

3. Reflect the muscles and identify the **tibial collateral ligament** of the knee (Fig. 6.33). Note that the tibial collateral ligament is attached to the medial meniscus through the joint capsule.

4. On the lateral side of the knee, cut the tendon of the biceps femoris muscle close to its distal attachment on the head of the fibula.

5. Reflect the biceps femoris muscle and identify the **fibular collateral ligament** of the knee. Note that the fibular collateral ligament is not attached to the external surface of the joint capsule (Fig. 6.33). Observe that the popliteus tendon passes between the fibular collateral ligament and the joint capsule. [G 409; L 145; N 506; R 446; C 438]

6. On the posterior surface of the knee, remove the popliteal vessels, the tibial nerve, and the common fibular nerve.

7. Detach the semimembranosus and semitendinosus tendons and reflect the muscles. Note the oblique popliteal ligament that sweeps superiorly and laterally from the tendon of the semimembranosus muscle. The oblique popliteal ligament reinforces the posterior surface of the knee joint capsule.

8. Free the plantaris muscle and both heads of the gastrocnemius muscle from the joint capsule. Detach the proximal attachments of these muscles close to the femur.

9. Remove the popliteus muscle. As you do so, note the presence of the arcuate popliteal ligament that spans across the superficial surface of the popliteus tendon. During removal of the popliteus muscle the posterior wall of the joint capsule will be opened. Clear away the remnants of the posterior wall of the joint capsule to expose the joint cavity

10. From the posterior view, identify the **posterior cruciate ligament** (Fig. 6.33A). Verify that the cruciate ligaments are located *outside* of the synovial cavity but are *inside* the joint capsule. [G 412; L 145; N 509; R 446; C 440]

11. On the anterior surface of the knee, identify the tendon of the quadriceps femoris muscle. Observe that the tendon has **patellar retinacula** that help to keep the patella centered. Inferior to the patella, identify the **patellar ligament**.

12. Make a transverse incision superior to the patella through the quadriceps femoris tendon. Carry the incision around the sides of the knee, stopping short of the collateral ligaments.

13. Reflect the patella and patellar ligament inferiorly (Fig. 6.33B). Confirm that the femur and the tibia remain attached to each other by **two collateral ligaments** and **two cruciate ligaments**. [G 411; L 145; N 507; R 447; C 436]

14. Verify that the cruciate ligaments cross each other (Fig. 6.33C). The **anterior cruciate ligament** at-

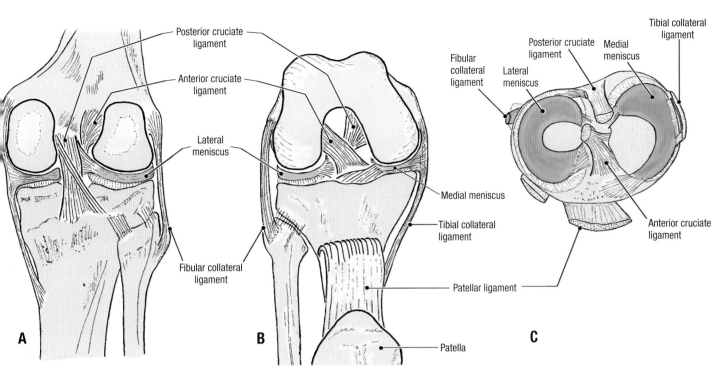

Figure 6.33. Right knee joint. **A.** Posterior view. **B.** Anterior view. **C.** Superior view.

taches to the tibia anteriorly. The **posterior cruciate ligament** attaches to the tibia posteriorly.

15. Extend the leg. With the leg in this position, observe:
    • The articular surfaces of the femur and tibia are in maximum contact.
    • The joint is "locked" in its most stable position.
    • The anterior cruciate ligament is taut and prohibits further extension.
16. Flex the leg. With the leg in this position, observe:
    • There is less contact between the articular surfaces of the femur and tibia.
    • Some rotation occurs in the knee joint.
    • The posterior cruciate ligament prevents the tibia from being pushed posteriorly.
    • The anterior cruciate ligament prevents the tibia from being pulled anteriorly.
17. Flex the leg and pull the tibia anteriorly. Note the tightness of the joint. Cut the anterior cruciate ligament. Now flex the leg and pull the tibia anteriorly. Feel the forward movement of the tibia. This forward movement indicates a ruptured anterior cruciate ligament and is an important clinical sign (anterior drawer sign).
18. Observe the **menisci** (Fig. 6.33C). Note that the **medial meniscus** is firmly attached to the tibial collateral ligament. In contrast, the **lateral meniscus** is not attached to the fibular collateral ligament.

CLINICAL CORRELATION

Knee Injuries

The medial meniscus is injured six to seven times more often than the lateral meniscus because the medial meniscus is firmly attached to the tibial collateral ligament.

Forced abduction and lateral rotation of the leg may result in the simultaneous injury of three structures: tibial collateral ligament, medial meniscus, and anterior cruciate ligament. The injury has been named the "unhappy triad." This injury is caused by a blow to the lateral side of the knee and is a common injury in contact sports.

ANKLE JOINT [G 454; L 146; N 527; R 450; C 452, 453]

1. Review the bony landmarks related to the ankle joint. On the distal end of the fibula identify the **lateral malleolus**. On the distal end of the tibia, identify the **medial malleolus**. On the talus, identify the **trochlea**. Review the tarsal bones.
2. Cut and reflect the tendons, vessels, and nerves that cross the anterior aspect of the ankle joint. Leave a 7.5-cm-long portion of the tibialis anterior tendon attached to the medial cuneiform and first metatarsal bone.
3. On the medial aspect of the ankle joint, cut and reflect the flexor digitorum longus muscle. Retract

the tendon of the tibialis posterior muscle anteriorly. Do not cut it.

4. Clean and define the **medial (deltoid) ligament of the ankle** (Fig. 6.34A). Identify its four parts:
   - **Posterior tibiotalar ligament**
   - **Tibiocalcaneal ligament**
   - **Tibionavicular ligament**
   - **Anterior tibiotalar ligament**

5. On the lateral side of the ankle, identify the tendons of the fibularis longus and fibularis brevis muscles. Open the superior and inferior fibular retinacula. Retract the tendons of the fibularis longus and fibularis brevis muscles anteriorly.

6. Clean and define the **lateral ligament of the ankle** (Fig. 6.34B). Identify its three parts:
   - **Posterior talofibular ligament**
   - **Calcaneofibular ligament**

- **Anterior talofibular ligament**

7. Dorsiflex and plantar flex the ankle joint. Observe that these are the only actions of the ankle joint.

Ankle Injuries

The ankle joint is the most frequently injured major joint in the body. The lateral ligament of the ankle is injured when the foot is forcefully inverted. The result is an ankle sprain with swelling around the lateral malleolus. In severe cases, the calcaneofibular and talofibular ligaments are torn, and the inferior tip of the lateral malleolus may be avulsed (pulled off).

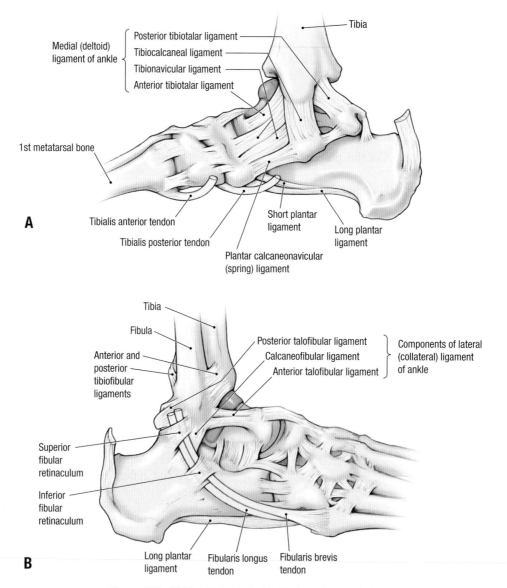

Figure 6.34. Right ankle joint. **A.** Medial view. **B.** Lateral view.

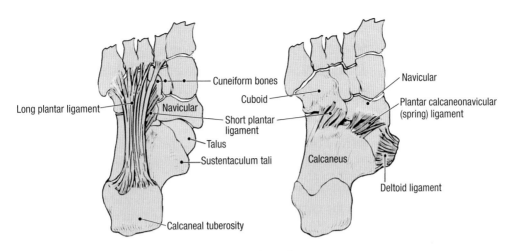

Figure 6.35. Plantar ligaments.

JOINTS OF INVERSION AND EVERSION

1. Study the movements of inversion and eversion of the foot in a suitable skeletal specimen (use caution—wired laboratory skeletons can be damaged). With one hand, immobilize the ankle joint by holding the talus stationary between the tibia and fibula. With the other hand, invert and evert the foot. Observe:
   - The talus remains fixed in the ankle joint.
   - The foot rotates about the inferior surface of the talus (subtalar joint) and anterior surface of the talus (talonavicular joint).

2. In the cadaver specimen, produce **eversion** by pulling on the tendons of the fibularis longus and fibularis brevis muscles. Produce **inversion** by pulling on the tendons of the tibialis anterior and tibialis posterior muscles simultaneously.

3. Observe that these movements occur in the **transverse tarsal joint** (calcaneocuboid and talonavicular joints) and the **subtalar joint**.

4. The longitudinal arch of the foot is supported by ligaments that span the tarsal bones. In the sole of the foot, remove the flexor digitorum brevis and quadratus plantae muscles. Observe the **long plantar ligament** and the **short plantar ligament** (Fig. 6.35). [G 464; L 147; N 528; R 449; C 455]

5. Remove the tendon of the tibialis posterior muscle where it crosses inferior to the talus. Identify the **plantar calcaneonavicular (spring) ligament** (Fig. 6.35). This ligament and the tibialis posterior tendon support the head of the talus and the longitudinal arch.

The study of head and neck anatomy provides a considerable intellectual challenge because the region is packed with small, important structures. These structures are associated with the proximal ends of the respiratory and gastrointestinal systems, the cranial nerves, and the organs of special sense. Dissection of the head and neck provides a special problem in that peripheral structures must be dissected long before their parent structure can be identified. A complete understanding of the region cannot be gained until the final dissection is completed.

The neck will be dissected before the head. The superficial aspects of the neck (superficial fascia, superficial veins, and cutaneous nerves) will be dissected first. Then, the neck will be dissected region by region and the regions will be defined as triangles. The vascular structures that go to the head as well as the endocrine glands in the neck will be dissected. The pharynx and larynx will be dissected after the head because they cannot be mobilized until after the head is dissected.

NECK

The neck is a region of transition between the head and the thorax. The major vessels that supply the head pass through the neck. The nerves that innervate the organs within the thorax and abdomen pass through the neck. Portions of several systems are located in the neck: gastrointestinal system (pharynx and esophagus), respiratory system (larynx and trachea), cardiovascular system (major vessels to the head and upper limbs), central nervous system (spinal cord), and endocrine system (thyroid and parathyroid glands). Finally, nerves and vessels to the upper limbs pass through the inferior part of the neck.

Skeleton of the Neck

The bones of the neck were first studied in Chapter 1, The Back. Use an articulated skeleton and your atlas to recall several characteristics of the cervical vertebrae. Cervical vertebrae have:

- Small bodies
- Relatively large vertebral foramina
- Bifid spinous processes
- Transverse processes that contain a transverse foramen (foramen transversarium)

Observe the following features of individual cervical vertebrae: [G 294; L 7, 8; N 17, 21; R 194; C 342]

- **Atlas (C1)**
  Anterior arch and tubercle
  Transverse process with transverse foramen
  Groove for vertebral artery
  Posterior arch and tubercle
  Superior articular surface for occipital condyle
  Note that the atlas does not have a body.
- **Axis (C2)**
  Dens
  Body
  Transverse process with transverse foramen
  Lamina
  Spinous process
  Superior articular facet for atlas
- **Vertebrae C3 to C7**
  Body
  Transverse process with transverse foramen
  Groove for spinal nerve
  Lamina
  Spinous process
  Note that C7 has the longest cervical spinous process (**vertebra prominens**).

POSTERIOR TRIANGLE OF THE NECK

Dissection Overview

Study a transverse section through the neck (Fig. 7.1). The posterior part of the neck contains the cervical vertebral column and the muscles that move it. The anterior part of the neck houses the cervical viscera. The cervical viscera include: [G 747; L 305; N 35; R 154; C 474]

- **Pharynx** and **esophagus** – the superior parts of the digestive tract

ATLAS REFERENCES
G = Grant's Atlas, 12th ed., page number
L = LWW Atlas of Anatomy, 1st ed., page number
N = Netter's Atlas, 4th ed., plate number
R = Color Atlas of Anatomy, 6th ed., page number
C = Clemente's Atlas, 5th ed., plate number

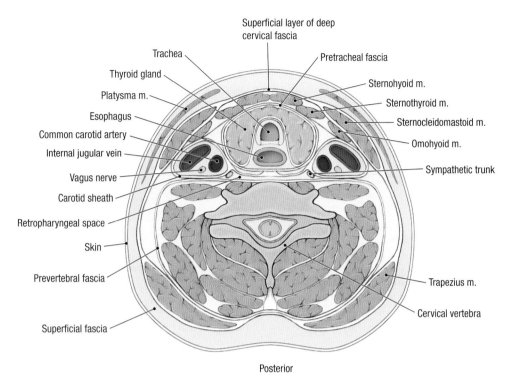

Superficial layer of deep cervical fascia

Trachea

Thyroid gland

Platysma m.

Esophagus

Common carotid artery

Internal jugular vein

Vagus nerve

Carotid sheath

Retropharyngeal space

Skin

Prevertebral fascia

Superficial fascia

Pretracheal fascia

Sternohyoid m.

Sternothyroid m.

Sternocleidomastoid m.

Omohyoid m.

Sympathetic trunk

Trapezius m.

Cervical vertebra

Posterior

Figure 7.1. Transverse section through the neck.

- **Larynx** and **trachea** – the superior parts of the respiratory tract
- **Thyroid gland** and **parathyroid glands**

The visceral part of the neck has the following boundaries:

- **Posterior** – the cervical vertebrae
- **Posterolateral** – the scalene muscles
- **Lateral** – the sternocleidomastoid muscle
- **Anterior** – the infrahyoid muscles

Large vessels and nerves lie lateral to the cervical viscera (Fig. 7.1). The **carotid artery** (**internal carotid artery** at more superior levels), **internal jugular vein**, and **vagus nerve** are contained within the **carotid sheath**.

The order of dissection will be as follows: The skin will be removed from the anterior and lateral neck. The platysma muscle will be studied and reflected. The external jugular vein will be identified. Several cutaneous branches of the cervical plexus (great auricular nerve, lesser occipital nerve, transverse cervical nerve, and supraclavicular nerves) will be dissected. The accessory nerve (cranial nerve XI) will be identified and followed from the sternocleidomastoid muscle to the trapezius muscle.

Dissection Instructions

SKIN REMOVAL

1. The skin is thin on the neck. Be careful when removing it.
2. Refer to Figure 7.2 and make an anterior midline skin incision from the jugular notch of the sternum (E) to the chin (F).
3. Make a second skin incision along the margin of the mandible from point F to just below the ear lobe (G).
4. Make a skin incision in the transverse plane from point G to the external occipital protuberance (H). If the back has been dissected, part of this incision has been made previously.
5. If the back has not been dissected, make a skin incision along the anterior border of the trapezius muscle from point H to the acromion (I).
6. If the thorax has not been dissected, make an incision along the anterior surface of the clavicle from point I to the jugular notch of the sternum (E).

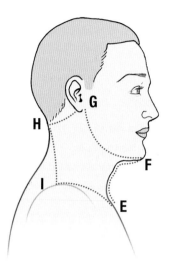

Figure 7.2. Skin incisions.

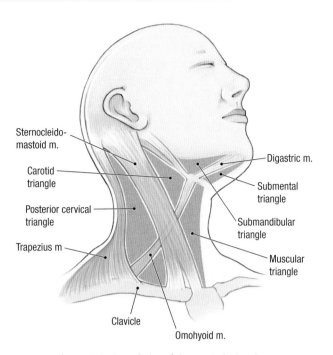

Figure 7.3. Boundaries of the cervical triangles.

7. Beginning at the anterior midline, reflect the skin in the lateral direction as far as the anterior border of the trapezius muscle. Detach the skin and place it in the tissue container.

POSTERIOR TRIANGLE OF THE NECK [G 752; L 297; N 26; R 174; C 476]

For descriptive purposes the neck is divided into an anterior triangle and a posterior triangle (Fig. 7.3). The **boundaries of the posterior triangle** of the neck are:

- **Anterior** – the posterior border of the sternocleidomastoid muscle
- **Posterior** – the anterior border of the trapezius muscle
- **Inferior** – the middle one-third of the clavicle
- **Superficial (roof)** – superficial layer of the deep cervical fascia
- **Deep (floor)** – muscles of the neck covered by prevertebral fascia

The cutaneous nerves for the shoulder and anterior neck pass to the surface through the posterior triangle of the neck. Therefore, these structures are dissected with the posterior cervical triangle even though they may distribute over the shoulder or anterior triangle. At the outset, note that the structures in the following dissection lie within the superficial fascia of the neck except the accessory nerve, which lies deep to the superficial layer of the deep cervical fascia.

1. Examine the **platysma muscle** in the superficial fascia (Fig. 7.4). The platysma muscle covers the lower part of the posterior triangle. At its inferior end, the platysma muscle passes superficial to the clavicle and attaches to the superficial fascia of the deltoid and pectoral regions. Superiorly, the platysma muscle is attached to the mandible, skin

of the cheek, angle of the mouth, and orbicularis oris muscle. It is innervated by the facial nerve.

2. Note that the supraclavicular nerves, the transverse cervical nerve, and the external jugular vein are in contact with the deep surface of the platysma muscle. Preserve them in the next dissection step.

3. Near the clavicle, use a probe to raise the inferior border of the platysma muscle. Carefully use sharp dissection to free the platysma muscle from the vessels and nerves on its deep surface and reflect the muscle superiorly as far as the mandible. Leave

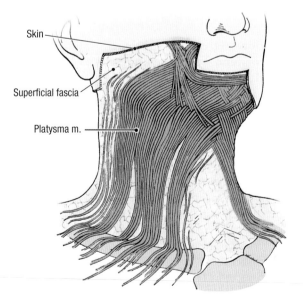

Figure 7.4. The platysma muscle.

the platysma muscle attached along the border of the mandible.

4. Identify the **external jugular vein** (Fig. 7.5). The external jugular vein is in the superficial fascia deep to the platysma muscle. The external jugular vein begins posterior to the angle of the mandible and crosses the superficial surface of the sternocleidomastoid muscle. About 3 cm superior to the clavicle, the external jugular vein pierces the superficial layer of the deep cervical fascia (roof of the posterior triangle) to drain into the subclavian vein. Follow the external jugular vein until it passes through the investing layer of deep cervical fascia. [G 754; L 306; N 31; R 178; C 477]

5. The skin of the neck and part of the posterior head is innervated by cutaneous nerves that are branches of the **cervical plexus.** The cutaneous nerves enter the superficial fascia near the midpoint of the posterior border of the sternocleidomastoid muscle (Fig. 7.5). Identify:

   • **Great auricular nerve** – crosses the superficial surface of the sternocleidomastoid muscle parallel to the external jugular vein. The great auricular nerve supplies the skin of the lower part of the ear and an area of skin extending from the angle of the mandible to the mastoid process.
   • **Lesser occipital nerve** – passes superiorly along the posterior border of the sternocleido-

mastoid muscle. The lesser occipital nerve supplies the part of the scalp that is immediately behind the ear.

   • **Transverse cervical nerve** – passes transversely across the sternocleidomastoid muscle and neck. It supplies the skin of the anterior triangle of the neck. If you have trouble identifying the transverse cervical nerve, it may have been removed with the platysma muscle.
   • **Supraclavicular nerves** – pass inferiorly to innervate the skin of the shoulder. Observe medial, intermediate, and lateral branches.

CLINICAL CORRELATION

Diaphragmatic Pain Referred to the Shoulder

The supraclavicular nerves and the phrenic nerve share a common origin from spinal cord segments C3 and C4. Irritation of the parietal pleura or parietal peritoneum covering the diaphragm produces pain that is carried by the phrenic nerve and referred to the area supplied by the supraclavicular nerves (shoulder region).

---

6. The **accessory nerve (XI)** courses from slightly superior to the midpoint of the posterior border of the sternocleidomastoid muscle to the anterior border of the trapezius muscle (Fig. 7.5). The accessory nerve lies deep to the superficial layer of the deep cervical fascia. Use blunt dissection to free the accessory nerve from the surrounding connective tissue. Note that branches of spinal nerves C3 and C4 join the accessory nerve in the posterior cervical triangle and these branches provide proprioceptive sensory innervation. The accessory nerve innervates the sternocleidomastoid muscle and the trapezius muscle. If the back has been dissected, confirm that the accessory nerve may be found on the deep surface of the trapezius muscle.

7. The inferior portion of the posterior triangle will be dissected with the root of the neck.

Dissection Review

1. Review Figure 7.1 and note that the platysma muscle, external jugular vein, and cutaneous nerves of the neck are all located in the superficial fascia. Of the structures just dissected, only the accessory nerve is located deep to the investing layer of deep cervical fascia.

2. Use an illustration to review the relationship of the platysma muscle to the cutaneous branches of the cer-

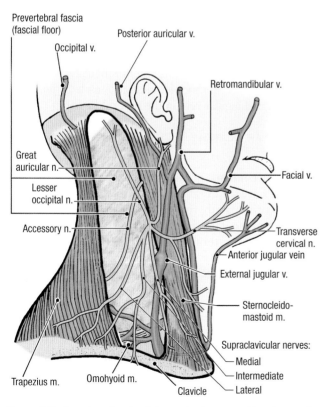

Figure 7.5. Posterior triangle of the neck. The external jugular vein lies superficial to the superficial layer of deep cervical fascia.

Prevertebral fascia (fascial floor)
Occipital v.
Posterior auricular v.
Retromandibular v.
Great auricular n.
Lesser occipital n.
Accessory n.
Facial v.
Transverse cervical n.
Anterior jugular vein
External jugular v.
Sternocleido- mastoid m.
Trapezius m.
Omohyoid m.
Clavicle
Supraclavicular nerves:
Medial
Intermediate
Lateral

vical plexus. Note that the transverse cervical nerve crosses the neck deep to the platysma muscle but that its branches pass through the muscle to reach the skin of the anterior neck.

3. Review the area of distribution of all cutaneous branches of the cervical plexus.

4. Review the course of the accessory nerve. Note that the accessory nerve is superficial in the neck where it is vulnerable to injury by laceration or blunt trauma.

5. Review the course of the occipital artery at the apex of the posterior triangle.

ANTERIOR TRIANGLE OF THE NECK [G 763; L 297; N 28; R 175; C 470]

Dissection Overview

The boundaries of the **anterior triangle of the neck** are (Fig. 7.3):

- **Anterior** – the median line of the neck
- **Posterior** – the anterior border of the sternocleidomastoid muscle
- **Superior** – the inferior border of the mandible
- **Superficial (roof)** – superficial layer of the deep cervical fascia
- **Deep (floor)** – larynx and pharynx

For descriptive purposes, the anterior triangle is divided by the digastric and omohyoid muscles into smaller triangles: **muscular**, **carotid**, **submandibular**, and **submental** (Fig. 7.3).

BONES AND CARTILAGES

Use an illustration to identify the bony and cartilaginous landmarks that will be used as reference structures (Fig. 7.6): [G 761; L 307; N 29; R 175; C 470]

- **Hyoid bone** – (Gr. *hyoideus*, U-shaped) at the angle between the floor of the mouth and the superior end of the neck
- **Thyrohyoid membrane** – stretching between the thyroid cartilage and hyoid bone
- **Thyroid cartilage** – (Gr. *thyreoeides*, shield) in the anterior midline of the neck

The order of dissection will be as follows: The superficial veins of the anterior triangle will be studied. The contents of each subdivision of the anterior triangle will be dissected in the following order: muscular triangle, carotid triangle, submandibular triangle, and submental triangle.

Dissection Instructions

SUPERFICIAL FASCIA [G 763; L 306; N 31; R 174; C 482]

1. The platysma muscle has been removed, revealing the **external jugular vein**. Follow the external jugular

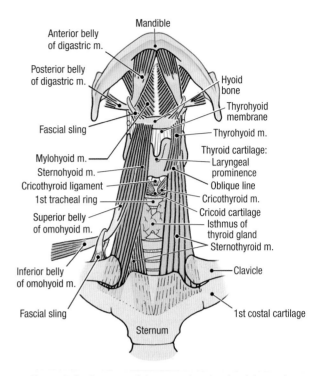

Figure 7.6. Contents of the muscular triangle of the neck.

vein superiorly and observe that it is formed by the joining of the posterior division of the **retromandibular vein** and the **posterior auricular vein** (Fig. 7.5).

2. In the superficial fascia near the anterior midline, note the **anterior jugular vein** (Fig. 7.5). It courses inferiorly near the midline to the suprasternal region where it penetrates the superficial layer of the deep cervical fascia. The anterior jugular vein passes deep to the sternocleidomastoid muscle to join the external jugular vein in the root of the neck.

MUSCULAR TRIANGLE [G 763; L 307, 308; N 29; R 175; C 470]

1. The contents of the **muscular triangle** of the neck are the infrahyoid muscles, the thyroid gland, and the parathyroid glands. The **boundaries of the muscular triangle** are (Fig. 7.3):
   - **Superolateral** – superior belly of the omohyoid muscle
   - **Inferolateral** – anterior border of the sternocleidomastoid muscle
   - **Medial** – median plane of the neck

2. In the midline of the neck, use a probe to break through the superficial layer of the deep cervical fascia and identify the **sternohyoid muscle** (Fig. 7.6). The inferior attachment of the sternohyoid muscle is the sternum and its superior attachment is the body of the hyoid bone. The sternohyoid muscle depresses the hyoid bone.

3. Lateral to the sternohyoid muscle, identify the **superior belly of the omohyoid muscle**. The superior belly is attached to the inferior border of the hyoid bone. The inferior belly of the omohyoid muscle attaches to the superior border of the scapula near the suprascapular notch. The omohyoid muscle depresses the hyoid bone.

4. Use blunt dissection to loosen the medial border of the sternohyoid muscle from the structures that lie deep to it. Use scissors to transect the sternohyoid muscle close to the hyoid bone and reflect the muscle inferiorly. If the thorax has been dissected previously, the sternohyoid muscle has been detached from the sternum. It should remain attached by deep fascia to other muscles. Conserve this deep fascial attachment so that the muscle is not removed.

5. Use a probe to raise the medial border of the superior belly of the omohyoid muscle and loosen it from deeper structures. Use scissors to transect the superior belly of the omohyoid muscle close to the hyoid bone and reflect it inferiorly.

6. Identify the **sternothyroid muscle** (Fig. 7.6). The inferior attachment of the sternothyroid muscle is the sternum and its superior attachment is the oblique line of the thyroid cartilage. The sternothyroid muscle depresses the larynx.

7. Identify the **thyrohyoid muscle**. The inferior attachment of the thyrohyoid muscle is the oblique line of the thyroid cartilage and its superior attachment is the hyoid bone. The thyrohyoid muscle elevates the larynx.

8. The **ansa cervicalis** innervates the four infrahyoid muscles. It will be identified later.

9. Gently retract the right and left sternothyroid muscles to widen the gap in the midline. Identify (Fig. 7.6): [G 759; L 308; N 31; R 175; C 484]
   - **Laryngeal prominence**
   - **Cricothyroid ligament**
   - **Cricoid cartilage**
   - **First tracheal ring**
   - **Isthmus of the thyroid gland**

CLINICAL CORRELATION

Tracheotomy

Tracheotomy (tracheostomy) is the creation of an opening into the trachea. As an emergency operation, it must be rapidly performed in cases with sudden obstruction of the airway (e.g., aspiration of a foreign body, edema of the larynx, or paralysis of the vocal folds). The opening is made in the midline between the infrahyoid muscles of the neck.

SUBMANDIBULAR TRIANGLE [G 763; L 312, 313; N 32; R 183; C 493]

1. The contents of the **submandibular triangle** are the submandibular gland, facial artery, facial vein, stylohyoid muscle, part of the hypoglossal nerve (XII), and lymph nodes. The **boundaries of the submandibular triangle** are (Fig. 7.3):
   - **Superior** – inferior border of the mandible
   - **Anteroinferior** – anterior belly of the digastric muscle
   - **Posteroinferior** – posterior belly of the digastric muscle
   - **Superficial (roof)** – superficial layer of deep cervical fascia
   - **Deep (floor)** – mylohyoid and hyoglossus muscles

2. Refer to a skull. On the temporal bone, identify the **mastoid process** and the **styloid process**.

3. Examine the **inner aspect of the mandible** and identify: [G 665; L 327; N 15; R 52; C 581]
   - **Digastric fossa**
   - **Mylohyoid line**
   - **Submandibular fossa**
   - **Mylohyoid groove**

4. On the cadaver, identify the submandibular gland and use a probe to define its borders. Note that a portion of the gland extends deep to the posterior border of mylohyoid muscle.

5. Use blunt dissection to separate the facial artery and vein from the submandibular gland. Note that the facial vein passes superficial to the submandibular gland and the facial artery courses deep to the gland.

6. Preserve the facial vessels and use scissors to remove the superficial part of the submandibular gland. Do not disturb the deep part of the gland.

7. Use blunt dissection to clean the superficial surface of the **anterior and posterior bellies of the digastric muscle** (Fig. 7.6). The anterior attachment of the anterior belly is the digastric fossa of the mandible. The anterior belly of the digastric muscle is innervated by the mylohyoid nerve, a branch of the mandibular division of the trigeminal nerve (V₃). The posterior attachment of the posterior belly is the mastoid process of the temporal bone and it is innervated by the facial nerve (VII). The two bellies attach to each other by an **intermediate tendon**. The intermediate tendon is attached to the body and the greater horn of the hyoid bone by a fibrous sling. The digastric muscle elevates the hyoid bone and depresses the mandible.

8. Identify the **tendon of the stylohyoid muscle**, which attaches to the body of the hyoid bone by straddling the intermediate tendon of the digastric muscle. The stylohyoid muscle is innervated by the facial nerve and it elevates the hyoid bone.

9. Use a probe to follow the **hypoglossal nerve (XII)** through the submandibular triangle. Observe that the hypoglossal nerve enters the submandibular triangle by passing deep to the posterior belly of the digastric muscle. It passes deep to the **mylohyoid muscle** within the submandibular triangle (Fig. 7.7).

SUBMENTAL TRIANGLE [G 758; L 307; N 31; R 174; C 492]

1. The contents of the **submental triangle** are the submental lymph nodes. The submental triangle is an unpaired triangle that crosses the midline. The **boundaries of the submental triangle** are (Fig. 7.3):
    *   **Right and left** – anterior bellies of the right and left digastric muscles
    *   **Inferior** – hyoid bone
    *   **Superficial (roof)** – superficial layer of the deep cervical fascia
    *   **Deep (floor)** – mylohyoid muscle
2. Use a probe to clean the superficial fascia from the surface of the right and left mylohyoid muscles. Each mylohyoid muscle has a proximal attachment on the mylohyoid line of the mandible and distal attachments on the hyoid bone and the mylohyoid raphe. The mylohyoid muscle supports the floor of the oral cavity.

CAROTID TRIANGLE [G 763; L 312, 313; N 32; R 182; C 478]

1. The contents of the **carotid triangle** are the carotid arteries (common, internal, and external), the branches of the external carotid artery, part of the hypoglossal nerve, and branches of the vagus

nerve (X). The **boundaries of the carotid triangle** are (Fig. 7.3):
*   **Inferomedial** – superior belly of the omohyoid muscle
*   **Inferolateral** – anterior border of the sternocleidomastoid muscle
*   **Superior** – posterior belly of the digastric muscle

2. Clean the anterior margin of the sternocleidomastoid muscle from its inferior end to its superior attachment. Use blunt dissection to free the anterior border of the muscle from the deep cervical fascia.
3. If the thorax has been dissected, the sternocleidomastoid muscle has already been detached from its inferior attachments. If the thorax has not been dissected, transect the sternocleidomastoid muscle about 5 cm superior to its attachments to the sternum and clavicle.
4. Reflect the sternocleidomastoid superiorly. Attempt to conserve the cutaneous branches of the cervical plexus that radiate from the posterior border of the sternocleidomastoid muscle. Use your fingers to free the sternocleidomastoid muscle from the deep cervical fascia as far superiorly as the mastoid process. *Release of the sternocleidomastoid up to the mastoid process is important to facilitate disarticulation of the head in a later dissection.*
5. Find the accessory nerve (XI) where it crosses the deep surface of the sternocleidomastoid muscle near the base of the skull. Trace the accessory nerve superiorly as far as possible. Note that the accessory nerve passes through the jugular foramen to exit the skull but this relationship is too far superior to be seen at this time.
6. To allow better access to deeper structures cut the common facial vein where it empties into the internal jugular vein. Transect the digastric muscle at its intermediate tendon and reflect the posterior belly.
7. Palpate the **tip of the greater horn of the hyoid bone** (Figs. 7.7 and 7.8). Find the hypoglossal nerve superior to the tip of the greater horn of the hyoid bone. Observe that a muscular branch of the occipital artery crosses superior to the hypoglossal nerve. The hypoglossal nerve carries axons of spinal nerve C1 that branch off as the **nerve to the thyrohyoid muscle**. [G 763; L 313; N 32; R 182; C 479]
8. Use blunt dissection to trace the **hypoglossal nerve** anteriorly. Verify that the hypoglossal nerve passes medial to the posterior belly of the digastric muscle and deep to the mylohyoid muscle (Fig. 7.7).
9. The **superior root of the ansa cervicalis** travels with the hypoglossal nerve (Fig. 7.8). The superior root of the ansa cervicalis is mainly composed of

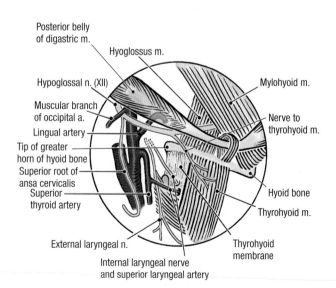

Posterior belly of digastric m.
Hyoglossus m.
Hypoglossal n. (XII)
Muscular branch of occipital a.
Lingual artery
Tip of greater horn of hyoid bone
Superior root of ansa cervicalis
Superior thyroid artery
External laryngeal n.
Internal laryngeal nerve and superior laryngeal artery
Mylohyoid m.
Nerve to thyrohyoid m.
Hyoid bone
Thyrohyoid m.
Thyrohyoid membrane

Figure 7.7. The carotid triangle of the neck. The tip of the greater horn of the hyoid bone is an important reference point.

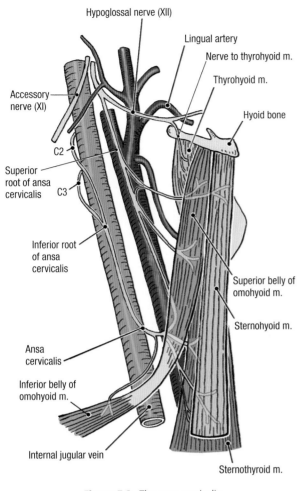

Hypoglossal nerve (XII)

Lingual artery

Nerve to thyrohyoid m.

Thyrohyoid m.

Accessory nerve (XI)

Hyoid bone

C2

Superior root of ansa cervicalis

C3

Inferior root of ansa cervicalis

Superior belly of omohyoid m.

Sternohyoid m.

Ansa cervicalis

Inferior belly of omohyoid m.

Internal jugular vein

Sternothyroid m.

Figure 7.8. The ansa cervicalis.

fibers from C1. The **inferior root of the ansa cervicalis** (C2, C3) passes around the carotid sheath to join the superior root. Thus, a loop (L. *ansa*, handle) is formed.

10. Clean the ansa cervicalis and trace its delicate branches to the lateral borders of the infrahyoid muscles (Fig. 7.8).

11. Use a probe to raise the posterior border of the thyrohyoid muscle and identify the **thyrohyoid membrane** that extends between the thyroid cartilage and the hyoid bone (Fig. 7.9). Find the **internal branch of the superior laryngeal nerve** where it passes through the thyrohyoid membrane. The internal branch of the superior laryngeal nerve supplies sensory fibers to the mucosa of the larynx.

12. Follow the internal branch of the superior laryngeal nerve proximally. It joins the **external branch of the superior laryngeal nerve** to form the **superior laryngeal nerve** (Fig. 7.9). The superior laryngeal nerve may be too far superior to be seen at this stage of the dissection.

13. Trace the external branch of the superior laryngeal nerve distally and observe that it innervates the **cricothyroid muscle**. It also innervates part of the inferior pharyngeal constrictor muscle.

14. While preserving the ansa cervicalis, use scissors to open the **carotid sheath**. The carotid sheath contains the common carotid artery, internal carotid artery, internal jugular vein, and vagus nerve (X).

15. Observe that the **internal jugular vein** is located lateral to the common carotid or internal carotid artery in the carotid sheath. Use an illustration to study its largest tributaries: **common facial vein, superior thyroid vein,** and **middle thyroid vein.** Use blunt dissection to separate the internal jugular vein from the common and internal carotid arteries.

16. To clear the dissection field, remove the tributaries of the internal jugular vein.

17. At the level of the superior border of the thyroid cartilage, find the origin of the **external carotid artery** (Fig. 7.9). Use blunt dissection to follow the external carotid artery superiorly until it passes on the medial side of (deep to) the posterior belly of the digastric muscle. Temporarily replace the posterior belly of the digastric muscle in its correct anatomical position to confirm this relationship. [G 766; L 314; N 34; R 183; C 479]

18. The external carotid artery has six branches in the carotid triangle (Fig. 7.9). Each branch has a companion vein that may be removed to clear the dissection field. At this time, identify five branches:

• **Superior thyroid artery** – arises from the anterior surface of the external carotid artery at the level of the superior horn of the thyroid cartilage. The superior thyroid artery descends to the superior pole of the lobe of the thyroid gland. The **superior laryngeal artery** is a branch of the superior thyroid artery, which pierces the thyrohyoid membrane together with the internal laryngeal nerve.

• **Lingual artery** – arises from the anterior surface of the external carotid artery at the level of the greater horn of the hyoid bone (Fig. 7.9). It passes deeply into the muscles of the tongue. Do not follow it at this time.

• **Facial artery** – arises from the anterior surface of the external carotid artery immediately superior to the lingual artery (Fig. 7.9). The facial artery crosses the inferior border of the mandible to enter the face. Do not follow it into the face at this time. In 20% of cases, the lingual and facial arteries arise from a common trunk.

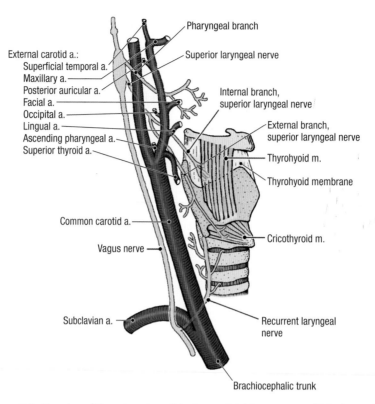

Figure 7.9. Branches of the external carotid artery and right vagus nerve (X) in the neck.

- **Occipital artery** – arises from the posterior surface of the external carotid artery and supplies part of the scalp (Fig. 7.9).
- **Posterior auricular artery** – arises from the posterior surface of the external carotid artery and passes posterior to the ear to supply part of the scalp.

19. Use blunt dissection to clean the **bifurcation of the common carotid artery**. Identify the **carotid sinus**, a dilation of the origin of the internal carotid artery. The wall of the carotid sinus contains pressoreceptors that monitor blood pressure. The carotid sinus is innervated by the glossopharyngeal nerve (IX) and the vagus nerve (X).

20. The **carotid body** is a small mass of tissue located on the medial aspect of the carotid bifurcation. The carotid body monitors changes in oxygen and carbon dioxide concentration of the blood. The carotid body is innervated by the glossopharyngeal nerve (IX) and the vagus nerve (X)

21. Identify the **internal carotid artery** and note that it has no branches in the neck.

22. The **ascending pharyngeal artery** is the sixth branch of the external carotid artery. It branches from the medial surface of the external carotid artery. Use your fingers to raise the external carotid artery and look for the origin of the ascending pharyngeal artery close to the carotid bifurcation.

23. Identify the **vagus nerve (X)** within the carotid sheath where it lies between and posterior to the vessels (Fig. 7.9). To see the vagus nerve, retract the internal jugular vein laterally and the common carotid artery medially.

Dissection Review

1. Replace the sternocleidomastoid muscle and the infrahyoid muscles in their correct anatomical positions. Review the attachments and actions of the infrahyoid muscles.

2. Review the cutaneous branches of the cervical plexus. Review the ansa cervicalis.

3. Use the dissected specimen to review the positions of the common carotid and internal carotid arteries, internal jugular vein, and vagus nerve within the carotid sheath.

4. Follow each branch of the external carotid artery through the regions dissected, noting their relationships to muscles, nerves, and glands.

5. Trace the branches of the superior laryngeal nerve distally and note their distribution.

6. Review the course of the hypoglossal nerve.

7. Review the ansa cervicalis and its relationship to the hypoglossal nerve and carotid sheath.

8. Note that the superior laryngeal nerve passes medial to the internal and external carotid arteries and the hypoglossal nerve passes lateral to the internal and external carotid arteries.

THYROID AND PARATHYROID GLANDS [G 768–771; N 74, 76; R 184; C 483]

Dissection Overview

The cervical viscera are the pharynx, esophagus, larynx, trachea, thyroid gland, and parathyroid glands. The thyroid gland and parathyroid glands lie between the infrahyoid muscles and the larynx and trachea, and these glands will be dissected now. The pharynx, esophagus, larynx, and trachea will be dissected after head disarticulation has been performed.

Dissection Instructions

1. Once again, reflect the sternocleidomastoid and sternohyoid muscles.
2. Observe the **thyroid gland**. [L 308, 309] The thyroid gland is located at vertebral levels C5 to T1. Laterally, the thyroid gland is in contact with the carotid sheath (Fig. 7.10B).
3. Identify the **right lobe** and **left lobe** of the **thyroid gland**. The two lobes are connected by the **isthmus**, which crosses the anterior surface of tracheal rings 2 and 3 (Fig. 7.10A).
4. Frequently, the thyroid gland has a **pyramidal lobe** that extends superiorly from the isthmus. The pyramidal lobe is a remnant of embryonic development that shows the route of descent of the thyroid gland.
5. Identify the **superior thyroid artery** where it enters the superior end of the lobe of the thyroid gland. Recall that the superior thyroid artery is a branch of the external carotid artery. The inferior thyroid artery will be dissected later.
6. The **superior and middle thyroid veins** are tributary to the internal jugular vein. The **right and left inferior thyroid veins** descend into the thorax on the anterior surface of the trachea. The right and left inferior thyroid veins drain into the right and left brachiocephalic veins, respectively.
7. Look for the **thyroidea ima artery** (L. *ima*, lowest). The thyroidea ima artery is a relatively rare (published reports place the incidence at 2% to 12% of the population) but clinically significant variant. When present, the thyroidea ima artery enters the thyroid gland from inferiorly, near the midline.
8. Use scissors to cut the isthmus of the thyroid gland. Use blunt dissection to detach the capsule of the thyroid gland from the tracheal rings. Spread the lobes widely apart.
9. On both sides of the cadaver, use blunt dissection to display the **recurrent laryngeal nerve** that

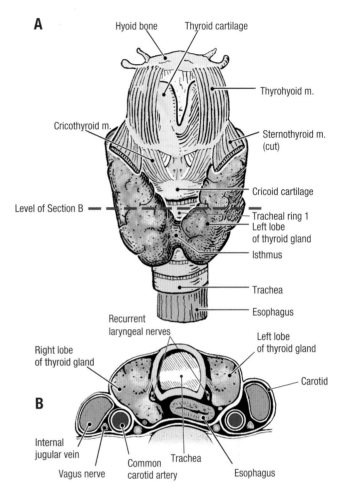

Figure 7.10. The relationships of the thyroid gland. **A.** Anterior view. Dashed line indicates the level of section. **B.** Transverse section.

passes immediately posterior to the lobe of the thyroid gland in the groove between the trachea and esophagus. Use an illustration to note the close relationship of the recurrent laryngeal nerve to the thyroid gland (Fig. 7.10B).

CLINICAL CORRELATION

Recurrent Laryngeal Nerve

If a recurrent laryngeal nerve is injured by a thyroid tumor or during thyroidectomy (removal of the thyroid gland), paralysis of the laryngeal muscles will occur on the affected side. The result is hoarseness of the voice.

10. Cut all blood vessels leading to or from the left lobe of the thyroid gland. Use a probe to free the left lobe from surrounding connective tissue and remove it.

11. Examine the posterior aspect of the left lobe of the thyroid gland and attempt to identify the **parathyroid glands**. The parathyroid glands are about 5 mm in diameter and may be darker in color than the thyroid gland. Usually, there are two parathyroid glands on each side of the neck but the number can vary from one to three.

CLINICAL CORRELATION

Parathyroid Glands

The parathyroid glands play an important role in the regulation of calcium metabolism. During thyroidectomy, these small endocrine glands are in danger of being damaged or removed. To maintain proper serum calcium levels, at least one parathyroid gland must be retained during surgery.

Dissection Review

1. Review the relationship of the thyroid gland to the infrahyoid muscles, carotid sheaths, larynx, and trachea.

2. Use an illustration and the dissected specimen to review the blood supply and venous drainage of the thyroid gland. Note that there are only two thyroid arteries (superior and inferior) but there are three thyroid veins (superior, middle, and inferior).

3. Review the relationship of the parathyroid glands to the thyroid gland. Use an embryology textbook to review the origin and migration of the thyroid and parathyroid glands during development.

ROOT OF THE NECK [G 772; L 309; N 33; R 184; C 480]

Dissection Overview

The **root (base) of the neck** is the junction between the thorax and the neck. The root of the neck is an important area because it lies superior to the **superior thoracic aperture**. All structures that pass between the head and thorax or the upper limb and thorax must pass through the root of the neck.

The order of dissection will be as follows: The branches of the subclavian artery will be dissected. The course of the vagus and phrenic nerves will be studied. The muscles that form the floor of the posterior cervical triangle will be studied. Some of these structures will be followed superiorly or inferiorly beyond the root of the neck.

Dissection Instructions

1. The clavicle has been cut at its midlength and the thoracic wall was removed during dissection of the thorax. Remove the anterior thoracic wall and set it aside.

2. Reflect superiorly the sternocleidomastoid muscle, sternohyoid muscle, and sternothyroid muscle.

3. Clean the inferior belly of the **omohyoid muscle**. Note that its inferior belly and superior belly are joined by an **intermediate tendon**. Review its attachments and action.

4. Use scissors to cut the fascial sling that binds the intermediate tendon of the omohyoid muscle to the clavicle.

5. Follow the **external jugular vein** through the investing layer of deep cervical fascia. Note that the external jugular vein is the only tributary of the subclavian vein. To expose the blood vessels in the root of the neck, remove the investing layer of deep cervical fascia that forms the roof of the lower part of the posterior cervical triangle.

6. Identify the **subclavian vein** (Fig. 7.11). Use blunt dissection to loosen the subclavian vein from structures that lie deep to it.

7. Follow the subclavian vein inferiorly to the point where it is joined by the **internal jugular vein** to form the **brachiocephalic vein**.

8. Identify the **subclavian artery**. Observe that the right subclavian artery is a branch of the brachiocephalic trunk and the left subclavian artery is a branch of the aortic arch. [G 774; L 309. 310; N 33; R 170, 184; C 491]

9. The subclavian artery has three parts that are defined by its relationship to the anterior scalene muscle (Fig. 7.12):
    - **First part** – from its origin to the medial border of the anterior scalene muscle
    - **Second part** – posterior to the anterior scalene muscle
    - **Third part** – between the lateral border of the anterior scalene muscle and the lateral border of the first rib

10. The **first part of the subclavian artery** has three branches:
    - **Vertebral artery** – courses superiorly between the anterior scalene muscle and the longus colli muscle (Fig. 7.12). Trace the vertebral artery superiorly until it passes into the transverse foramen of vertebra C6.
    - **Internal thoracic artery** – arises from the anteroinferior surface of the subclavian artery and passes inferiorly to supply the anterior thoracic wall (Fig. 7.12).

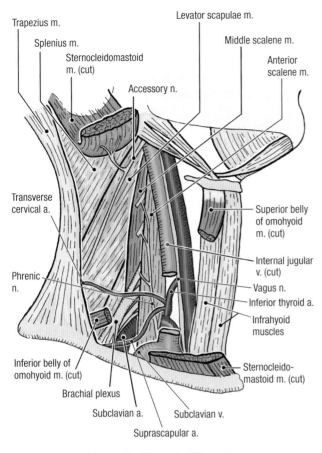

Figure 7.11. The root of the neck.

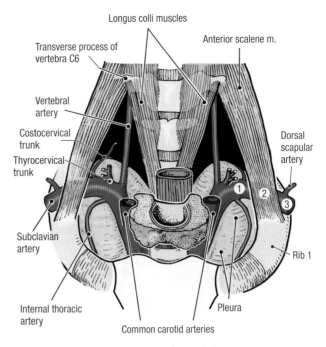

Figure 7.12. Branches of the subclavian artery.

- **Thyrocervical trunk** – arises from the antero-superior surface of the subclavian artery (Fig. 7.12). The thyrocervical trunk has three branches:

  Transverse cervical artery – crosses the root of the neck about 2 to 3 cm superior to the clavicle and deep to the omohyoid muscle (Fig. 7.13). It supplies the trapezius muscle.

  Suprascapular artery – passes laterally and posteriorly to the region of the suprascapular notch (Fig. 7.13). It passes superior to the transverse scapular ligament and supplies the supraspinatus and infraspinatus muscles.

  Inferior thyroid artery – passes medially toward the thyroid gland. Trace the inferior thyroid artery toward the thyroid gland. Usually, the inferior thyroid artery passes posterior to the **cervical sympathetic trunk**. The **ascending cervical artery** is a branch of the inferior thyroid artery.

11. The **second part of the subclavian artery** has one branch, the **costocervical** trunk (Fig. 7.12). The costocervical trunk arises from the posterior surface of the second part of the subclavian artery. Use your fingers to elevate the subclavian artery from the surface of the first rib and use blunt dissection to look for the costocervical trunk passing posteriorly above the cupula of the pleura. The costocervical trunk divides into the **deep cervical artery** and the **supreme intercostal artery**. The supreme intercostal artery gives rise to posterior intercostal arteries 1 and 2.

12. The **third part of the subclavian artery** has one branch, the **dorsal scapular artery**. The dorsal scapular artery passes between the superior and middle trunks of the brachial plexus to supply the muscles of the scapular region (Fig. 7.13). In about 30% of cases the dorsal scapular artery arises from the transverse cervical artery instead of from the subclavian artery.

13. Find the **thoracic duct**, which ascends from the thorax into the neck. The thoracic duct is posterior to the esophagus at the level of the superior thoracic aperture, and then it arches anteriorly and to the left to join the venous system near the junction of the **left subclavian vein** and the **left internal jugular vein** (Fig. 7.13). The thoracic duct is usually a single structure, which has the diameter of a small vein, but it may be represented by several smaller ducts. [G 773; L 309; N 206; R 182; C 168]

14. On the right side of the neck, several small lymphatic vessels join with lymph vessels from the right upper limb and right side of the thorax to form the **right lymphatic duct**. The right lymphatic duct drains into the junction of the right subclavian and right internal jugular veins.

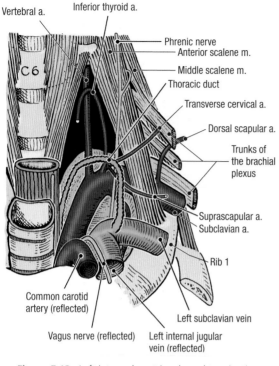

Figure 7.13. Left interscalene triangle and termination of the thoracic duct.

15. On both sides of the neck, find the **vagus nerve** in the carotid sheath and follow it into the thorax. Note that the vagus nerve passes posterior to the root of the lung. [G 772; L 309; N 32; R 184; C 481]

16. The right vagus nerve passes anterior to the subclavian artery, where it gives off the **right recurrent laryngeal nerve**. The left vagus nerve passes on the left side of the aortic arch, where it gives off the **left recurrent laryngeal nerve**.

17. Follow the right and left recurrent laryngeal nerves superiorly along the lateral surface of the trachea and esophagus. Trace them as far as the first tracheal ring. Do not follow them into the larynx at this time.

18. Verify that the **phrenic nerve** crosses the anterior surface of the anterior scalene muscle (Fig. 7.13). Follow the phrenic nerve into the thorax and confirm that it passes anterior to the root of the lung.

19. Identify the cervical portion of the **sympathetic trunk**. Note that the inferior cervical sympathetic ganglion is located in the root of the neck. Verify that the cervical sympathetic trunk is continuous with the thoracic sympathetic trunk.

20. Examine the muscles that form the floor of the posterior cervical triangle. Identify the **splenius capitis**, the **levator scapulae**, and the **anterior, middle, and posterior scalene muscles**. [G 773; L 310; N 33; R 185; C 480]

21. Use blunt dissection to define the borders of the **anterior scalene** and **middle scalene muscles**. The anterior and middle scalene muscles attach to the first rib. The first rib and the adjacent borders of the anterior and middle scalene muscles form the boundaries of the **interscalene triangle**. Observe (Fig. 7.13):
    - The **subclavian artery** and the **roots of the brachial plexus** pass between the posterior scalene muscle and the anterior scalene muscle (through the interscalene triangle).
    - The **subclavian vein, transverse cervical artery**, and **suprascapular artery** cross the anterior surface of the anterior scalene muscle.
    - The **phrenic nerve** descends vertically across the anterior surface of the anterior scalene muscle.

22. Use blunt dissection to clean the **roots of the brachial plexus** at the level of the interscalene triangle. Identify the parts of the **supraclavicular portion of the brachial plexus: roots, trunks, and divisions**.

23. If the upper limb has been dissected previously, follow the suprascapular nerve as far laterally as the suprascapular notch of the scapula where it is joined by the suprascapular artery.

CLINICAL CORRELATION

Interscalene Triangle

The **interscalene triangle** becomes clinically significant when anatomical variations (additional muscular slips, an accessory cervical rib, or exostosis on the first rib) narrow the interval. As a result, the subclavian artery and/or roots of the brachial plexus may be compressed, resulting in ischemia and nerve dysfunction in the upper limb.

Dissection Review

1. Replace the anterior thoracic wall in its correct anatomical position. Replace the infrahyoid muscles and sternocleidomastoid muscle in their correct anatomical positions. Review the boundaries of the posterior cervical triangle. Review the attachments of the infrahyoid muscles. Review the distribution of the cutaneous branches of the cervical plexus.

2. Remove the anterior thoracic wall. Review the origin and course of the brachiocephalic artery, left common carotid artery, and left subclavian artery in the superior mediastinum.

3. Review the three parts and the branches of the subclavian artery.

4. Review the distribution of the transverse cervical, suprascapular, and dorsal scapular arteries to the superficial muscles of the back and scapulohumeral muscles.

5. Use an illustration to review the course of the vertebral artery from its origin on the first part of the subclavian artery to the cranial cavity.

HEAD

The dissection of the head is foremost a dissection of the course and distribution of the cranial nerves and the branches of the external carotid artery. All of the cranial nerves and many blood vessels pass through openings in the skull. Therefore, the skull is an important tool with which to organize the study of the soft tissues of the head and neck. Parts of the skull will be studied as needed and details will be added as the dissection proceeds.

Skull

All parts of the skull are fragile, but the bones of the orbit are exceptionally delicate. The medial wall of the orbit is very easily broken. Never hold a skull by placing your fingers into the orbits.

ANTERIOR VIEW OF THE SKULL [G 610; L 298; N 2; R 22; C 514]

Examine the skull from an anterior view and identify (Fig. 7.14):

- **Frontal bone**
   Glabella
   Superciliary arch
   Supraorbital notch (foramen)
- **Nasal bone**
- **Zygomatic bone**
- **Maxilla**
   Frontal process
   Infraorbital foramen
   Anterior nasal spine
   Alveolar process
- **Nasal septum**
- **Mandible**
   Alveolar process
   Mental foramen
   Mental protuberance

Parts of several bones combine to form the following features (Fig. 7.14):

- **Nasion** – the junction between the frontal and nasal bones

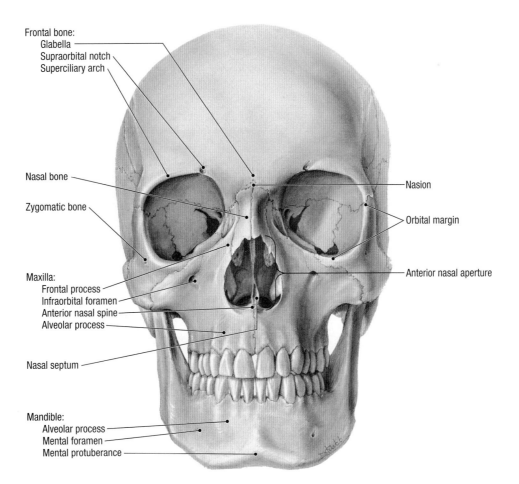

Figure 7.14. The skull, anterior view.

- **Orbital margin** – formed by three bones (frontal, maxillary, and zygomatic)
- **Anterior nasal aperture** – bounded by the nasal bones and maxillae

LATERAL VIEW OF THE SKULL [G 612; L 299; N 4; R 21; C 515]

Examine the skull from a lateral view and identify (Fig. 7.15):

- **Parietal bone**
    Superior temporal line
    Inferior temporal line
- **Frontal bone**
- **Sphenoid bone**
    Greater wing
- **Zygomatic bone**
    Frontal process
    Temporal process
- **Temporal bone**
    Squamous part
    External acoustic meatus

       Mastoid process
       Zygomatic process
- **Occipital bone**
    External occipital protuberance
- **Sutures**
    Lambdoid
    Squamosal
    Coronal
- **Pterion** – the junction of the frontal bone, parietal bone, greater wing of sphenoid bone, and squamous part of temporal bone
- **Mandible** (Fig. 7.16) [G 664; L 327; N 15; R 52; C 581]
    Ramus
        Coronoid process
        Mandibular notch
        Condylar process
            Head (condyle)
            Neck
Angle
Body
Mental foramen
Inferior border

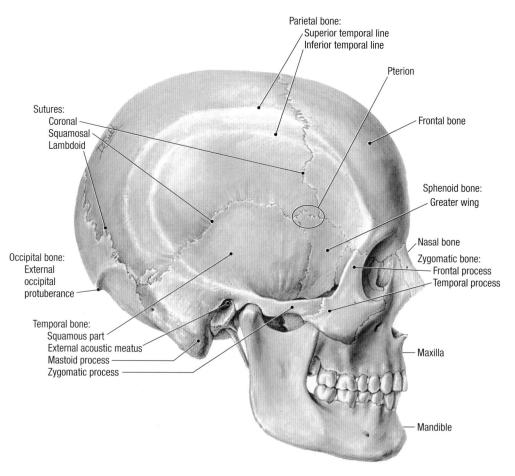

Figure 7.15. The skull, lateral view.

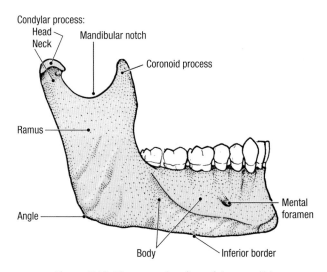

Figure 7.16. The external surface of the mandible.

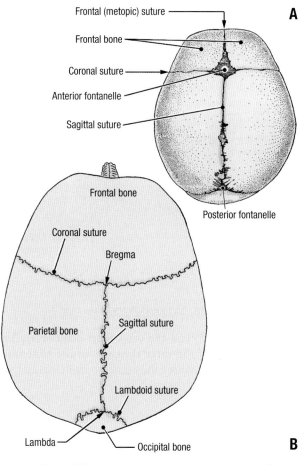

Figure 7.17. Superior view of the calvaria of the skull. **A.** Infant skull. **B.** Adult.

SUPERIOR VIEW OF THE SKULL [G 614; L 300; N 7; R 29; C 516]

The **calvaria** is the skull cap that is formed by parts of the frontal, parietal, and occipital bones. Examine the external surface of the calvaria and identify (Fig. 7.17):

- **Frontal (metopic) suture** – between the ossification centers of the frontal bone, usually obliterated in the adult
- **Coronal suture** – between the frontal bone and the two parietal bones
- **Sagittal suture** – between the two parietal bones
- **Bregma** – the point where the sagittal and coronal sutures meet
- **Lambdoid suture** – between the occipital bone and the two parietal bones
- **Lambda** – the point where the sagittal and lambdoid sutures meet

FACE

Surface Anatomy

Palpate the following structures on the head of the cadaver (Fig. 7.18):

- **Vertex**
- **Supraorbital margin**
- **Nasal bones**
- **Alveolar process of the maxilla**
- **Mental protuberance of the mandible**
- **Zygomatic arch**
- **Zygomatic bone**
- **Angle of the mandible**

Dissection Overview

The skin of the face receives sensory innervation from three divisions (branches) of the trigeminal nerve (V). Two cervical spinal nerves complete the cutaneous innervation of the head (Fig. 7.19).

- **Ophthalmic division (V₁)** – skin of the forehead, upper eyelids, and nose
- **Maxillary division (V₂)** – skin of the lower eyelid, cheek, and upper lip
- **Mandibular division (V₃)** – skin of the lower face and part of the side of the head
- **Cervical spinal nerves 2 and 3** – skin of the back of the head and the area around the ear

In contrast, all of the muscles of facial expression receive motor innervation from the **facial nerve (VII)**. [G 631; L 325; N 24; C 499]

The order of dissection will be as follows: The skin of the face will be removed to expose the muscles of facial expression. The parotid duct and gland will be identified. Branches of the facial nerve will be identified as they emerge from the anterior border of the parotid gland. Several facial muscles will be identified. Two important sphincter muscles will receive particular attention: the or-

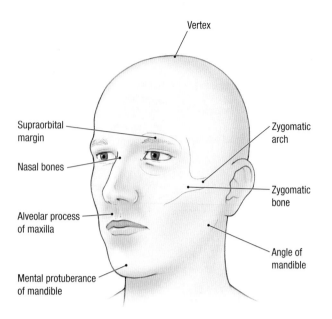

Figure 7.18. Surface anatomy of the face.

bicularis oris (mouth) and the orbicularis oculi (eye). The terminal branches of the three divisions of the trigeminal nerve will be exposed where they emerge from openings in the skull.

Dissection Instructions

SKIN INCISIONS

The skin of the face is very thin. It is firmly attached to the cartilage of the nose and ears but it is mobile over other parts of the face. This mobility permits the action of the muscles of facial expression. The muscles of facial expression are attached to the skin superficially and the bones of the skull deeply. They act as sphincters and dilators for the openings of the eyes, mouth, and nostrils.

1. Place the cadaver in the supine position and refer to Figure 7.20.
2. In the midline, make a skin incision that begins on the forehead at about the level of the hairline (A) passes through the nasion (B) and continues to the mental protuberance (C). Encircle the mouth at the margin of the lips.
3. On the lateral surface of the head, make a skin incision from point A to the upper part of the ear, then passing anterior to the ear down to the level of the ear lobe. This incision should end at the incision that was made when dissecting the neck (D).
4. Starting at the nasion (B), make an incision that encircles the orbital margin. Extend the incision from the lateral angle of the eye to the incision near the ear.
5. An incision was made from the mental protuberance (C) along the inferior border of the mandible to point D when the neck was dissected.
6. Beginning at the midline, remove the skin of the forehead. Note that the skin adheres to tough subcutaneous connective tissue. Leave this connective tissue intact and do not remove the frontalis muscle.
7. Remove the skin of the lower face, beginning at the midline and proceeding laterally. The superficial fascia of the face is thick and contains the muscles of facial expression.
8. Detach the skin along the incision line from the forehead to the angle of the mandible (A to D) and place it in the tissue container.

SUPERFICIAL FASCIA OF THE FACE [G 626; L 324, 325; N 23; R 76; C 494]

The superficial fascia of the face contains the parotid gland, part of the submandibular gland, muscles of facial expression, branches of the facial nerve, branches of the trigeminal nerve, and the facial artery and vein. The muscles of facial expression are attached to the skin, and these attachments have been severed during skin removal. The goal of this stage of the dissection is to identify some of the muscles of facial expression and

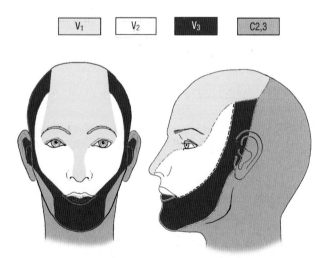

Figure 7.19. Cutaneous nerve distribution of the head and neck.

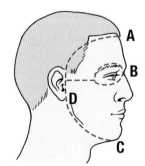
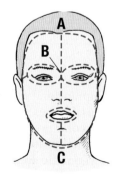

Figure 7.20. Skin incisions.

follow branches of the facial nerve posteriorly into the parotid gland.

1. A small part of the **platysma muscle** extends into the face along the inferior border of the mandible (Fig. 7.21). Recall that the inferior attachment of the platysma muscle is the superficial fascia of the upper thorax and that it forms a sheet of muscle that covers the anterior neck. Use blunt dissection to define the superior attachment of the muscle on the inferior border of the mandible, skin of the cheek, and angle of the mouth.
2. Identify the **masseter muscle**. It is a muscle of mastication, which will be dissected later.
3. Identify the **parotid duct** (Fig. 7.21). The parotid duct is approximately the diameter of a probe handle and it crosses the lateral surface of the masseter muscle about 2 cm inferior to the zygomatic arch. Use blunt dissection to follow the parotid duct anteriorly as far as the anterior border of the masseter muscle where the duct turns deeply, pierces the buccinator muscle of the cheek, and drains into the oral cavity.

FACIAL NERVE [G 627; L 325; N 25; R 76, 78; C 500]

1. Use a probe to follow the parotid duct posteriorly and identify the anterior margin of the **parotid gland**.
2. Study the branches of the facial nerve in an illustration (Fig. 7.21). Note that several small branches course parallel to the parotid duct. Using blunt dissection, locate one of these branches superior or inferior to the parotid duct.
3. Use a probe to follow the branch toward the anterior margin of the parotid gland. Move the probe parallel to the branch as you dissect through the superficial fascia.
4. At the anterior border of the parotid gland, extend your dissection field superiorly and inferiorly to locate other branches of the facial nerve. Identify the following:
   - **Temporal branch** – crosses the zygomatic arch
   - **Zygomatic branch** – crosses the zygomatic bone
   - **Buccal branches** – cross the superficial surface of the masseter muscle
   - **Mandibular branch** – parallels the inferior margin of the mandible
   - **Cervical branch** – crosses the angle of the mandible to enter the neck
5. The parotid gland has very tough connective tissue that will not yield to a probe. To follow the branches of the facial nerve into the parotid gland, use the point of a scalpel blade as a probe.
6. Follow the branches of the facial nerve into the parotid gland. Superficial to the nerves, remove the parotid gland piece by piece. Within the parotid gland the nerve branches join to form the **parotid plexus**. Follow the nerve branches poste-

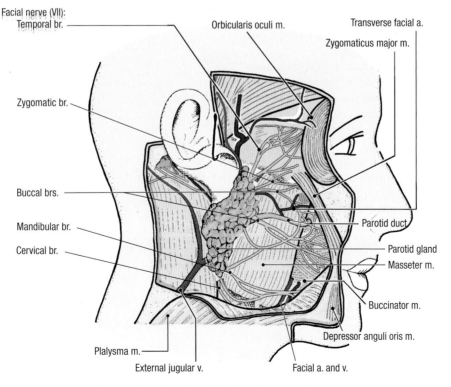

Figure 7.21. Dissection of the lateral aspect of the face.

riorly until they combine into one or two nerves, just anterior to the ear lobe.

7. Use a probe to define the anterior border of the **masseter muscle**. Anterior to the masseter muscle is the **buccal fat pad**. Use blunt dissection to remove the buccal fat pad and expose the **buccinator muscle**. Verify that the **parotid duct** pierces the buccinator muscle.

8. Observe that two nerves enter the buccinator muscle:
   • **Buccal branch of the facial nerve** – crosses the superficial surface of the masseter muscle and provides motor innervation to the buccinator muscle.
   • **Buccal nerve**, a branch of the mandibular division of the trigeminal nerve (V_3) – emerges from deep to the masseter muscle. The buccal nerve does not supply motor innervation to the buccinator muscle; it pierces the buccinator muscle to provide sensory innervation to the mucosa of the cheek. The buccal nerve also provides sensory innervation to the skin of the cheek.

FACIAL ARTERY AND VEIN [G 626; L 326; N 23; R 79; C 501]

The facial artery and vein follow a winding course across the face and they may pass either superficial or deep to the muscles of facial expression.

1. Find the **facial artery** where it crosses the inferior border of the mandible at the anterior edge of the masseter muscle (Fig. 7.21). The facial vein should be located posterior to the facial artery. At this location, the facial artery and vein are covered only by skin and the platysma muscle.

2. Preserve the facial vessels. Cut the platysma muscle along the inferior border of the mandible and detach it from the angle of the mouth. Place the platysma muscle in the tissue container.

3. Follow the facial artery inferiorly and note that the facial artery passes deep to the submandibular gland in the neck, then becomes superficial where it crosses the inferior border of the mandible. The facial vein travels a more superficial course relative to the submandibular gland and may have been cut when the gland was removed earlier.

4. Use a probe to trace the facial artery superiorly toward the angle of the mouth. Observe that the facial artery has several loops or bends in this part of its course. Near the angle of the mouth, the facial artery gives off the **inferior labial** and **superior labial arteries**.

5. Continue to trace the facial artery as far as the lateral side of the nose, where its name changes to **angular artery**.

6. The **facial vein** receives tributaries that correspond to the branches of the facial artery. The angular vein has a clinically important anastomotic connection with the ophthalmic veins in the orbit, which will be detailed when the orbit is dissected.

MUSCLES AROUND THE ORBITAL OPENING [G 626; L 324, 325; N 26; R 58; C 494]

1. At only 1 to 2 mm in thickness, the skin of the eyelids is the thinnest skin in the body. Carefully skin the upper and lower eyelids.

2. Identify the **orbicularis oculi muscle**, which encircles the **palpebral fissure** (opening of the eyelid) (Fig. 7.22). Identify:
   • **Orbital part** – surrounds the orbital margin and is responsible for the tight closure of the eyelid
   • **Palpebral part** – a thinner portion, which is contained in the eyelids and is responsible for blinking of the eyelid

3. Note that the medial attachment of the orbicularis oculi muscle is the medial orbital margin, the medial palpebral ligament, and the lacrimal bone. The lateral attachment of the orbicularis oculi muscle is the skin around the orbital margin. It is innervated by the temporal and zygomatic branches of the facial nerve.

MUSCLES AROUND THE ORAL OPENING [G 626, 630; L 324, 325; N 26; R 58; C 495]

1. Several muscles alter the shape of the mouth and lips. Use a probe to define some of these muscles (Fig. 7.22):

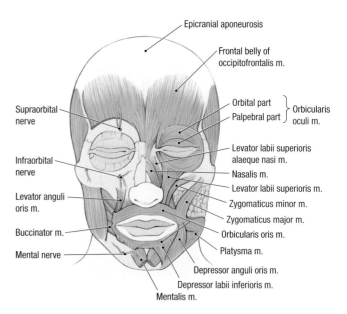

Figure 7.22. Muscles of the face.

- **Levator labii superioris muscle** – has a superior attachment to the maxilla just below the orbital margin and an inferior attachment to the upper lip. It elevates the upper lip.
- **Zygomaticus major muscle** – has a lateral attachment to the zygomatic bone and a medial attachment to the angle of the mouth. It draws the angle of the mouth superiorly and posteriorly.
- **Orbicularis oris muscle** – has medial attachments to the maxilla, mandible, and skin in the median plane and a lateral attachment to the angle of the mouth. The orbicularis oris muscle is the sphincter of the mouth.
- **Buccinator muscle** – has proximal attachments to the pterygomandibular raphe and the lateral surfaces of the alveolar processes of the maxilla and mandible. The distal attachment of the buccinator muscle is the angle of the mouth. It compresses the cheek against the molar teeth, keeping food on the occlusal surfaces during chewing.
- **Depressor anguli oris muscle** – has an inferior attachment to the mandible and a superior attachment to the angle of the mouth. It depresses the corner of the mouth.

2. The muscles described above are innervated by the zygomatic, buccal, and mandibular branches of the facial nerve.

Facial Nerve

Bell's palsy is a sudden loss of control of the muscles of facial expression on one side of the face. The patient presents with drooping of the mouth and inability to close the eyelid on the affected side.

SENSORY NERVES OF THE FACE [G 630; L 324; N 24; R 73; C 501]

1. Use an illustration to summarize the sensory nerves of the face (Fig. 7.23):
   - **Supraorbital nerve** – a branch of the ophthalmic division of the trigeminal nerve (V$_1$) that passes through the supraorbital notch (foramen). It will be dissected later.
   - **Infraorbital nerve** – a branch of the maxillary division of the trigeminal nerve (V$_2$) that passes through the infraorbital foramen.
   - **Mental nerve** – a branch of the mandibular division of the trigeminal nerve (V$_3$) that passes through the mental foramen.

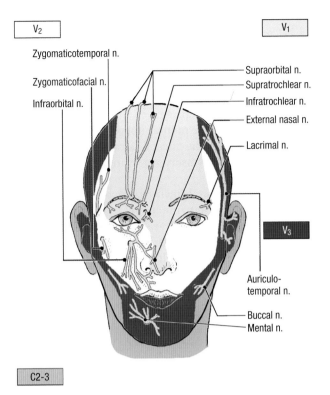

Figure 7.23. Sensory nerves of the face.

2. The supraorbital nerve passes through the supraorbital notch (foramen) and will be seen when the scalp is studied.
3. The infraorbital nerve emerges from the infraorbital foramen to supply sensory innervation to the inferior eyelid, side of the nose, and upper lip. On the right side, use blunt dissection to define the borders of the levator labii superioris muscle. Transect the muscle close to the infraorbital margin and reflect it inferiorly to expose the infraorbital nerve (V$_2$).

Dental Anesthesia

Study the infraorbital foramen and infraorbital canal in the skull. For purposes of dental anesthesia, the infraorbital nerve may be infiltrated where it emerges from the infraorbital foramen. The needle is inserted through the oral mucosa deep to the upper lip and directed superiorly.

4. In the midline, make an incision through the entire thickness of the lower lip, extending as far inferiorly as the mental protuberance. On the right side, make a second incision parallel to the first. The second incision should begin at the angle of the mouth and end at the margin of the mandible. Reflect the flap of lip inferiorly.

5. Cut through the mucous membrane where it reflects from the lip to the gums. Use blunt dissection to peel the flap of lip from the bone and locate the **mental foramen** (L. *mentum*, chin). The mental foramen is located approximately 3 cm from the median plane.

6. Observe that the **mental nerve, artery, and vein** emerge from the mental foramen. The mental nerve supplies sensory innervation to the lower lip and chin.

7. There are several smaller branches of the trigeminal nerve that innervate the facial region (lacrimal, infratrochlear, zygomaticofacial, zygomaticotemporal, etc.). Do not dissect these branches. The auriculotemporal nerve (a branch of V₃) will be dissected later.

Dissection Review

1. Use the dissected specimen to trace the branches of the facial nerve from the parotid plexus to the muscles of facial expression.
2. Review the attachments, action, and innervation of each muscle that was identified in this dissection.
3. Use a skull and the dissected specimen to review the branches of the trigeminal nerve that were dissected and the openings in the bones that they pass through.
4. Use an illustration and the dissected specimen to review the origin and course of the facial artery and vein.

PAROTID REGION

Dissection Overview

The parotid region (parotid bed) is the area occupied by the parotid gland and the vessels and nerves that pass through it. The parotid gland develops as an evagination of the oral mucosa and it surrounds the posterior edge of the ramus of the mandible. Therefore, the parotid gland is in close contact with nerves, vessels, muscles, bones, and ligaments in the region. The superficial portion of the parotid gland was removed to expose the branches of the facial nerve. The goal of this dissection is to remove the remainder of the parotid gland piece by piece, preserving the nerves and vessels that pass through it.

The order of dissection will be as follows: The branches of the facial nerve will be reviewed and then followed posteriorly toward the stylomastoid foramen. Parotid tissue will be removed during this process. The facial nerve will be transected near the lobe of the ear and reflected anteriorly to preserve its branching pattern. The retromandibular vein will be followed superiorly through the parotid

gland as more parotid tissue is removed. The external carotid artery will then be followed superiorly as additional parotid tissue is removed. Finally, remnants of the parotid gland will be removed in a final cleanup step.

SKELETON OF THE PAROTID REGION

Refer to a skull and identify (Fig. 7.24):

- **Temporal bone** [G 664; L 327; N 4; R 21; C 515]
  Mandibular fossa
  External acoustic meatus
  Styloid process
  Stylomastoid foramen
  Mastoid process
- **Mandible** [G 654; L 327; N 15; R 52; C 581]
  Head
  Neck
  Angle
  Ramus

Use the skull and an illustration to define the **boundaries of the parotid bed** (Fig. 7.25B): [G 662; L 326; N 34; R 77; C 499]

- **Posterior** – mastoid process and posterior belly of the digastric muscle
- **Anterior** – medial pterygoid muscle, ramus of the mandible, and masseter muscle
- **Medial** – styloid process and associated muscles (stylopharyngeus, styloglossus, and stylohyoid)
- **Posterosuperior** – floor of the external acoustic meatus

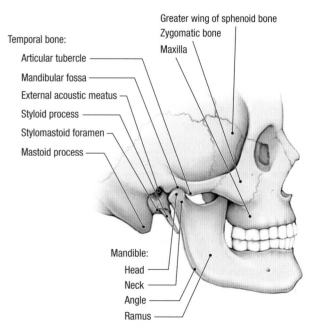

Temporal bone:
- Articular tubercle
- Mandibular fossa
- External acoustic meatus
- Styloid process
- Stylomastoid foramen
- Mastoid process

Greater wing of sphenoid bone
Zygomatic bone
Maxilla

Mandible:
- Head
- Neck
- Angle
- Ramus

Figure 7.24. Skeleton of the parotid region in lateral view.

A

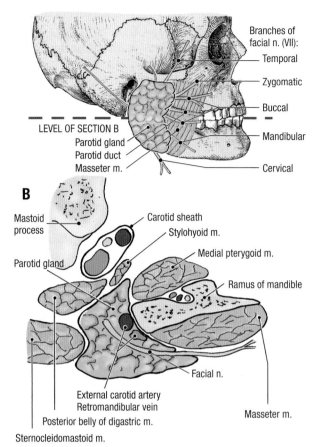

Branches of
facial n. (VII):

Temporal

Zygomatic

Buccal

Mandibular

Cervical

LEVEL OF SECTION B
Parotid gland
Parotid duct
Masseter m.

B

Mastoid
process

Parotid gland

Carotid sheath

Stylohyoid m.

Medial pterygoid m.

Ramus of mandible

Facial n.

External carotid artery
Retromandibular vein

Masseter m.

Posterior belly of digastric m.

Sternocleidomastoid m.

Figure 7.25. Topographic relations of the parotid gland.
A. Lateral view. Dashed line indicates the level of section B.
B. Transverse section through the parotid bed.

Dissection Instructions

1. Review the course of the parotid duct. The parotid duct enters the oral vestibule lateral to the second maxillary molar tooth.
2. Review the branches of the facial nerve: temporal, zygomatic, buccal, mandibular, and cervical (Fig. 7.25A). [G 662; L 326; N 25; R 77; C 501]
3. The parotid gland is enclosed within the **parotid sheath**. The parotid sheath and the stroma of the parotid gland are continuous with the superficial layer of the deep cervical fascia. This tough connective tissue will not yield to probe dissection. To dissect into the parotid gland, use the tip of a scalpel blade as you would normally use a probe.
4. Trace the facial nerve branches posteriorly toward the lobe of the ear. Remove small pieces of the parotid gland and place them in the tissue container. The branches of the parotid plexus will unite to form the **facial nerve**.
5. Follow the facial nerve as far as possible toward the **stylomastoid foramen**. Cut the facial nerve,

leaving a short stump emerging from the stylomastoid foramen. Reflect the parotid plexus and all of its branches anteriorly.

6. Cut the **parotid duct** at the anterior margin of the parotid gland and reflect the duct anteriorly. Do not disturb its passage through the buccinator muscle.
7. Identify the **auriculotemporal nerve**, a branch of the mandibular division of the trigeminal nerve (V_3). The auriculotemporal nerve passes between the head of the mandible and the external acoustic meatus. It crosses the zygomatic process of the temporal bone to innervate the skin of the anterior side of the ear and temporal region. As the auriculotemporal nerve passes through the parotid gland, it delivers postganglionic parasympathetic nerve fibers from the otic ganglion.
8. In the neck, find the **external jugular vein**. [L 313] Use blunt dissection to follow the external jugular vein superiorly to the point where it is formed by the joining of the posterior auricular vein and the retromandibular vein.
9. Use blunt dissection to follow the retromandibular vein superiorly until it enters the parotid gland. Switch to the scalpel dissection technique and remove small pieces of parotid tissue as you follow the retromandibular vein through the parotid gland.
10. Trace the retromandibular vein to the point where it is formed by the joining of the **maxillary vein** and the **superficial temporal vein**. Do not follow the maxillary vein, as it will be dissected later.
11. Follow the **superficial temporal vein** superiorly through the parotid gland until it crosses the superficial surface of the zygomatic arch.
12. Return to the neck and find the **external carotid artery**. Use blunt dissection to follow the external carotid artery to the inferior border of the parotid gland. [G 663; L 313, 314; N 34; R 79; C 510]
13. Switch to the scalpel dissection technique and follow the external carotid artery superiorly into the parotid gland. The external carotid artery passes superiorly along the posterior edge of the ramus of the mandible (Fig. 7.25B). Posterior to the neck of the mandible, the external carotid artery divides into its two terminal branches, the **maxillary artery** and the **superficial temporal artery**. Do not follow the maxillary artery, as it will be dissected later.
14. Use the scalpel dissection technique to clean the **superficial temporal artery**. The superficial temporal artery crosses the zygomatic process of the temporal bone just anterior to the external acoustic meatus. At this location, the superficial temporal artery is anterior to the auriculotempo-

ral nerve. The superficial temporal artery supplies the lateral part of the scalp.

15. Clean the lateral surface of the **posterior belly of the digastric muscle** and the **stylohyoid muscle**. Use the scalpel technique to remove all other remnants of the parotid gland.

Parotid Gland

Because of the close relationship between the parotid gland and the external acoustic meatus, swelling of the parotid gland (as occurs in mumps) pushes the ear lobe superiorly and laterally. During parotidectomy (surgical excision of the parotid gland), the facial nerve is in danger of being injured. If the facial nerve is damaged, the facial muscles are paralyzed.

Dissection Review

1. Replace the facial nerve in its correct anatomical position and approximate the cut ends.
2. Replace the parotid duct in its correct anatomical position.
3. Use an illustration, a skull, and the dissected specimen to review the course of the facial nerve from the internal acoustic meatus to the facial muscles.
4. Review the superficial venous drainage of the lateral side of the head and neck, beginning with the superficial temporal veins and ending with the subclavian vein in the root of the neck.
5. Review the origin, course, and branches of the external carotid artery.
6. Review the boundaries of the parotid bed.

SCALP [G 636; L 344; R 85; C 520]

Dissection Overview

The scalp consists of five layers that are firmly bound together (Fig. 7.26):

- **Skin**
- **Connective tissue** – dense subcutaneous tissue containing the vessels and nerves of the scalp
- **Aponeurosis** (epicranial aponeurosis) – connecting the frontalis muscle to the occipitalis muscle
- **Loose connective tissue** – permits the scalp to move over the calvaria
- **Pericranium** – the periosteum of the cranial bones

As an aid to memory, note that the first letters of the names of the five layers spell the word *scalp*.

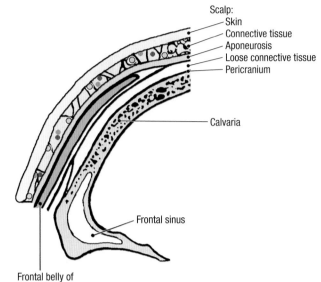

Figure 7.26. Layers of the scalp.

Scalp

The connective tissue layer of the scalp contains collagen fibers that attach to the external surface of the blood vessels. When a blood vessel of the scalp is cut, the connective tissue holds the lumen open, resulting in profuse bleeding.

If an infection occurs in the scalp, it can spread within the loose connective tissue layer. Therefore, the loose connective tissue layer is often called the "dangerous area." From the "dangerous area," the infection may pass into the cranial cavity through emissary veins.

The order of dissection will be as follows: The five layers of the scalp will be reflected as one. The muscles of the scalp will be examined on the cut surface of the scalp.

Dissection Instructions

1. These cuts should be made through the entire scalp and the scalpel should contact the bones of the calvaria.
2. Refer to Figure 7.27 and make a midline cut from the nasion (C) to the vertex (A). Extend this cut to the external occipital protuberance (G).
3. Make a cut in the coronal plane from the vertex (A) to the ear (D). Duplicate this cut on the opposite side of the head.
4. Beginning at the vertex, use forceps to grasp one corner of the cut scalp and insert a chisel between

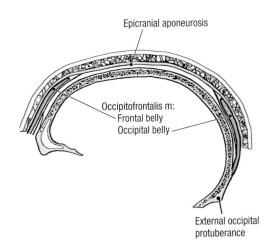

Figure 7.29. The occipitofrontalis muscle in sagittal section.

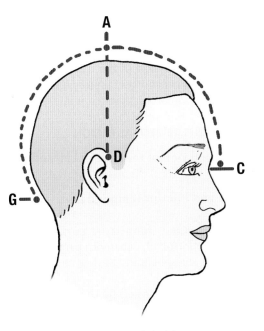

Figure 7.27. Scalp incisions.

the scalp and the calvaria. Use the chisel to loosen the scalp from the calvaria.

5. Once the flap of scalp is raised, grasp the flap with both hands and pull it inferiorly.

6. Reflect all four flaps of scalp down to the level that a hatband would occupy (Fig 7.28). Do not detach the flaps.

7. Examine the cut edge of the scalp and identify the **occipitofrontalis muscle** (Fig. 7.29). The inferior attachment of the occipital belly is the occipital bone and its superior attachment is the epicranial aponeurosis. The superior attachment of the frontal belly is the epicranial aponeurosis and its inferior attachment is the skin of the forehead and eyebrows. Both muscles are innervated by the fa-

cial nerve (VII). [G 629, 634; L 325; N 23, 26; R 59, 63; C 498, 500]

8. Pull the anterior scalp flap inferiorly to expose the supraorbital margin. Identify the **supraorbital nerve and vessels** where they exit the supraorbital notch and enter the deep surface of the scalp (Fig. 7.28).

9. Use an illustration to observe that nerves and vessels are contained within the flaps of the scalp (Fig. 7.30). Note that the nerves and vessels enter the scalp from more inferior regions.

10. On the lateral surface of the calvaria, note that the scalp has been separated from the fascia that covers the **temporalis muscle (temporal muscle)**.

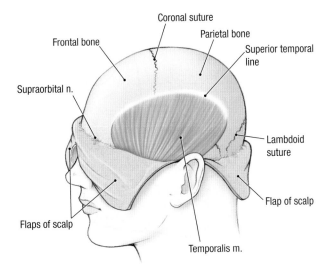

Figure 7.28. How to reflect the scalp.

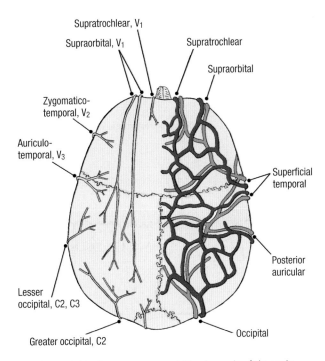

Figure 7.30. Sensory nerves and blood vessels of the scalp.

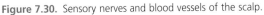

Dissection Review

1. Replace the flaps of scalp in their correct anatomical positions.
2. Use an illustration to review the course of nerves and vessels that supply the scalp.
3. Use a skull and the dissected specimen to review the course of the supraorbital nerve through the supraorbital notch.
4. Use an illustration to study the course of the greater occipital nerve from the cervical region to the posterior surface of the head.
5. Recall the attachments of the occipitofrontalis muscle and review its two bellies in the sagittal scalp cut.

TEMPORAL REGION

Dissection Overview

The **temporal region** consists of two fossae: temporal and infratemporal. The **temporal fossa** is located superior to the zygomatic arch and it contains the temporalis muscle. The **infratemporal fossa** is inferior to the zygomatic arch and deep to the ramus of the mandible. The infratemporal fossa contains the medial and lateral pterygoid muscles, branches of the mandibular division of the trigeminal nerve (V_3), and the maxillary vessels and their branches. The infratemporal and temporal fossae are in open communication with each other through the area between the zygomatic arch and the lateral surface of the skull.

The dissection will proceed as follows: The masseter muscle will be studied. The zygomatic arch will be detached and the masseter muscle will be reflected with the arch attached to it. The temporalis muscle will be studied. The coronoid process of the mandible will be detached and the temporalis muscle will be reflected with the coronoid process attached to it. The superior part of the ramus of the mandible will then be removed and the maxillary artery will be traced across the infratemporal fossa. The branches of the mandibular division of the trigeminal nerve will be dissected. The medial and lateral pterygoid muscles will be studied and the temporomandibular joint will be dissected.

SKELETON OF THE TEMPORAL REGION

Refer to a lateral view of the skull and identify the following (Figs. 7.15 and 7.24): [G 664; L 327; N 4; R 21; C 515]

- **Superior and inferior temporal lines** – on the parietal bone.
- **Temporal fossa** – formed by parts of four cranial bones: parietal, frontal, squamous part of temporal, and greater wing of sphenoid. Review the location of the pterion.
- **Zygomatic arch** – formed by **the zygomatic process of the temporal bone** and the **temporal process of the zygomatic bone.**
- **Mandibular fossa and articular tubercle** – on the temporal bone (Fig. 7.24).

From a lateral view of the mandible, identify (Fig. 7.31A): [G 664; L 327; N 15; R 52; C 581]

- **Head**
- **Neck**
- **Mandibular notch**
- **Coronoid process**
- **Ramus**
- **Angle**

On the **internal surface of the mandible**, identify (Fig. 7.31B):

- **Lingula** – for the attachment of the sphenomandibular ligament

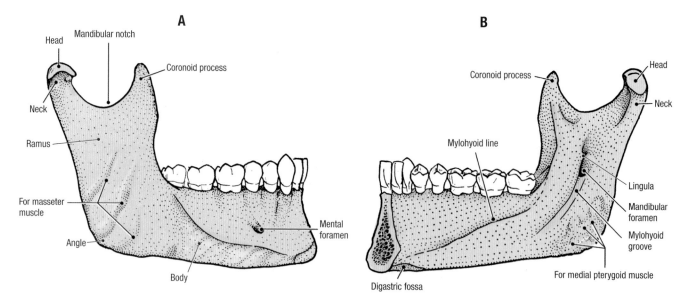

Figure 7.31. Mandible. **A.** External surface. **B.** Internal surface.

- **Mandibular foramen** – for the inferior alveolar nerves and vessels
- **Mylohyoid groove** – for the mylohyoid nerve and vessels

Remove the mandible from the skull and view the bones of the infratemporal fossa from the lateral perspective. Identify (Fig. 7.32): [G 665; L 327; N 4; C 541]

- **Pterygomaxillary fissure** – between the lateral plate of the pterygoid process and the maxilla
- **Inferior orbital fissure** – between the greater wing of the sphenoid bone and the maxilla
- **Infratemporal surface** of the maxilla
- **Greater wing of the sphenoid bone** – contains the **foramen ovale** and the **foramen spinosum**
- **Lateral plate of the pterygoid process** of the sphenoid bone
- **Pterygopalatine fossa** – at the superior end of the pterygomaxillary fissure
- **Sphenopalatine foramen** – an opening in the medial wall of the pterygopalatine fossa that enters the nasal cavity

Reposition the mandible on the skull and identify the **boundaries of the infratemporal fossa**:

- **Lateral** – ramus of the mandible
- **Anterior** – the infratemporal surface of the maxilla
- **Medial** – lateral plate of the pterygoid process
- **Roof** – greater wing of the sphenoid bone

Dissection Instructions

MASSETER MUSCLE AND REMOVAL OF THE ZYGOMATIC ARCH

1. Reflect the facial nerve branches and the parotid duct anteriorly.
2. Clean the lateral surface of the **masseter muscle**. The superior attachment of the masseter muscle is the inferior border of the zygomatic arch and its inferior attachment is the lateral surface of the ramus of the mandible. The masseter muscle elevates the mandible (closes the jaw) and protrudes the mandible. It is innervated by the masseteric branch of the mandibular division of the trigeminal nerve (V_3). [G 666; L 328; N 54; R 56; C 499]
3. Cut the temporal fascia along the superior temporal line and use a scalpel to peel it inferiorly. Observe that the temporalis muscle is attached to the deep surface of the temporal fascia. Cut the temporal fascia along the superior border of the zygomatic arch and remove the fascia completely.
4. Insert a probe deep to the zygomatic arch as close to the orbit as possible (Fig. 7.33, arrow 1). Use a saw to cut through the zygomatic bone to the probe.
5. Insert the probe deep to the zygomatic arch near the anterior border of the head of the mandible (Fig. 7.33, arrow 2). Use a saw to cut through the zygomatic arch to the probe.
6. Reflect the masseter muscle and the attached portion of the zygomatic arch in the inferior direction. Use a scalpel to detach the masseter muscle from the superior part of the ramus of the mandible, but leave the masseter muscle attached to the inferior part of the ramus, near the angle. During reflection, the masseteric nerve and vessels will be cut.

TEMPORAL REGION [G 666; L 328; N 54; R 56; C 499]

1. On a skull, identify the boundaries of the temporal fossa (Fig. 7.15):
   - **Superior and posterior** – superior temporal line

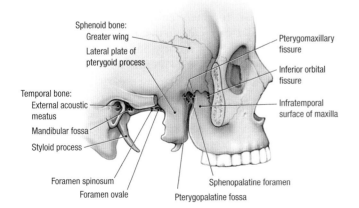

Figure 7.32. Skeleton of the infratemporal region.

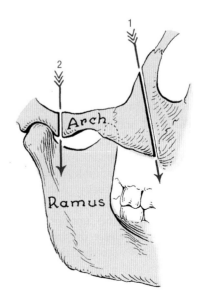

Figure 7.33. How to cut the zygomatic arch.

- **Anterior** – frontal and zygomatic bones
- **Inferior** – zygomatic arch superficially and in-fratemporal crest of the sphenoid bone deeply
- **Deep** – parts of the frontal, parietal, temporal, and sphenoid bones
- **Superficial** – temporal fascia

2. Note that the temporal vessels and the auriculotemporal nerve are located in the scalp, superficial to the temporal fascia. The primary content of the temporal fossa is the temporalis muscle.

3. Identify the **temporalis (temporal) muscle**. Observe:
   - The temporalis muscle was attached to the deep surface of the temporal fascia.
   - The inferior attachment of the temporalis muscle is the coronoid process of the mandible.
   - Fibers of the anterior portion of the temporalis muscle have a vertical direction (elevation of the mandible).
   - Fibers of the posterior portion of the temporalis muscle have a more horizontal direction (retraction of the mandible).

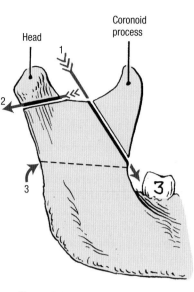

Figure 7.34. How to cut the mandible.

INFRATEMPORAL FOSSA [G 668; L 329; N 40; R 80; C 512]

1. On a skull, identify the boundaries of the infratemporal fossa:
   - **Superior**:
     Zygomatic arch superficially
     Infratemporal crest of the sphenoid bone deeply
   - **Anterior** – alveolar border of maxilla
   - **Lateral** – ramus of mandible
   - **Medial** – lateral plate of the pterygoid process

2. *Wear eye protection for all steps that require the use of bone cutters.*

3. The ramus of the mandible must be removed to view the contents of the infratemporal fossa. *The ramus of the mandible must be removed on both sides of the head to permit the head to be bisected in a later dissection step.*

4. The first step is to remove the coronoid process and reflect the temporalis muscle with the coronoid process attached. Insert a probe through the mandibular notch and push it anteroinferiorly toward the third mandibular molar tooth (Fig. 7.34, arrow 1). Keep the probe in close contact with the deep surface of the mandible. Use a saw to cut through the coronoid process to the probe.

5. Reflect the coronoid process together with the temporalis muscle in the superior direction. Use blunt dissection to release the temporalis muscle from the skull and note that the deep temporal nerves (branches of the mandibular division of the trigeminal nerve) enter the muscle from its deep surface. The deep temporal nerves provide motor

innervation to the temporalis muscle and they are accompanied by deep temporal arteries.

6. Insert a probe medial to the neck of the mandible (Fig. 7.34, arrow 2). Use a saw to cut through the neck of the mandible.

7. Use bone cutters to carefully nibble away the superior part of the mandible, beginning at the mandibular notch and proceeding inferiorly as far as the level of the lingula (Fig. 7.34, line 3). Make small cuts and stay on the lateral side of muscles, nerves, and vessels.

8. Deep to the mandible, identify the **inferior alveolar nerve** and **vessels** (Fig. 7.35B). Clean the inferior alveolar nerve and follow it to the mandibular foramen. Note that the mylohyoid nerve arises from the inferior alveolar nerve just before it enters the mandibular foramen.

9. The inferior alveolar nerve and vessels enter the mandibular foramen and pass distally in the **mandibular canal**. Note that the inferior alveolar nerve provides sensory innervation to the **mandibular teeth**. The **mental nerve** is a branch of the inferior alveolar nerve, which passes through the mental foramen to innervate the chin and lower lip.

10. Identify the **lingual nerve**. The lingual nerve is located just anterior to the inferior alveolar nerve. The lingual nerve passes medial to the third mandibular molar tooth and it innervates the mucosa of the anterior two-thirds of the tongue and floor of the oral cavity.

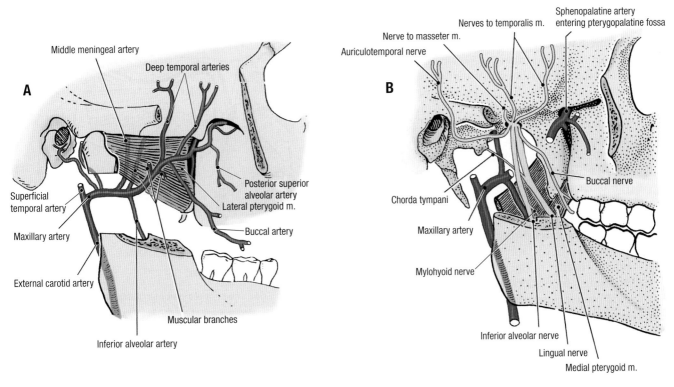

Figure 7.35. Arteries and nerves of the infratemporal fossa. **A.** Branches of the maxillary artery. **B.** Branches of the mandibular division of the trigeminal nerve (V3).

CLINICAL CORRELATION

Dental Anesthesia

A mandibular nerve block is produced by injecting an anesthetic agent into the infratemporal fossa. Understand from your dissection that the mandibular nerve block will anesthetize not only the mandibular teeth, but also the lower lip, the chin, and the tongue.

11. Identify the **maxillary artery** where it arises from the bifurcation of the external carotid artery (Fig. 7.35A). The maxillary artery crosses either the superficial surface (two-thirds) or the deep surface (one-third) of the lateral pterygoid muscle. If the maxillary artery in your specimen passes deep to the lateral pterygoid muscle, perform step 15 first and then return to step 12. [G 669, 670; L 330; N 40; R 80; C 513]

12. Use blunt dissection to trace the maxillary artery through the infratemporal fossa. The maxillary artery has 15 branches. Identify only the following five (Fig. 7.35A):
    - **Middle meningeal artery** – arises medial to the neck of the mandible and courses superiorly, passing through a split in the auriculotemporal nerve. The middle meningeal artery

passes through the foramen spinosum, enters the middle cranial fossa, and supplies the dura mater.
    - **Deep temporal arteries (anterior and posterior)** – pass superiorly and laterally across the roof of the infratemporal fossa at bone level and enter the deep surface of the temporalis muscle.
    - **Masseteric artery** (cut in a previous dissection step) – courses laterally and passes through the mandibular notch to enter the deep surface of the masseter muscle.
    - **Inferior alveolar artery** – enters the mandibular foramen with the inferior alveolar nerve.
    - **Buccal artery** – passes anteriorly to supply the cheek.

13. Identify the **lateral pterygoid muscle** (Fig. 7.35A). The lateral pterygoid muscle has two heads. The anterior attachment of the superior head is the infratemporal surface of the greater wing of the sphenoid bone. The anterior attachment of the inferior head is the lateral surface of the lateral plate of the pterygoid process. The posterior attachments of the lateral pterygoid muscle are the articular disc within the capsule of the temporomandibular joint and the neck of the mandible. The lateral pterygoid muscle depresses the mandible (opens the jaw). [G 672; L 329; N 55; R 57; C 512]

14. Inferior to the lateral pterygoid muscle, identify the **medial pterygoid muscle** (Fig. 7.35B). The lingual nerve and inferior alveolar nerve pass between the inferior border of the lateral pterygoid muscle and the medial pterygoid muscle and can be used as guides to separate the two muscles. The proximal attachments of the medial pterygoid muscle are the maxilla and the medial surface of the lateral plate of the pterygoid process. The distal attachment of the medial pterygoid muscle is the inner surface of the ramus of the mandible. The medial pterygoid muscle elevates the mandible (closes the jaw).

15. Remove the **lateral pterygoid muscle** to see the deeper part of the infratemporal fossa. Define the inferior border of the lateral pterygoid muscle by inserting a probe between it and the medial pterygoid muscle. Use scissors to cut the lateral pterygoid muscle close to its posterior attachments to the neck of the mandible and the articular disc. Remove the muscle in a piecemeal fashion to preserve superficially positioned nerves and vessels.

16. Use a probe to follow the **inferior alveolar nerve** and the **lingual nerve** to the foramen ovale in the roof of the infratemporal fossa. Identify the **chorda tympani**, which joins the posterior side of the lingual nerve (Fig. 7.35B).

17. Follow the maxillary artery toward the **pterygopalatine fossa**. Before entering the pterygopalatine fossa the maxillary artery divides into four branches: posterior superior alveolar artery, infraorbital artery, descending palatine artery, and sphenopalatine artery. At this time, identify only the **posterior superior alveolar artery**, which enters the infratemporal surface of the maxilla (Fig. 7.35A). The other branches will be dissected later.

TEMPOROMANDIBULAR JOINT [G 675; L 328; N 16; R 54; C 505]

1. Identify the capsule of the **temporomandibular joint**. The joint capsule is loose and its lateral surface is reinforced by the **temporomandibular ligament**.

2. Insert the point of a scalpel into the temporomandibular joint close to the mandibular fossa and open the **superior synovial cavity** of the joint (Fig. 7.36). Remove the head of the mandible along with the articular disc.

3. Examine the isolated specimen and note that the tendon of the lateral pterygoid muscle is attached to the neck of the mandible and the articular disc (Fig. 7.36). Cut the articular capsule to open the **inferior synovial cavity** and observe the shape and variable thickness of the articular disc.

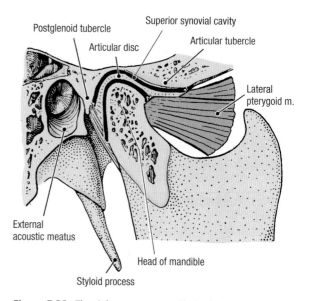

Figure 7.36. The right temporomandibular joint in lateral view.

4. Two types of movements occur in the temporomandibular joint. In the superior synovial cavity, gliding movements occur between the articular disc and the articular tubercle (protrusion and retraction). In the inferior synovial cavity, hinge movements occur between the head of the mandible and the articular disc.

5. Place your fifth digit in the cartilaginous portion of your external acoustic meatus. Palpate the head of the mandible as you perform hinge movements of the mandible and protrude and retract your mandible.

Dissection Review

1. Review the attachments and actions of the four muscles of mastication (masseter, temporalis, medial pterygoid, and lateral pterygoid).

2. Use an atlas illustration to study the origin of the mandibular division of the trigeminal nerve (V_3) at the trigeminal ganglion and trace it to the foramen ovale. Follow the mandibular division of the trigeminal nerve through the foramen ovale into the infratemporal fossa. Review the sensory and motor branches of the mandibular division.

3. Follow the external carotid artery from its origin near the hyoid bone to the infratemporal fossa.

4. Review the course of the superficial temporal artery and the maxillary artery. Follow the branches of the maxillary artery that were identified in dissection to their regions of supply.

5. Note the relationship of the middle meningeal artery to the auriculotemporal nerve.

6. Use an illustration and the dissected specimen to preview the terminal branches of the maxillary artery.

INTERIOR OF THE SKULL

Dissection Overview

Many schools remove the brain before the cadaver is placed on the dissection table. If the brain has been removed in your specimen, skip ahead to the section entitled Cranial Meninges. If you must remove the brain yourself, proceed with the following instructions.

The bones of the calvaria provide a protective covering for the cerebral hemispheres. To view the internal features of the cranial cavity, the calvaria must be removed. In addition, a wedge of occipital bone will be removed to open the dissection field and make removal of the brain easier.

The order of dissection will be as follows: The scalp and temporalis muscle will be reflected inferiorly. The calvaria will be cut with a saw and removed. A wedge of occipital bone will be removed. The dura mater will be examined and then opened to reveal the arachnoid mater and pia mater.

Dissection Instructions

REMOVAL OF THE CALVARIA

1. The cadaver should be in the supine position. Reflect the scalp inferiorly.
2. Use a scalpel to detach the temporalis muscle from the calvaria and reflect the temporalis muscle inferiorly. Fold it down over the reflected scalp (Fig. 7.37).
3. Observe the **pericranium** that covers the calvaria. Use a scalpel or chisel to scrape the bones of the calvaria clean of periosteum and muscle fibers.
4. Place a rubber band around the circumference of the skull (Fig. 7.37, dashed line). Anteriorly, the

rubber band should be about 2 cm superior to the supraorbital margin. Posteriorly, the rubber band should be about 2 cm superior to the external occipital protuberance. Use the rubber band as a guide to mark the circumference of the calvaria with a pencil line.

5. Refer to a skull. Remove the calvaria and note that the bones of the calvaria have three layers:
   - **Outer lamina** – compact bone
   - **Diploë** – spongy bone between the outer and inner laminae
   - **Inner lamina** – compact bone
6. Use a saw to cut along the pencil line. The saw cut should pass through the outer lamina of the calvaria but not completely through the bone. Moist red bone indicates that the saw is within the diploë. Be particularly careful when cutting the squamous part of the temporal bone, which is very thin. If you saw through the inner lamina, you may damage the underlying dura mater or the brain.
7. While sawing, turn the body alternately from supine to prone and back to supine as you work your way around the skull. After making a complete circumferential cut, break the inner lamina of the calvaria by repeatedly inserting a chisel into the saw cut and striking the chisel gently with a mallet. Continue with this procedure until the calvaria can be pried loose.
8. Remove the calvaria by prying it from the dura mater with the handle of a forceps or a chisel blade. Work from anterior to posterior and do not use more force than is necessary. Violent pulling may result in tearing of the dura and damage to the brain.

REMOVAL OF A WEDGE OF OCCIPITAL BONE

1. Place the cadaver in the prone position and refer to Figure 7.38.
2. Use a scalpel to detach the semispinalis capitis muscle, splenius capitis muscle, obliquus capitis superior muscle, and rectus capitis posterior major and minor muscles from the occipital bone.
3. Identify the **posterior atlanto-occipital membrane**, which spans the interval between the **atlas** (C1) and the **occipital bone**. Use a scalpel to incise the posterior atlanto-occipital membrane transversely from the left vertebral artery to the right vertebral artery. Preserve the **vertebral arteries**.
4. Use a scalpel or chisel to scrape the occipital bone clean of remaining muscle fibers and pericranium.
5. Review the following landmarks on a skull (Fig. 7.38): [G 614; L 300; N 4; R 21; C 515]
   - **Mastoid process**
   - **External occipital protuberance**
   - **Lambdoid suture**

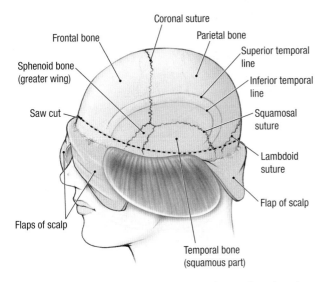

Figure 7.37. How to reflect the temporalis muscle and mark the calvaria for sawing.

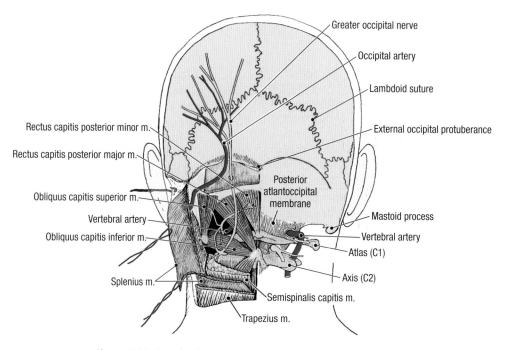

Figure 7.38. Muscles that must be removed to cut an occipital wedge.

6. On the skull, note the point where the lambdoid suture meets the saw cut where the calvaria was removed. Transfer this point to the cadaver specimen and mark the location with a pencil (Fig. 7.39, point A).

7. On the skull, examine the internal surface of the **occipital bone** and identify (Fig. 7.40): [G 619; L 302; N 9; R 30; C 531]
   • **Foramen magnum**
   • **Groove for the superior sagittal sinus**

• **Grooves for the transverse sinuses**
• **Fossae for the cerebellum (2)** – inferior to the grooves for the transverse sinuses
• **Fossae for the occipital poles of the cerebral hemispheres (2)** – superior to the grooves for the transverse sinuses

8. On the external surface of the skull, identify the lateral margin of the foramen magnum and transfer this point to the cadaver specimen (Fig. 7.39, point B). On the right and left sides of the cadaver,

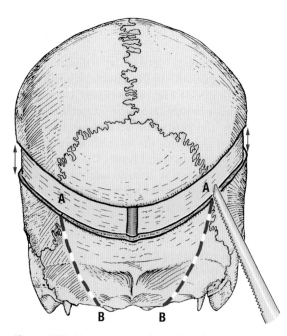

Figure 7.39. How to remove the wedge of occipital bone. Make one saw cut on each side from A to B.

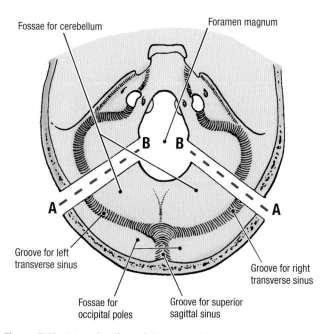

Figure 7.40. Internal surface of the occipital bone. Demarcation of the wedge-shaped area that is to be removed from the occipital bone.

connect points A and B with a pencil line to define the wedge of occipital bone that will be removed in the cadaver.

9. Use a saw to cut along the pencil lines. As in the removal of the calvaria, do not cut through the inner lamina of compact bone. Extend the saw cut into the foramen magnum but preserve the vertebral arteries. Loosen the wedge of bone with chisel and mallet and remove it, leaving the dura mater intact (Fig. 7.41).

CRANIAL MENINGES [G 636; L 344; N 102; R 84; C 520]

1. The brain is covered with three membranes called meninges (Gr. *meninx*, membrane). From outside to inside they are (Fig. 7.42):
   - **Dura mater** – the outer tough membrane
   - **Arachnoid mater** – the intermediate membrane
   - **Pia mater** – a delicate membrane that is closely applied to the surface of the brain
2. The **dura mater** (L. *dura mater*, hard mother) consists of two layers, an external **periosteal layer** and an internal **meningeal layer** (Fig. 7.42). The two dural layers are indistinguishable except where they separate to enclose the dural venous sinuses.
3. Identify the **superior sagittal sinus** and the right and left **transverse sinuses** (Fig. 7.41). [G 637; L 342, 343; N 100; C 521]

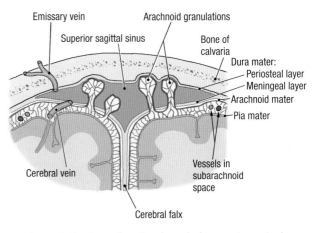

Figure 7.42. Coronal section through the superior sagittal sinus showing the meninges.

4. Use scissors to make a longitudinal incision in the superior sagittal sinus (Fig. 7.43) and verify that:
   - Its inner surface is smooth because it is lined by endothelium.
   - Its caliber increases from anterior to posterior (direction of venous blood flow).
   - It has lateral expansions called **lateral venous lacunae.**
   - **Arachnoid granulations** may be seen in the lateral venous lacunae (Fig. 7.42). The arachnoid granulations return cerebrospinal fluid (CSF) to the venous system.
5. Examine the surface of the dura mater that covers the cerebral hemispheres and observe the branches of the **middle meningeal artery**. The middle meningeal artery supplies the dura mater and adjacent calvaria. Note that the **anterior branch** of the middle meningeal artery crosses the inner surface of the **pterion**, where it may tunnel through the bone. Fractures through the pterion may result in tearing of the middle meningeal artery.

CLINICAL CORRELATION

Epidural Hematoma

When the middle meningeal artery is torn in a head injury, blood accumulates between the skull and the dura mater (epidural hematoma).

6. Examine the inner surface of the removed calvaria. Identify the following features: [L 300; N 7; C 517]
   - **Groove for the superior sagittal sinus**
   - **Granular foveolae** – shallow depressions caused by the arachnoid granulations
   - **Grooves for the branches of the middle meningeal artery**

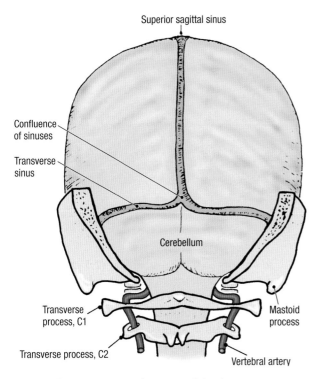

Figure 7.41. Posterior aspect of the dura mater.

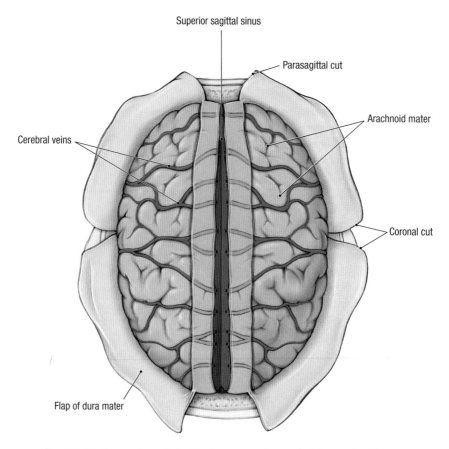

Superior sagittal sinus

Parasagittal cut

Arachnoid mater

Cerebral veins

Coronal cut

Flap of dura mater

Figure 7.43. Dura mater reflected to show a superior view of the arachnoid mater.

7. Use scissors to make a parasagittal cut through the dura mater about 2 cm lateral to the midline (Fig. 7.43). Cut only the dura mater, not the arachnoid mater. This cut should be lateral and parallel to the lateral edge of the superior sagittal sinus. Extend the cut to the frontal bone anteriorly and to the transverse sinus posteriorly. Duplicate the parasagittal cut on the opposite side of the cadaver.

8. Make a coronal cut through the dura mater from the midpoint of the parasagittal cut (near the vertex) to just above the ear (Fig. 7.43). Repeat on the opposite side of the midline.

9. The result of these cuts is a median strip of dura mater containing the superior sagittal sinus and four flaps of dura mater that are similar in position to the scalp flaps (Fig. 7.43). Fold the dural flaps inferiorly over the cut edge of the skull. Use scissors to detach any small adhesions or blood vessels that constrain the flaps.

10. Observe the **arachnoid mater** (Gr. *arachnoeides*, like a cobweb—in reference to the spider web–like connective tissue strands in the subarachnoid space). The arachnoid mater loosely covers the brain and spans across the fissures and sulci. In the living person, the arachnoid mater is closely applied to the internal meningeal layer of the dura mater with no space between (Fig. 7.42). [G 637; L 344; N 102; R 84]

11. Observe the **cerebral veins** that are visible through the arachnoid mater. The cerebral veins empty into the superior sagittal sinus. At the point where the cerebral veins enter the sinus, they may be torn in cases of head trauma.

CLINICAL CORRELATION

Subdural Hematoma

As a complication of head injury, cerebral veins may bleed into the potential space between the dura mater and the arachnoid mater. When this happens, the blood accumulates between the dura mater and arachnoid mater (a "subdural space" is created), and this condition is called a subdural hematoma.

12. Use scissors to make a small cut (2.5 cm) through the arachnoid mater over the lateral surface of the brain. Use a probe to elevate the arachnoid mater and observe the **subarachnoid space**. In the living person, the subarachnoid space is a real space that contains cerebrospinal fluid.

13. Through the opening in the arachnoid mater, observe the **pia mater** (L. *pia mater*, tender mother)

on the surface of the brain. The pia mater faithfully follows the contours of the brain, passing into all sulci and fissures. The pia mater cannot be removed from the surface of the brain.

Dissection Review

1. Review the bones that form the calvaria.
2. Review the external features of the cranial dura mater and note that the external periosteal layer is attached to the skull.
3. Review the features of the spinal dura mater and compare it to the cranial dura mater.
4. Review the extradural (epidural) space in the vertebral canal and recall that it contains fat and the internal vertebral venous plexus. Under normal conditions there is no extradural space in the cranial cavity.
5. Compare and contrast the features of an epidural hematoma and a subdural hematoma.

REMOVAL OF THE BRAIN

Dissection Overview

If the brain has been removed from your cadaver, skip ahead to the section entitled Dural Infoldings and Dural Venous Sinuses.

The internal meningeal layer of the dura mater forms inwardly projecting folds (dural infoldings) that serve as incomplete partitions of the cranial cavity. Three of these folds (cerebral falx, cerebellar tentorium, and cerebellar falx) extend inward between parts of the brain. These infoldings must first be cut before the brain can be removed.

The order of dissection will be as follows: The brain will be removed intact, along with the arachnoid mater and pia mater. The dura mater will be left in the cranial cavity, where the dural infoldings will be studied.

Dissection Instructions

1. Use a skull to identify the following features (Fig 7.44): [G 619; L 302; N 9; R 30; C 531]
   - **Crista galli**
   - **Cribriform plate**
   - **Anterior clinoid process**
   - **Posterior clinoid process**
   - **Superior border of the petrous part of the temporal bone**
   - **Internal acoustic meatus**
   - **Jugular foramen**
   - **Hypoglossal canal**
   - **Foramen magnum**
   - **Groove for the sigmoid sinus**
   - **Groove for the transverse sinus**

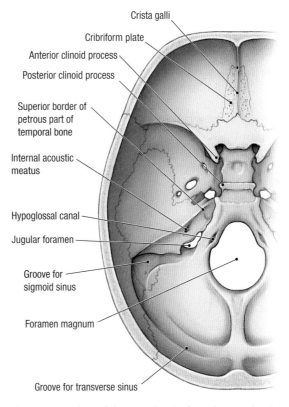

Figure 7.44. Floor of the cranial cavity from the superior view.

2. In the midline, use your fingers to gently retract one cerebral hemisphere 1 or 2 cm laterally and observe the **cerebral falx** (L. *falx*, sickle) between the cerebral hemispheres (Fig. 7.45). The cerebral falx is attached to the **crista galli** at its anterior end and the **cerebellar tentorium** at its posterior end. [G 638; L 342, 343; N 103; R 87; C 523]
3. Use your hand to gently lift the frontal lobes (anterior part of the brain) and use scissors to cut the cerebral falx where it is attached to the crista galli.
4. Use scissors to cut the cerebral veins where they enter the superior sagittal sinus (Fig. 7.43) so that the veins will remain on the surface of the brain. Grasp the cerebral falx near the crista galli and pull it superiorly and posteriorly from between the cerebral hemispheres. At its posterior end, the cerebral falx will remain attached to the cerebellar tentorium.
5. On the right side, gently lift the occipital lobe (posterior part of brain) and observe the **cerebellar tentorium**. Beginning anteriorly, use a scalpel to cut the cerebellar tentorium as close to bone as possible. Sever the cerebellar tentorium from the posterior clinoid process and then from the superior border of the petrous part of the temporal bone (Fig. 7.44). The cut should continue to the posterolateral end of the superior border of the petrous part of the temporal bone, near the groove

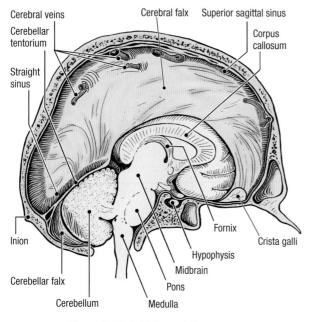

Figure 7.45. Infoldings of dura mater.

for the sigmoid sinus. Repeat the cut on the left side of the cadaver.

6. Pull the cerebral falx and cerebellar tentorium posteriorly from between the cerebral hemispheres and cerebellum. This procedure will tear the **great cerebral vein** (Fig. 7.46).

7. With the dural infoldings detached, the brain may be gently moved to expose the cranial nerves and vessels that are located on its inferior surface.

8. Use your fingers to gently elevate the frontal lobes. Use a probe to lift the olfactory bulb from the cribriform plate on each side of the crista galli.

9. Use a scalpel to cut the following structures bilaterally: optic nerve, internal carotid artery, and oculomotor nerve. Cut the stalk of the pituitary gland in the midline.

10. Raise the brain slightly higher and cut the following structures bilaterally: trochlear nerve, trigeminal nerve, and abducent nerve.

11. Elevate the cerebrum and brainstem still further and cut the following structures bilaterally: facial and vestibulocochlear nerves near the internal acoustic meatus; glossopharyngeal, vagus, and accessory nerves near the jugular foramen; and hypoglossal nerve near the hypoglossal canal.

12. Sever the two vertebral arteries where they enter the skull through the foramen magnum and use a scalpel to cut the cervical spinal cord as low in the foramen magnum (or cervical vertebral canal) as you can reach.

13. Support the brain with the palm of one hand under the frontal lobes and your fingers extending down the ventral surface of the brainstem. Insert the tip of your middle finger into the cut that was made across the cervical spinal cord to support the brainstem and cerebellum. Roll the brain, brainstem, and cerebellum posteriorly and out of the cranial cavity in one piece.

14. The brain should be stored in a bath of preservative fluid.

DURAL INFOLDINGS AND DURAL VENOUS SINUSES

Dissection Overview

The two layers of the dura mater separate in several locations to form dural venous sinuses. The dural venous sinuses collect venous drainage from the brain and conduct it out of the cranial cavity.

The order of dissection will be as follows: The dura mater will be repositioned to recreate its three-dimensional morphology during life. The infoldings of the dura mater and the associated dural venous sinuses will be identified.

Dissection Instructions

DURAL INFOLDINGS [G 638; L 343; N 103; R 87; C 522]

1. Return the dura mater to its correct anatomical position.

2. On the right side of the head, open the two flaps of dura mater and identify the **cerebral falx (falx**

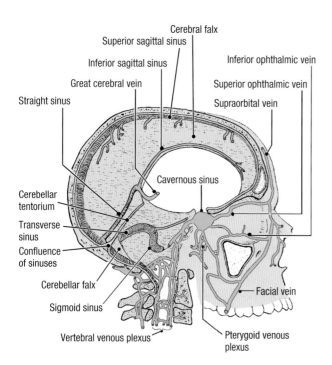

Figure 7.46. Dural venous sinuses.

cerebri) (Fig. 7.46). In the living person, the cerebral falx lies between the cerebral hemispheres. The cerebral falx is attached to the crista galli, the calvaria on both sides of the groove for the superior sagittal sinus, and the cerebellar tentorium.

3. Identify the **cerebellar tentorium** (**tentorium cerebelli**; L. *tentorium*, tent) (Fig. 7.45). The cerebellar tentorium is attached to the clinoid processes of the sphenoid bone, the superior border of the petrous portion of the temporal bone, and the occipital bone on both sides of the groove for the transverse sinus. The opening in the cerebellar tentorium is called the **tentorial notch (tentorial incisure)**, and the brainstem passes through it. In the living person, the cerebellar tentorium is between the cerebral hemispheres and the cerebellum.

4. Identify the **cerebellar falx (falx cerebelli)**, which is located inferior to the cerebellar tentorium in the midline (Fig. 7.46). Note that the cerebellar falx is attached to the inner surface of the occipital bone and that it is located between the cerebellar hemispheres.

DURAL VENOUS SINUSES [G 639; L 342, 343; N 104; R 87; C 522]

1. Review the position of the **superior sagittal sinus** (Fig. 7.46). Note that the superior sagittal sinus begins near the crista galli and ends near the cerebellar tentorium by draining into the **confluence of sinuses**.

2. Identify the **inferior sagittal sinus**, which is in the inferior margin of the cerebral falx (Fig. 7.46). The inferior sagittal sinus begins anteriorly and ends near the cerebellar tentorium by draining into the straight sinus. Note that the inferior sagittal sinus is much smaller in diameter than the superior sagittal sinus.

3. The **straight sinus** is located in the line of junction of the cerebral falx and the cerebellar tentorium. At its anterior end, the straight sinus receives the inferior sagittal sinus and the **great cerebral vein**. The straight sinus drains into the confluence of sinuses.

4. Review the position of the **transverse sinuses** (right and left). Each transverse sinus carries venous blood from the confluence of sinuses to the sigmoid sinus. Use a scalpel to open the lumen of the transverse sinus.

5. Identify the **sigmoid sinus**. The sigmoid sinus begins at the lateral end of the transverse sinus and ends at the jugular foramen. Use a scalpel to open the lumen of the sigmoid sinus and trace it to the jugular foramen. The **internal jugular vein** is formed at the external surface of the jugular foramen.

6. Observe the floor of the cranial cavity. Note that the dura mater covers all of the bones and provides openings through which the cranial nerves pass. There are small dural venous sinuses located between the layers of the dura mater in the floor of the cranial cavity. Use an atlas illustration to study the following dural venous sinuses: [G 639; L 342; N 104; R 87; C 532]
   - **Sphenoparietal sinus**
   - **Cavernous sinus**
   - **Superior petrosal sinus**
   - **Inferior petrosal sinus**
   - **Basilar plexus**

Dissection Review

1. Review the infoldings of the dura mater and obtain a three-dimensional understanding of their arrangement.
2. Naming all venous structures encountered along the way, trace the route of a drop of blood from:
   - A cerebral vein to the internal jugular vein
   - The sphenoparietal sinus to the sigmoid sinus
   - The great cerebral vein to the internal jugular vein

GROSS ANATOMY OF THE BRAIN

Dissection Overview

The study of brain anatomy is highly specialized and is usually reserved for a neuroscience course. The description that is provided here is intended to relate the major features of the external surface of the brain to the parts of the skull that will be studied in subsequent dissections. An additional goal of this study is to establish a mental picture of the continuity of the arteries and nerves of the brain with those same structures that are left behind in the cranial fossae after brain removal.

Dissection Instructions

1. Examine the **lateral surface of the brain** and identify (Fig. 7.47): [G 722; L 348; N 105; R 92]
   - **Frontal lobe**
   - **Central sulcus**
   - **Parietal lobe**
   - **Occipital lobe**
   - **Lateral sulcus**
   - **Temporal lobe**
2. Identify the **cerebellum** and the **brainstem**.
3. Refer to a skull and identify the **three cranial fossae: anterior, middle**, and **posterior** (Fig. 7.47).

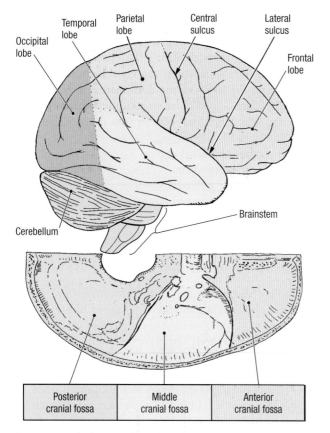

Occipital lobe / Temporal lobe / Parietal lobe / Central sulcus / Lateral sulcus / Frontal lobe / Brainstem / Cerebellum

Posterior cranial fossa | Middle cranial fossa | Anterior cranial fossa

Figure 7.47. The brain and its relationship to the three cranial fossae.

Use the cadaver specimen and the brain to verify the following: [N 9; C 531]

- The **frontal lobe** is located in the **anterior cranial fossa.**
- The **temporal lobe** is located in the **middle cranial fossa.**
- The **cerebellum** is located in the **posterior cranial fossa.**
- The **occipital lobe** is located superior to the cerebellar tentorium.
- The **brainstem** becomes continuous with the cervical spinal cord at the **foramen magnum.**

4. Examine the inferior surface of the brain and note that it is covered by arachnoid mater. Use a probe to peel back the arachnoid mater and expose the arteries. Observe the arteries and note the following (Fig. 7.48): [G 646; L 347, 351; N 139; R 93; C 526, 527]

- Two vertebral arteries and two internal carotid arteries supply the brain.
- Each **vertebral artery** gives rise to one **posterior inferior cerebellar artery (PICA).**
- The two vertebral arteries combine to form the **basilar artery.**
- The **basilar artery** gives off the **anterior inferior cerebellar artery,** the **superior cerebel-**

lar artery, and several **pontine branches.**

- The basilar artery terminates by branching into two **posterior cerebral arteries.**
- Each posterior cerebral artery gives off a **posterior communicating artery** that anastomoses with the **internal carotid artery.**
- After giving off the **ophthalmic artery,** each internal carotid artery terminates by dividing into a **middle cerebral artery** and an **anterior cerebral artery.**
- The anterior cerebral arteries are joined across the midline by the **anterior communicating artery.**
- The **cerebral arterial circle** is formed by the posterior cerebral, posterior communicating, internal carotid, anterior cerebral, and anterior communicating arteries.

5. On the inferior surface of the brain, identify the **12 cranial nerves** by name and by number (Fig. 7.48):

- **Olfactory bulb and tract (I)**
- **Optic (II)**
- **Oculomotor (III)**
- **Trochlear (IV)**
- **Trigeminal (V)**
- **Abducent (VI)**
- **Facial (VII)**
- **Vestibulocochlear (VIII)**
- **Glossopharyngeal (IX)**
- **Vagus (X)**
- **Accessory (XI)**
- **Hypoglossal (XII)**

Dissection Review

1. Review the parts of the brain and the cranial fossae in which they are found.
2. Review the infoldings of the dura mater and their relationship to the cerebral hemispheres and cerebellum.
3. Review the formation of the cerebral arterial circle.
4. Recall the origins of the internal carotid and vertebral arteries and the route that each takes to enter the cranial cavity.

CRANIAL FOSSAE

Dissection Overview

The order of dissection will be as follows: The bones of the floor of the cranial cavity will be studied and the boundaries of the cranial fossae will be identified. The vessels and the nerves of each cranial fossa will be studied. Because the floor of the cranial cavity is covered by dura mater, the dissection is much easier if a skull is held beside the cadaver specimen during dissection to permit direct observation of the foramina.

Nerves

Vessels

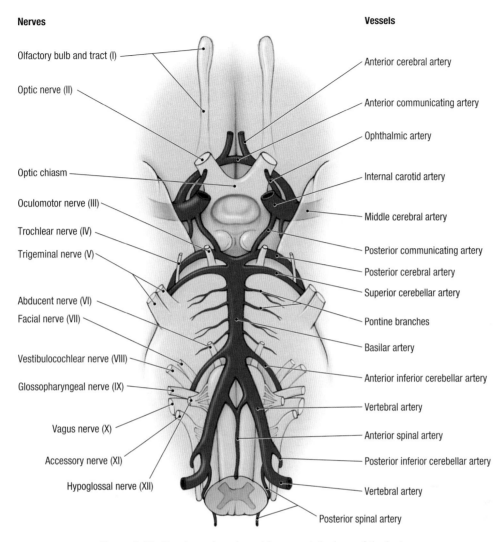

Olfactory bulb and tract (I)

Optic nerve (II)

Optic chiasm

Oculomotor nerve (III)

Trochlear nerve (IV)

Trigeminal nerve (V)

Abducent nerve (VI)

Facial nerve (VII)

Vestibulocochlear nerve (VIII)

Glossopharyngeal nerve (IX)

Vagus nerve (X)

Accessory nerve (XI)

Hypoglossal nerve (XII)

Anterior cerebral artery

Anterior communicating artery

Ophthalmic artery

Internal carotid artery

Middle cerebral artery

Posterior communicating artery

Posterior cerebral artery

Superior cerebellar artery

Pontine branches

Basilar artery

Anterior inferior cerebellar artery

Vertebral artery

Anterior spinal artery

Posterior inferior cerebellar artery

Vertebral artery

Posterior spinal artery

Figure 7.48. Blood vessels and cranial nerves at the base of the brain.

SKELETON OF THE CRANIAL BASE

Use a skull to identify (Fig. 7.49): [G 618, 619; L 302; N 9; R 30; C 531]

- **Ethmoid bone**
  Crista galli
  Cribriform plate
- **Frontal bone**
  Orbital part
- **Sphenoid bone**
  Lesser wing
  Sphenoidal crest
  Superior orbital fissure
  Anterior clinoid process
  Sphenoidal limbus
  Optic canal
  Hypophyseal fossa
  Posterior clinoid process
  Greater wing
    Foramen rotundum
    Foramen ovale
    Foramen spinosum

- **Temporal bone**
  Squamous part
  Petrous part
    Superior border (petrous ridge)
  Groove for the sigmoid sinus
  Internal acoustic meatus
- **Occipital bone**
  Clivus
  Jugular foramen
  Hypoglossal canal
  Groove for the sigmoid sinus
  Foramen magnum
  Groove for the transverse sinus
  Internal occipital protuberance

Identify the **foramen lacerum,** which is formed by portions of the greater wing of the sphenoid bone and the temporal bone.

The **anterior cranial fossa** is separated from the **middle cranial fossa** by the right and left sphenoidal crests and the sphenoidal limbus. The middle cranial fossa is separated from the **posterior cranial fossa** by the superior border of

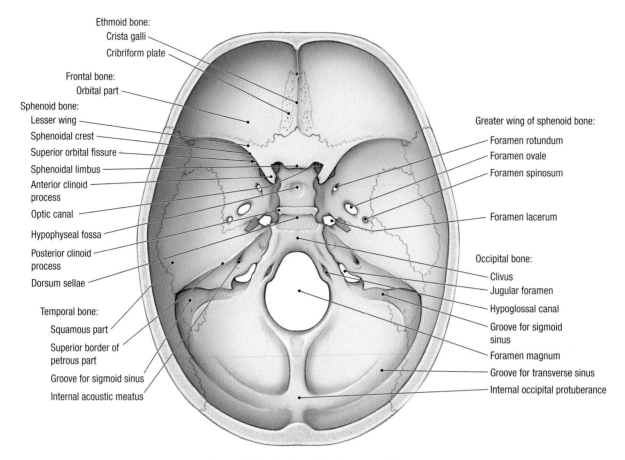

Figure 7.49. Features of the three cranial fossae.

the petrous part of the right and left temporal bones and the dorsum sellae. The cerebellar tentorium is attached to the superior border of the petrous part of the temporal bone and it forms the roof of the posterior cranial fossa.

Dissection Instructions

ANTERIOR CRANIAL FOSSA [G 640; L 346; N 104; R 64; C 532]

1. On the right side of the cadaver only, use a probe to loosen the dura mater along the cut edge of the frontal bone. Grasp the dura mater with your fingers and pull it posteriorly as far as the lesser wing of the sphenoid bone. Use scissors to detach the dura mater along the sphenoidal crest and along the midline and place it in the tissue container.
2. Note that the sphenoparietal venous sinus is located along the sphenoidal crest and that its lumen may now be visible where you detached the dura mater.
3. Identify the three bones that participate in the formation of the **anterior cranial fossa**: sphenoid bone, ethmoid bone, and orbital part of the frontal bone (Fig. 7.49). Note that the orbital part of the frontal bone forms the roof of the orbit.

4. Before the brain was removed, the cerebral falx was attached to the crista galli and the frontal lobe of the brain rested on the orbital part of the frontal bone. The olfactory bulb rested on the cribriform plate and the fibers of the **olfactory nerve (I)** passed through the openings of the cribriform plate to enter the nasal cavity (Fig. 7.50).

MIDDLE CRANIAL FOSSA [G 640, 644; L 346, 355; N 104; R 69; C 532]

1. Recall that the **middle cranial fossa** contains the temporal lobe of the brain.
2. Observe the dura mater that covers the floor of the middle cranial fossa. The dura mater hides all of the openings in the skull and the nerves and vessels that pass through them (Fig. 7.50).
3. Identify the **middle meningeal artery** that can be seen through the dura mater (Fig. 7.50). It appears as a dark line extending laterally from the deepest point of the middle cranial fossa. The middle meningeal artery enters the middle cranial fossa by passing through the **foramen spinosum**.
4. Grasp the dura mater along the sphenoidal crest and peel it posteriorly as far as the superior border of the petrous part of the temporal bone. Note

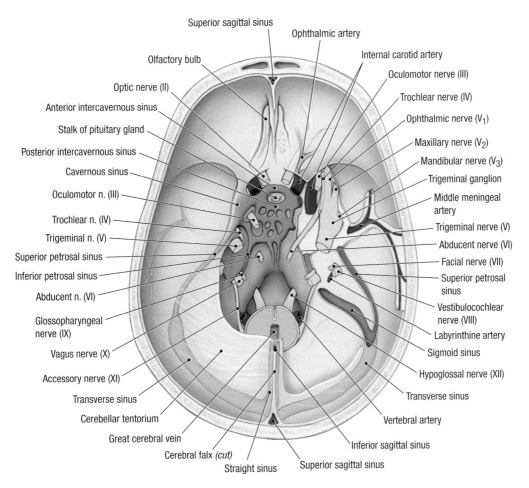

Figure 7.50. Nerves and vessels in the cranial fossae.

that the middle meningeal artery adheres to the external surface of the dura mater. Use a probe to tease the proximal part of middle meningeal artery away from the dura mater and leave it in the skull.

5. Use scissors to detach the dura mater along the superior border of the petrous part of the temporal bone and place it in the tissue container. Do not cut the cranial nerves that cross the anterior end of the superior border of the petrous part of the temporal bone (oculomotor, trigeminal, trochlear, and abducent). Note that the lumen of the **superior petrosal sinus** can be seen along the line of the cut (Fig. 7.50).

6. Observe that the floor of the middle cranial fossa is formed by two bones: sphenoid and temporal (Fig. 7.49).

7. Identify the **optic nerve (II)** (Fig. 7.50). The optic nerve passes through the **optic canal** to enter the orbit. The optic nerve is surrounded by a sleeve of dura mater as it exits the middle cranial fossa.

8. Use a probe to identify the **superior orbital fissure** that is located inferior to the lesser wing of the sphenoid bone (Fig. 7.49). Three cranial nerves and part of a fourth exit the middle cranial fossa by passing through the superior orbital fissure:

- **Oculomotor nerve (III)** – passes over the superior border of the petrous part of the temporal bone and passes anteriorly within the lateral wall of the cavernous sinus.
- **Trochlear nerve (IV)** – courses anteriorly within the lateral wall of the cavernous sinus immediately inferior to the oculomotor nerve (Fig. 7.50). The trochlear nerve is a very small nerve that enters the dura mater at the anterior end of the tentorial notch. It may have been cut during brain removal but should be intact farther anteriorly.
- **Ophthalmic division of the trigeminal nerve (V$_1$)** – arises from the trigeminal ganglion and passes anteriorly within the lateral wall of the cavernous sinus inferior to the trochlear nerve (Fig. 7.50).
- **Abducent nerve (VI)** – enters the dura mater over the clivus of the occipital bone (Fig. 7.50). The abducent nerve passes anteriorly within the cavernous sinus in close relationship to the lateral surface of the internal carotid artery.

9. Use a probe to clean the nerves that pass through the superior orbital fissure. Note that three of these nerves are located within the lateral wall of

the cavernous sinus (III, IV, V₁) and one is within the cavernous sinus (VI) (Fig. 7.51).

10. Identify the **trigeminal nerve (V)** (Fig. 7.50). It is the largest cranial nerve and is easily found where it crosses the superior border of the petrous part of the temporal bone.

11. Follow the trigeminal nerve anteriorly and identify the **trigeminal ganglion**. Use a probe to define the three divisions (nerves) that arise from the anterior border of the trigeminal ganglion (ophthalmic [V₁], maxillary [V₂], and mandibular [V₃]). Note that these three divisions are named according to their region of distribution and are numbered from superior to inferior as they arise from the trigeminal ganglion.

12. Identify the **maxillary division of the trigeminal nerve (V₂)** and follow it anteriorly to the **foramen rotundum**, where it exits the middle cranial fossa (Fig. 7.50). The maxillary division courses within the lateral wall of the cavernous sinus just inferior to the ophthalmic division of the trigeminal nerve (V₁) (Fig. 7.51).

13. Identify the **mandibular division of the trigeminal nerve (V₃)** and follow it inferiorly to the **foramen ovale**, which is where it exits the middle cranial fossa (Fig. 7.50).

14. Return to the area of the cavernous sinus and use a probe to retract the cranial nerves. Identify **the internal carotid artery** (Fig. 7.50). The internal carotid artery enters the cranial cavity by passing through the **carotid canal**. It makes an S-shaped bend in the cavernous sinus and emerges near the optic nerve. Cranial nerves III, IV, V₁, V₂, and VI cross the lateral side of the internal carotid artery. Among this group of nerves, the abducent nerve (VI) is most closely related to the internal carotid artery (Fig. 7.51).

15. Identify the region of the **hypophyseal fossa**. The hypophyseal fossa is covered by the **sellar diaphragm (diaphragma sellae),** which is a dural infolding (Fig. 7.51). The stalk of the pituitary gland passes through an opening in the sellar diaphragm. The pituitary gland is still contained within the hypophyseal fossa.

16. Anterior and posterior to the stalk of the pituitary gland are two small dural venous sinuses called the **anterior and posterior intercavernous sinuses** (Fig. 7.50). The intercavernous sinuses connect the right and left cavernous sinuses across the midline. Do not attempt to dissect the intercavernous sinuses.

17. Use an atlas illustration to identify all of the veins and venous sinuses that drain into or out of the cavernous sinus. [G 639; L 342; N 104; R 87; C 532]

CLINICAL CORRELATION

Cavernous Sinus

In fractures of the base of the skull, the internal carotid artery may rupture within the cavernous sinus. The release of arterial blood into the cavernous sinus creates an abnormal reflux of blood from the cavernous sinus into the ophthalmic veins. As a result, the orbit is engorged and the eyeball is protruded and is pulsating in synchrony with the radial pulse (pulsating exophthalmos).

POSTERIOR CRANIAL FOSSA [G 640, 642; L 346; N 104; R 67; C 532]

1. Recall that the posterior cranial fossa contains the cerebellum and the brainstem. At the foramen magnum, the brainstem becomes continuous with the cervical spinal cord. The features of the posterior cranial fossa will be studied with the dura mater intact.

2. Identify the **facial nerve (VII)** and the **vestibulocochlear nerve (VIII)** where they enter the internal acoustic meatus (Fig. 7.50). Do not follow them into the bone at this time.

3. The jugular foramen is inferior to the internal acoustic meatus (Fig. 7.49). Identify the rootlets of

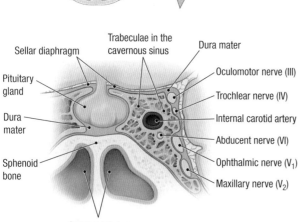

Figure 7.51. Coronal section through the cavernous sinus.

the **glossopharyngeal nerve (IX)**, the **vagus nerve (X)**, and the **accessory nerve (XI)** where they enter the jugular foramen. Because cranial nerves IX and X are formed by rootlets, it is difficult to distinguish one nerve from the other as they enter the jugular foramen. However, the **cervical root of the accessory nerve** can be positively identified because it enters the posterior cranial fossa through the foramen magnum and crosses the inner surface of the occipital bone (Fig. 7.50).

4. Identify the **hypoglossal nerve (XII)** where it enters the **hypoglossal canal** (Fig. 7.50).

5. Review the course of the transverse sinus and sigmoid sinus. Observe that the sigmoid sinus ends at the jugular foramen posterior to the exit point of cranial nerves IX, X, and XI.

6. On the left (undissected) side of the cranial cavity, identify the cranial nerves in order from anterior to posterior (Fig. 7.50).

Dissection Review

1. Review the bones that form the floor of the cranial cavity.

2. Read an account of the dural venous sinuses and review them in the cadaver.

3. Summarize the cranial nerves, review the course of each cranial nerve, and name the opening through which each passes to exit the cranial cavity. In the skull, review the openings (foramina and fissures) through which the cranial nerves pass.

4. If the brain is still available, hold it beside the cranial cavity so that you can see its ventral surface, and review the cranial nerves and severed vessels on both the brain and the cadaver.

ORBIT

Dissection Overview

The orbit contains the eyeball and extraocular muscles. The eyeball is about 2.5 cm in diameter and occupies the anterior half of the orbit. The posterior half of the orbit contains fat, extraocular muscles, branches of cranial nerves, and blood vessels. Some vessels and nerves pass through the orbit to reach the scalp and face.

The order of dissection will be as follows: The bones of the orbit will be studied. On the right side only, the floor of the anterior cranial fossa will be removed and the right orbit will be dissected from a superior approach. Cranial nerves III, IV, V$_1$, and VI will be followed through the superior orbital fissure into the orbit and the extraocular muscles will be identified. The left orbit will be dissected from an anterior approach. On the left side only, the anatomy of the eyelid will be studied and then the eyeball

will be removed. The attachments of the extraocular muscles will be studied.

SKELETON OF THE ORBIT

The bones of the orbit form a four-sided pyramid. The base of the pyramid is the orbital margin and the apex of the pyramid is the optic canal. Viewed from above, the medial walls of the two orbits are parallel to each other and about 2.5 cm apart. The lateral walls of the two orbits form a right angle to each other.

Refer to a skull and identify the bones that participate in the formation of the walls of the orbit (Fig. 7.52): [G 650; L 352; N 2; R 46; C 540]

- **Frontal bone**
  - **Supraorbital notch**
  - **Orbital surface**
  - **Lacrimal fossa**
- **Ethmoid bone**
- **Lacrimal bone**
  - **Posterior lacrimal crest**
  - **Lacrimal groove**
- **Maxilla**
  - **Anterior lacrimal crest**
  - **Infraorbital groove**
  - **Infraorbital foramen**
- **Zygomatic bone**
- **Sphenoid bone**
  - **Optic canal**
  - **Lesser wing**
  - **Superior orbital fissure**
  - **Greater wing**

On the medial wall of the orbit, identify the **anterior** and **posterior ethmoidal foramina**.

Identify the **inferior orbital fissure**, which is a gap between the maxilla and the greater wing of the sphenoid bone. Note that the lateral wall of the orbit is stout and strong but the part of the ethmoid bone that forms the medial wall is paper thin and for this reason it is called the **lamina papyracea**. Examine a coronal section through the orbit and note the following relationships (Fig. 7.53):

- **Roof of the orbit** – is related to the anterior cranial fossa
- **Floor of the orbit** – is related to the maxillary sinus
- **Medial wall of the orbit** – is related to the ethmoidal cells

The bones of the orbit are lined with periosteum called **periorbita**. At the optic canal and the superior orbital fissure, the periorbita is continuous with the dura mater of the middle cranial fossa.

SURFACE ANATOMY OF THE EYEBALL, EYELIDS, AND LACRIMAL APPARATUS

Use a mirror or recruit the assistance of your lab partner to inspect the living eye. Identify: [G 650, 651; L 353; N 81; C 538]

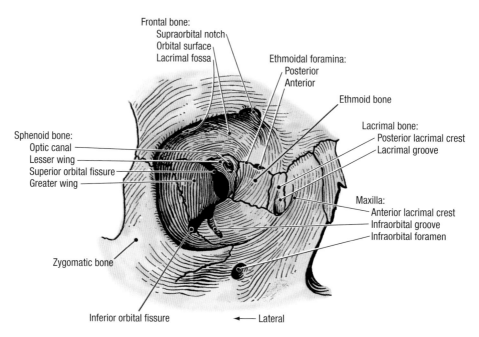

Figure 7.52. Walls of the right orbit, anterior view.

- **Eyelashes (cilia)**
- **Palpebral fissure (rima)** – the opening between the eyelids
- **Medial and lateral palpebral commissures** – where the upper and lower eyelids join

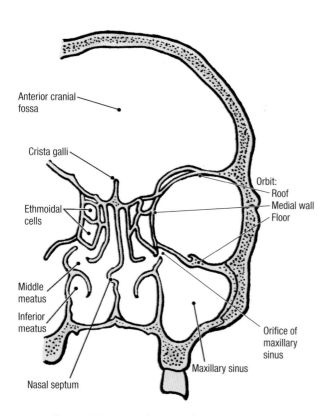

Figure 7.53. Coronal section of the skull to show the relationships of the orbit.

- **Medial and lateral angles (canthi)** – the medial and lateral corners of the eye
- **Sclera** – the whitish posterior five-sixths of the exterior coat of the eyeball
- **Cornea** – the transparent anterior one-sixth of the exterior coat of the eyeball
- **Iris** – the colored diaphragm seen through the cornea
- **Pupil** – the aperture in the center of the iris

In the medial angle of the eye, observe:

- **Lacrimal caruncle** – a pink fleshy bump
- **Lacrimal lake** – the area surrounding the lacrimal caruncle
- **Lacrimal papilla** – a small bump on the medial end of each eyelid
- **Lacrimal puncta** – a small opening at the apex of each lacrimal papilla

Evert the lower lid slightly and observe:

- **Margin of the eyelid** – flat and thick
- **Eyelashes (cilia)** – arranged in two or three irregular rows

Use an illustration to study the following features and relate them to the living eye: [G 655; L 353; N 81; R 132; C 545]

- **Bulbar conjunctiva** – the membrane that lines the surface of the eyeball
- **Palpebral conjunctiva** – the membrane that lines the inner surface of the eyelid
- **Superior and inferior conjunctival fornices** (L. *fornix*, arch) – the regions where the bulbar conjunctiva becomes continuous with the palpebral conjunctiva
- **Conjunctival sac** – the potential space between the bulbar conjunctiva and the palpebral conjunctiva

Dissection Instructions

EYELID AND LACRIMAL APPARATUS [G 651, 655; L 352, 353; N 81, 82; R 142; C 542, 543]

1. Dissect the eyelid and lacrimal gland only in the left eye.
2. Review the attachments of the **orbicularis oculi muscle**. Use a probe to raise the lateral part of the **orbital portion of the orbicularis oculi muscle** and reflect the muscle medially.
3. Raise the thin **palpebral portion of the orbicularis oculi muscle** off the underlying **tarsal plate** and reflect the muscle medially.
4. The **orbital septum** is a sheet of connective tissue that is attached to the periosteum at the margin of the orbit and to the tarsal plates (Figs. 7.54 and 7.55). The orbital septum separates the superficial fascia of the face from the contents of the orbit.
5. Identify the **tarsal plates**, which give shape to the eyelids (Fig. 7.54). **Tarsal glands** are embedded in the posterior surface of each tarsal plate. Tarsal glands drain by small orifices that are located posterior to the eyelashes. Tarsal glands secrete an oily substance onto the margin of the eyelid that prevents the overflow of lacrimal fluid (tears).

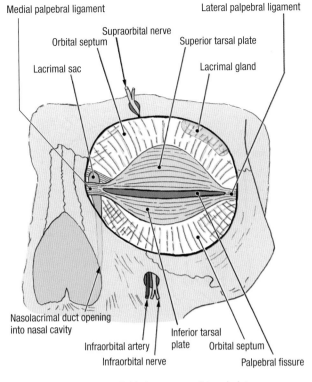

Figure 7.54. Orbital septum and tarsal plates.

CLINICAL CORRELATION

Tarsal Glands

If the duct of a tarsal gland becomes obstructed, a chalazion (cyst) will develop. A chalazion will be located between the tarsal plate and the conjunctiva. In contrast, a hordeolum (stye) is the inflammation of a sebaceous gland associated with the follicle of an eyelash.

---

6. The **lacrimal gland** occupies the lacrimal fossa in the frontal bone (Fig. 7.54). To find the lacrimal gland, use a scalpel to cut through the orbital septum adjacent to the orbital margin in the superolateral quadrant of the left orbit. Pass a probe through the incision and free the lacrimal gland from the lacrimal fossa. Note that the lacrimal gland drains into the superior conjunctival fornix by 6 to 10 short ducts (Fig. 7.56).
7. Use a skull to identify the **lacrimal groove** at the medial side of the orbital margin. Observe that the **anterior lacrimal crest** of the maxilla forms the anterior border of the lacrimal groove. The **medial palpebral ligament** is attached to the anterior lacrimal crest and the **lacrimal sac** lies posterior to the medial palpebral ligament (Fig. 7.54).

8. Two **lacrimal canaliculi** drain lacrimal fluid from the medial angle of the eye into the lacrimal sac. The **nasolacrimal duct** extends inferiorly from the lacrimal sac and enters the inferior meatus of the nasal cavity (Fig. 7.56).
9. Lacrimal fluid flows from the lacrimal gland across the eyeball to the medial angle of the eye.

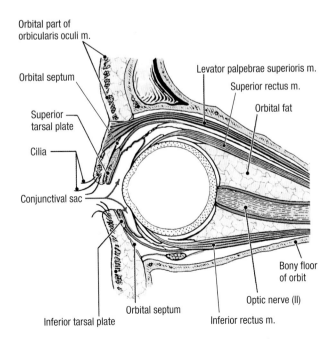

Figure 7.55. Parasagittal section through the orbit.

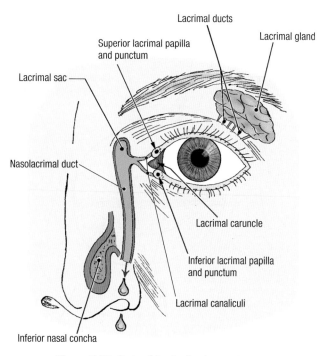

Figure 7.56. Parts of the lacrimal apparatus.

During crying, excess lacrimal fluid cannot be emptied through the lacrimal canaliculi and tears overflow the lower eyelids. Increased drainage of tears into the nasal cavity results in sniffling, which is characteristic of crying.

RIGHT ORBIT FROM THE SUPERIOR APPROACH [G 652; L 356–358; N 86; R 140; C 546]

1. Dissect only the right orbit from the superior approach. *Wear eye protection for all steps that require the use of bone cutters.*
2. In the floor of the anterior cranial fossa, tap the orbital part of the frontal bone with the handle of a chisel until the bone cracks. Use bone cutters to pick out the bone fragments and enlarge the opening in the **roof of the orbit**. Remove the roof of the orbit as far anteriorly as the superior orbital margin.
3. The frontal bone contains the **frontal sinus** that may extend into the roof of the orbit. Medially, the **ethmoidal cells** may extend into the roof of the orbit. If either situation occurs in your cadaver, you must remove the mucous membrane that lines the sinus and remove a second layer of thin bone to open the orbit.
4. Identify the membrane just inferior to the roof of the orbit. This is the **periorbita**, which lines the bones of the orbit.
5. Push a probe posteriorly between the roof of the orbit and the periorbita. The probe should pass inferior to the lesser wing of the sphenoid bone,

through the superior orbital fissure, and into the middle cranial fossa. Use the probe to break the lesser wing of the sphenoid bone.

6. Use bone cutters to remove the fragments of the lesser wing of the sphenoid bone. Chip away the roof of the optic canal and remove the anterior clinoid process (Fig. 7.57).
7. Examine the periorbita and note that the frontal nerve may be visible through it. Use scissors to incise the periorbita from the apex of the orbit to the midpoint of the superior orbital margin. Use forceps to lift the periorbita off deeper structures and make a transverse incision through the periorbita, close to the superior orbital margin. Use a probe to tease open the flaps of periorbita and use scissors to remove them.
8. The use of a fine probe and fine forceps is recommended from this point onward in the dissection.
9. Three nerves enter the apex of the orbit by passing superior to the extraocular muscles:
   • **Frontal nerve** (a branch of V_1) – courses from the apex of the orbit toward the superior orbital margin (Fig. 7.57). Trace the frontal nerve anteriorly and observe that it divides into the **supratrochlear nerve** and the **supraorbital nerve**.
   • **Lacrimal nerve** (a branch of V_1) – passes through the superior orbital fissure lateral to the frontal nerve and courses along the lateral

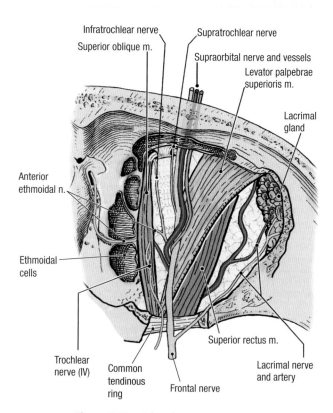

Figure 7.57. Right orbit in superior view.

wall of the orbit. The lacrimal nerve is much smaller than the frontal nerve (Fig. 7.57). Follow the lacrimal nerve anterolaterally toward the lacrimal gland.

- **Trochlear nerve** – passes through the superior orbital fissure medial to the frontal nerve (Fig. 7.57). Follow the trochlear nerve to the superior border of the **superior oblique muscle**, which it innervates. The trochlear nerve usually enters the superior border of the superior oblique muscle in its posterior one-third.

10. While preserving the nerves, use forceps to pick out lobules of fat and expose the superior surface of the **levator palpebrae superioris muscle** (Figs. 7.55 and 7.57). The levator palpebrae superioris muscle attaches to the upper eyelid, which it elevates.

11. Transect the levator palpebrae superioris muscle as far anteriorly as possible and reflect it posteriorly.

12. Identify the **superior rectus muscle** that lies immediately inferior to the levator palpebrae superioris muscle (Figs. 7.55 and 7.57). Clean the superior rectus muscle and observe that it is attached to the eyeball by a thin, broad tendon.

13. Transect the superior rectus muscle close to the eyeball and reflect it posteriorly (Fig. 7.58). Note that a branch of the superior division of the **oculomotor nerve (III)** reaches the inferior surface of the superior rectus muscle. A branch of the superior division passes around the medial side of the superior rectus muscle to innervate the levator

palpebrae superioris muscle. [G 652; L 357; N 86; R 141; C 548]

14. On the medial side of the orbit, identify the **superior oblique muscle** and trace it anteriorly (Fig. 7.58). Observe that the tendon of the superior oblique muscle passes through the trochlea (L. *trochlea*, pulley), bends at an acute angle, and attaches to the posterolateral portion of the eyeball.

15. On the lateral side of the orbit, identify the **lateral rectus muscle** (Fig. 7.58). The lateral rectus muscle arises by two heads from the **common tendinous ring**. The common tendinous ring surrounds the optic canal and part of the superior orbital fissure, and it is the posterior attachment of the four rectus muscles. The optic nerve (II), nasociliary nerve, oculomotor nerve (III), and abducent nerve (VI) pass through the common tendinous ring.

16. Use scissors to cut the common tendinous ring between the attachments of the superior rectus and lateral rectus muscles. All structures passing through the common tendinous ring are now exposed.

17. Identify the **abducent nerve (VI)**. The abducent nerve passes between the two heads of the lateral rectus muscle, turns laterally, and enters the medial surface of the lateral rectus muscle. Find the abducent nerve on the medial surface of the lateral rectus muscle near the apex of the orbit (Fig. 7.58).

18. Identify the **nasociliary nerve**, which is a branch of V$_1$ (Fig. 7.58). Trace the nasociliary nerve through the orbit and note that it is much smaller than the frontal nerve. The nasociliary nerve crosses superior to the optic nerve and gives off several **long ciliary nerves** to the posterior part of the eyeball.

19. Follow the nasociliary nerve toward the medial wall of the orbit. Use forceps to pick out the fat that fills the intervals between muscles, nerves, and vessels.

20. Identify the **anterior ethmoidal nerve**, which is a small branch of the nasociliary nerve that passes through the anterior ethmoidal foramen. The anterior ethmoidal nerve supplies part of the mucous membrane in the nasal cavity. Its terminal branch is the **external nasal nerve** that innervates the skin at the tip of the nose.

21. In the middle cranial fossa, identify the **oculomotor nerve** within the lateral wall of the cavernous sinus. Follow the oculomotor nerve to the superior orbital fissure where it branches into two divisions:

- **Superior division** – innervates the levator palpebrae superioris and the superior rectus muscles

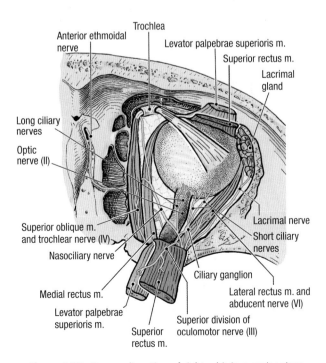

Figure 7.58. Deeper dissection of right orbit in superior view.

- **Inferior division** – innervates the medial rectus, inferior rectus, and inferior oblique muscles

22. The **ciliary ganglion** is a parasympathetic ganglion located between the optic nerve and the lateral rectus muscle. It is approximately 2 mm in diameter and is located about 1 cm anterior to the apex of the orbit (Fig. 7.58). Note that short ciliary nerves connect the ciliary ganglion to the posterior surface of the eyeball. Study the autonomic function of the ciliary ganglion.

23. Use an atlas illustration to study the course of the **superior ophthalmic vein** in the orbit. At the medial angle of the eye, the superior ophthalmic vein anastomoses with the angular vein, which is a tributary of the facial vein. [G 656; L 356; N 85; C 509]

CLINICAL CORRELATION

Ophthalmic Veins

Anastomoses between the angular vein and the superior and inferior ophthalmic veins are of clinical importance. Infections of the upper lip, cheeks, and forehead may spread through the facial and angular veins into the ophthalmic veins and then into the cavernous sinus. Thrombosis of the cavernous sinus may result, leading to involvement of the abducent nerve and dysfunction of the lateral rectus muscle.

---

24. Identify the **optic nerve (II)** (Fig. 7.58). The optic "nerve" is actually a brain tract and it is surrounded by the three meningeal layers: dura mater, arachnoid mater, and pia mater.

25. Identify the **ophthalmic artery** where it branches from the internal carotid artery (Fig. 7.59). In its course through the orbit, note that the ophthalmic artery usually crosses superior to the optic nerve and reaches the medial wall of the orbit. Use a probe to gently tease out the posterior ciliary arteries that supply the eyeball.

26. The **medial rectus**, **inferior rectus**, and **inferior oblique muscles** are not easily seen from the superior approach. They will be identified from the anterior approach.

LEFT ORBIT FROM THE ANTERIOR APPROACH [G 651; L 354; N 83; R 135; C 550]

1. Use a probe to explore the **conjunctival sac**. Verify that the conjunctiva is attached to the sclera.

2. To facilitate the dissection, remove both eyelids and the orbital septum. Examine the orbit from the anterior view and note:
   - The **lacrimal gland** is located superolaterally.
   - The **trochlea** is located superomedially.
   - The proximal attachment of the **inferior oblique muscle** is located inferomedially.

3. Review the attachments of the extraocular muscles on the eyeball. The four rectus muscles attach to

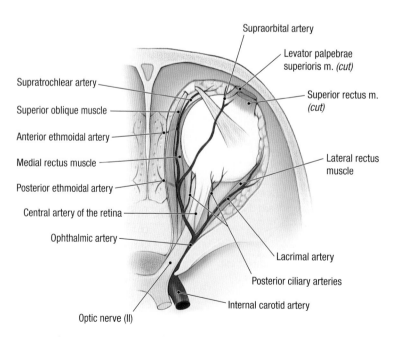

Figure 7.59. Branches of the ophthalmic artery in the right orbit.

the sclera near the cornea (Fig. 7.60). The two oblique muscles attach to the sclera on the posterior half of the eyeball.

4. Use a probe to pick up the tendon of each rectus muscle and transect it with scissors (Fig. 7.60).
5. Use forceps to grasp the lateral rectus muscle. Pull anteriorly to adduct the eyeball (turn it medially). Insert scissors into the orbit on the lateral side of the eyeball and cut the optic nerve.
6. Pull the eyeball farther anteriorly and transect the superior and inferior oblique tendons near the surface of the eyeball and remove the eyeball from the orbit.
7. Study the orbit (Fig. 7.61). Use forceps to pick out lobules of fat from the posterior portion of the orbit. Find the nerve to the inferior oblique muscle and follow it posteriorly to the **inferior division of the oculomotor nerve (III)**. [G 646; L 354; N 83; R 136; C 553]
8. Trace the four rectus muscles to their attachments on the **common tendinous ring**.
9. Identify the structures that pass through the common tendinous ring: the **optic nerve (II) and central artery of the retina, superior and inferior divisions of the oculomotor nerve (III), abducent nerve (VI)**, and **nasociliary nerve** (Fig. 7.61).
10. Examine the cut surface of the optic nerve and try to identify the central artery of the retina, which may be seen as a dark spot on the cut surface.
11. In most cases, the eyeball that is removed from the cadaver is poorly preserved. However, if the eyeball is in dissectible condition, use a new scalpel blade to cut it in half in the coronal plane. Remove the vitreous body.
12. Note the following features of the eyeball: [G 660; L 359; N 87; R 133; C 554]
    • **Fibrous (outer) layer** – sclera (posterior five-sixths) and cornea (anterior one-sixth)

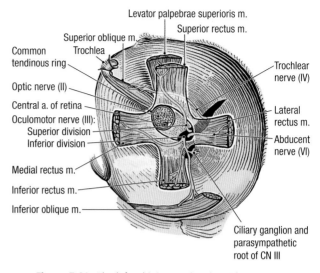

Figure 7.61. The left orbit in anterior view. The common tendinous ring and its relationship to the four rectus muscles and cranial nerves II, III, IV, and VI.

• **Vascular (middle) layer** – choroid, ciliary body, and iris
• **Inner layer** – retina, partially detached in the cadaver
• **Macula** – only seen in well-preserved specimens
• **Optic disc** – where the optic nerve and retinal vessels enter or leave
• **Lens** – may be replaced by a prosthetic implant

Dissection Review

1. Use a skull to review the bones that form the margin of the orbit, the walls of the orbit, and the openings at the apex of the orbit. Examine the middle cranial fossa and review the optic canal and superior orbital fissure.
2. Use the dissected specimen to review the nerves that course along the lateral wall of the cavernous sinus and pass through the superior orbital fissure to reach the apex of the orbit. Review the orbital course and function of each of these cranial nerves.
3. Review the course of the internal carotid artery through the cavernous sinus and note its relationship to the optic nerve near the optic canal. Note the origin of the ophthalmic artery and its course through the optic canal.
4. Review the course of the optic nerve through the optic canal to the eyeball.
5. Review the attachments of each of the six extraocular muscles. Use the cadaver specimen to find each of the extraocular muscles.
6. Use an illustration to review the movements of the eyeball and relate each movement to the extraocular muscles that are responsible.

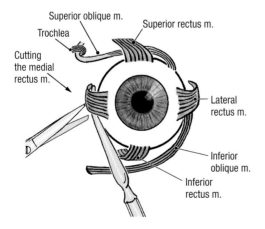

Figure 7.60. How to transect the muscles of the left eye.

7. Review the ciliary ganglion and note the origin of its preganglionic parasympathetic axons and the course of its postganglionic axons to the eyeball. State the function of the two smooth muscles that are innervated by the ciliary ganglion.

CRANIOVERTEBRAL JOINTS AND DISARTICULATION OF THE HEAD

Dissection Overview

The head must be detached from the vertebral column to allow a posterior approach to the cervical viscera. The joints between the skull and the first cervical vertebra (craniovertebral joints) are the logical site for separation of the head from the vertebral column.

The order of dissection will be as follows: The retropharyngeal space will be opened from the base of the skull to the superior thoracic aperture. The ligaments of the craniovertebral joints will be cut. The atlanto-occipital joints (left and right) will be disarticulated and the prevertebral muscles will be cut where they cross the atlanto-occipital joints.

SKELETON OF THE SUBOCCIPITAL REGION

Refer to a skeleton and identify the following: [G 295, 299; L 7, 8; N 17, 21, 22; R 200; C 343, 344]

- **Atlas (C1)** (Fig. 7.62)
  Anterior arch
  Superior articular facet
  Transverse process
  Posterior arch
  Anterior tubercle
- **Axis (C2)**
  Dens

- **Occipital bone** (Fig. 7.63)
  Occipital condyle
  Pharyngeal tubercle
  Foramen magnum
- **Atlanto-occipital joint** – between the occipital condyle and the superior articular facet of the atlas
- **Transverse ligament of the atlas** – holds the dens to the anterior arch of the atlas (Fig. 7.62)

Dissection Instructions

RETROPHARYNGEAL SPACE

1. Review the structures that pass through the foramen magnum: brainstem, vertebral arteries (left and right), and cervical roots of the accessory nerves (left and right). Review the hypoglossal nerve (XII) where it enters the hypoglossal canal. Review the structures that enter the jugular foramen: glossopharyngeal nerve (IX), vagus nerve (X), accessory nerve (XI), and sigmoid sinus.
2. Reflect the sternocleidomastoid muscle on both sides, taking care to separate each muscle from deeper structures all the way to the mastoid process.
3. Insert the fingers of both hands posterior to the carotid sheaths (Fig. 7.64, arrow). Push your fingers medially until they meet posterior to the cer-

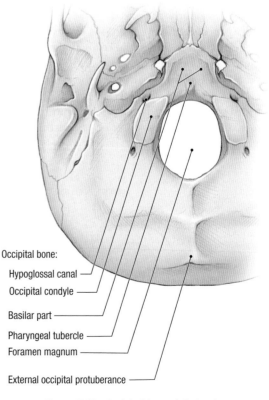

Occipital bone:
Hypoglossal canal
Occipital condyle
Basilar part
Pharyngeal tubercle
Foramen magnum
External occipital protuberance

Figure 7.63. Occipital bone, inferior view.

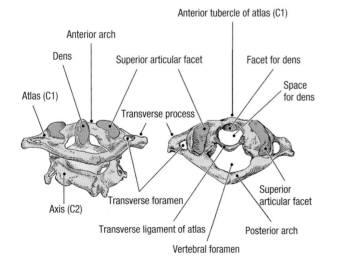

Anterior tubercle of atlas (C1)
Anterior arch
Dens
Superior articular facet
Facet for dens
Space for dens
Atlas (C1)
Transverse process
Axis (C2)
Transverse foramen
Transverse ligament of atlas
Vertebral foramen
Superior articular facet
Posterior arch

Figure 7.62. Skeleton and ligaments of the atlantoaxial joint.

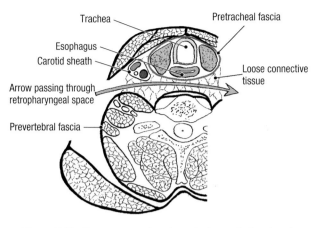

Figure 7.64. Transverse section through the neck showing the retropharyngeal space.

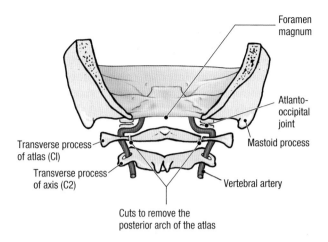

Figure 7.65. Atlanto-occipital joint in posterior view.

vical viscera. Your fingers are now in the **retropharyngeal space**.

4. To separate the viscera from the vertebral column, work your fingers superiorly as far as the basilar part of the occipital bone. This is the superior limit of the retropharyngeal space. Work your fingers inferiorly toward the superior thoracic aperture. Note that the retropharyngeal space extends into the thorax.

CRANIOVERTEBRAL JOINTS

1. Turn the cadaver to the prone position. A wedge-shaped portion of the occipital bone was removed earlier (Fig. 7.65).
2. Use bone cutters to remove the posterior arch of the atlas (Fig. 7.65). Open the spinal dura mater and remove the cervical spinal cord.
3. Strip the dura mater from the anterior border of the foramen magnum and identify the **tectorial membrane** (Fig. 7.66). The tectorial membrane is continuous with the posterior longitudinal ligament. Superior to the anterior border of the foramen magnum, cut the tectorial membrane and reflect it inferiorly as far as possible (Fig. 7.66). [G 299; N 22; R 201; C 344]
4. Anterior to the tectorial membrane, identify the **cruciate ligament of the atlas** (Fig. 7.66). The cruciate ligament has three parts:
   • **Superior longitudinal band**
   • **Transverse ligament of the atlas**
   • **Inferior longitudinal band**
5. Use a scalpel to cut the superior longitudinal band and the transverse ligament of the atlas. Retract the cruciate ligament and identify the left and right **alar ligaments** (Fig. 7.66). The alar ligaments extend from the dens to the lateral margins of the foramen magnum and they control lateral rotation and side-to-side movements of the head.

6. Use a scalpel to cut the alar ligaments close to the dens. Note that the rotation of the head is now very easy and extensive.

DISARTICULATION OF THE HEAD

1. Use a scalpel to open the capsule of the **atlanto-occipital joint** on both sides (Fig. 7.65). Force a chisel into each atlanto-occipital joint and disarticulate it.
2. Turn the cadaver to the supine position. Retract the cervical viscera and contents of the carotid sheath anteriorly. [G 775; L 310; N 30; C 488]

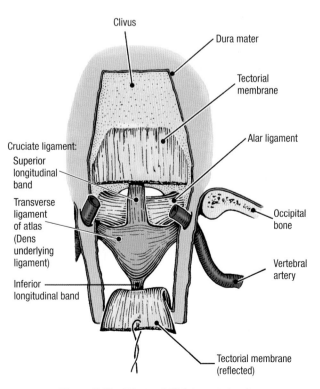

Figure 7.66. Atlantoaxial joint, posterior view.

3. Identify the **sympathetic trunk** and the **superior cervical sympathetic ganglion** on the anterior surface of the cervical vertebral column. On the left side identify the **internal carotid nerve,** which passes from the superior end of the superior cervical ganglion to the internal carotid artery. Sever the internal carotid nerve just superior to the superior cervical ganglion and leave the sympathetic trunk attached to the vertebral column. On the right side, leave the internal carotid nerve intact and reflect the sympathetic trunk and the superior cervical ganglion with the head and cervical viscera.

4. Protect cranial nerves IX, X, XI, and XII where they emerge from the base of the skull near the internal jugular vein. Insert a scalpel blade between the transverse process of the atlas and the occipital bone and sever the **rectus capitis lateralis muscle** on each side (Fig. 7.67). Repeat this cut on the opposite side of the neck.

5. More medially, sever the **rectus capitis anterior** and **longus capitis muscles**. Repeat this cut on the opposite side of the neck. Cut across the median plane just superior to the anterior arch of the atlas. Forcefully push the head anteriorly to detach it from the vertebral column.

6. Inspect the base of the skull from the posterior perspective and look for remnants of the C1 vertebra attached to the atlanto-occipital joint. If remnants of the C1 vertebra are present, use bone cutters to remove them.

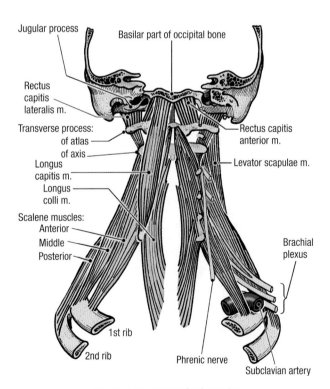

Figure 7.67. Prevertebral muscles.

PREVERTEBRAL AND LATERAL VERTEBRAL REGIONS
[G 774; L 310; N 130; R 184; C 481]

1. On the anterior surface of the cervical vertebral column, examine the **prevertebral fascia.** The prevertebral fascia covers the prevertebral muscles (longus colli and longus capitis muscles) and the lateral vertebral muscles (anterior, middle, and posterior scalene muscles).

2. On the left side of the cervical vertebral column, study the **sympathetic trunk.** Identify the **superior**, **middle**, and **inferior cervical sympathetic ganglia**. Observe the **gray rami communicantes** that connect the sympathetic ganglia with the ventral rami of cervical spinal nerves. Frequently, the inferior cervical ganglion is fused with the first thoracic ganglion to form the **cervicothoracic (stellate) ganglion**.

3. Identify the **longus colli, longus capitis,** and **anterior scalene muscles** (Fig. 7.67). Review the contributions to the brachial plexus made by the ventral rami of spinal nerves C5 to C8.

4. Follow the vertebral artery into the transverse foramen of vertebra C6 and observe where it emerges from the transverse foramen of the atlas (C1). Appreciate that the vertebral artery is well protected within the transverse foramina.

Dissection Review

1. Use a skull to review the anatomy of the occipital bone.
2. In the cadaver, review the structures that pass through the foramen magnum, hypoglossal canal, and jugular foramen.
3. Use a skeleton to study the atlantoaxial and atlanto-occipital joints.
4. Review the course of the sympathetic trunk from the upper thorax to the base of the skull.
5. Review the origin and relationships of the roots of the brachial plexus.

PHARYNX

Dissection Overview

The airway crosses the digestive tract in the pharynx. The pharynx extends from the base of the skull to the inferior border of the cricoid cartilage (vertebral level C6). The **pharyngeal wall** consists of three layers. From outside inward these layers are:

- **Buccopharyngeal fascia** – the adventitia of the pharynx that is continuous with the connective tissue that covers the buccinator muscle

- **Muscular layer** – composed of an outer circular part and an inner longitudinal part
- **Mucous membrane**

The order of dissection will be as follows: The external surface of the pharynx will be dissected from the posterior direction. The pharyngeal plexus of nerves will be identified and the borders of the pharyngeal constrictor muscles will be defined. The stylopharyngeus muscle and glossopharyngeal nerve will be identified. The contents of the carotid sheath will be examined and cranial nerves IX, X, XI, and XII will be followed from the base of the skull to their regions of distribution. The sympathetic trunk will be studied.

Dissection Instructions

MUSCLES OF THE PHARYNGEAL WALL [G 787, 788; L 315, 316; N 67; R 167; C 586, 588]

1. The cadaver should be in the supine position. Push the head anteroinferiorly and let the chin rest on the thorax. Use a probe to clean the buccopharyngeal fascia from the posterior surface of the pharynx.
2. Identify the **inferior pharyngeal constrictor muscle**. The anterior attachments of the inferior pharyngeal constrictor muscle are the oblique line of the thyroid cartilage and the lateral surface of the cricoid cartilage (Fig. 7.68B). The posterior attachment of the inferior pharyngeal constrictor muscle is the **pharyngeal raphe** (Fig. 7.68A).

Beginning near the thyroid cartilage, use blunt dissection to clean the superior border of the inferior pharyngeal constrictor muscle.

3. Identify the **middle pharyngeal constrictor muscle**. The anterior attachments of the middle pharyngeal constrictor muscle are the greater horn of the hyoid bone and the inferior portion of the stylohyoid ligament (Fig. 7.68B). The posterior attachment of the middle pharyngeal constrictor muscle is the pharyngeal raphe. Note that the inferior part of the middle pharyngeal constrictor muscle lies deep to the inferior pharyngeal constrictor muscle. Use blunt dissection to clean the superior border of the middle pharyngeal constrictor muscle.
4. Superior to the middle pharyngeal constrictor muscle, identify the **superior pharyngeal constrictor muscle**. The anterior attachment of the superior pharyngeal constrictor muscle is the **pterygomandibular raphe** and its posterior attachments are the pharyngeal raphe and **pharyngeal tubercle** of the occipital bone (Fig. 7.68A). Note that the inferior part of the superior pharyngeal constrictor muscle lies deep to the middle pharyngeal constrictor muscle.
5. Use blunt dissection to define the superior border of the superior pharyngeal constrictor muscle. The **pharyngobasilar fascia** is the dense connective tissue membrane that attaches the superior edge of the superior constrictor to the base of the skull.

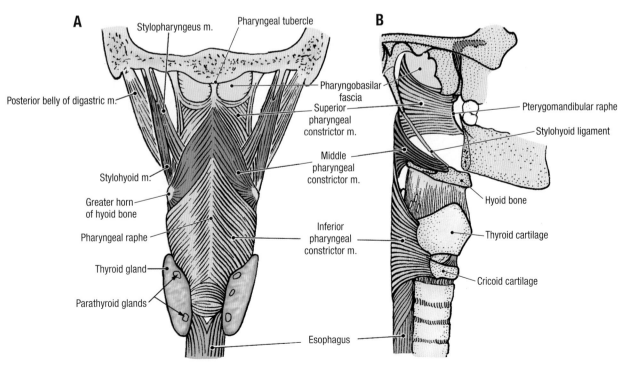

Figure 7.68. Muscles of the pharynx. **A.** Posterior view. **B.** Lateral view.

6. The **stylopharyngeus muscle** is attached to the medial surface of the styloid process superiorly and to the inner aspect of the pharyngeal wall inferiorly. It enters the pharyngeal wall by passing between the superior and middle pharyngeal constrictor muscles (Fig. 7.68A). The stylopharyngeus muscle is innervated by the glossopharyngeal nerve (IX).

7. To find the stylopharyngeus muscle, first palpate the greater horn of the hyoid bone. One finger's width above the greater horn of the hyoid bone, use blunt dissection to find the stylopharyngeus muscle where it passes between the superior pharyngeal constrictor muscle and the middle pharyngeal constrictor muscle.

8. Use a probe to clean the posterior and lateral surfaces of the stylopharyngeus muscle. Identify the **glossopharyngeal nerve (IX)** that crosses the posterior and lateral surfaces of the stylopharyngeus muscle to enter the pharynx (Fig. 7.69A). [G 786; L 316; N 71; R 165; C 589]

9. Examine the inferior part of the inferior constrictor muscle (Fig. 7.69B). Note that the most inferior fibers of the inferior constrictor muscle are continuous with the circular fibers of the esophagus.

10. Identify the **pharyngeal plexus of nerves** (Fig. 7.69A). The pharyngeal plexus is located on the posterolateral aspect of the pharynx. Note that the pharyngeal plexus receives branches from the:
    - Glossopharyngeal nerve – sensory to the pharyngeal mucosa
    - Vagus nerve – motor to the pharyngeal constrictor muscles
    - Superior cervical sympathetic ganglion – vasomotor

11. Identify the **contents of the carotid sheath** from the posterior view (Fig. 7.69A). Follow the internal carotid artery superiorly as far as possible. Note that the internal jugular vein is lateral to the internal carotid artery.

12. Identify the **glossopharyngeal nerve (IX)**, **vagus nerve (X)**, and **accessory nerve (XI)** where they exit the jugular foramen medial to the internal jugular vein (Fig. 7.69A):
    - **Glossopharyngeal nerve (IX)** – passes between the internal and external carotid arteries as it approaches the stylopharyngeus muscle.
    - **Vagus nerve** – lies posterior to the internal carotid artery and internal jugular vein in the carotid sheath. Trace the vagus nerve from the base of the skull to the thorax. The **superior**

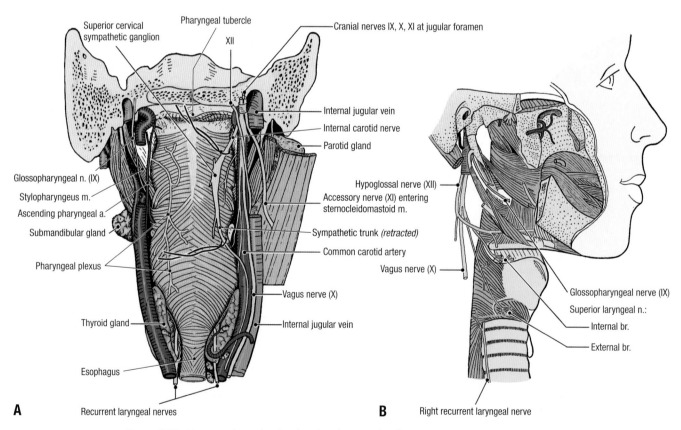

Figure 7.69. Nerves and vessels related to the pharyngeal wall. **A.** Posterior view. **B.** Lateral view.

laryngeal nerve arises from the vagus nerve about 2.5 cm inferior to the base of the skull. Trace the branches of the superior laryngeal nerve to the larynx (Fig. 7.69B). The **pharyngeal branch of the vagus nerve** arises near the base of the skull. Follow the pharyngeal branch to the pharyngeal plexus.

- **Accessory nerve (XI)** – usually passes between the internal jugular vein and the internal carotid artery to reach the deep surface of the sternocleidomastoid muscle (Fig. 7.69A).

13. Identify the **hypoglossal nerve (XII)** in the submandibular triangle and follow it posteriorly and superiorly as far as the base of the skull (Fig. 7.69B). Note that the hypoglossal nerve passes lateral to the internal and external carotid arteries.

14. On the right side of the cadaver, verify that the **superior cervical sympathetic ganglion** and the **sympathetic trunk** are posterior and medial to the carotid sheath (Fig. 7.69A). Identify the internal carotid nerve that passes from the superior end of the superior cervical ganglion to the internal carotid artery.

BISECTION OF THE HEAD

1. Use a scalpel to cut the posterior wall of the pharynx in the midline. Start at the superior end of the esophagus and cut through the pharyngeal raphe up to the pharyngeal tubercle. [L 317]
2. Use a scalpel to divide the uvula and the soft palate in the median plane.
3. Turn the specimen and use a scalpel to cut through the upper lip in the midline.
4. The skull must be sawed just lateral to the median plane. The nasal septum may not be in the median plane, so you must examine each nasal cavity and decide on which side the saw cut should be made in order to avoid the nasal septum.
5. On the chosen side, use a scalpel to cut through the cartilages of the external nose parallel to the nasal septum.
6. Examine a skull and study the bones through which you must cut:
   - **Nasal bone** and **frontal bone**
   - **Cribriform plate** of the ethmoid bone
   - **Body of the sphenoid bone**
   - **Hard palate**
   - **Basilar part of the occipital bone** as far as the **foramen magnum**
7. Saw through the skull from superior to inferior. Begin lateral to the crista galli (the side of the saw blade should touch the crista galli) and keep the blade close to the nasal septum. Cut through the nasal and frontal bones, ethmoid bone, body of the sphenoid, dorsum sellae, basilar part of the occip-

ital bone, and hard palate. Stop when the saw has passed into the foramen magnum. Do not cut the tongue or mandible at this time.

8. The two superior halves of the head should separate from each other. The tongue should be exposed.

INTERNAL ASPECT OF THE PHARYNX [G 808; L 318, 319; N 63; R 155; C 587]

1. The lumen of the pharynx communicates anteriorly with three cavities: nose, mouth, and larynx (Fig. 7.70). Identify the parts of the pharynx: **nasopharynx**, **oropharynx**, and **laryngopharynx**.
2. The **nasopharynx** lies posterior to the nose and superior to the soft palate (Fig. 7.70). Identify the **posterior nasal aperture** (**choana**) that is the transition region from the nasal cavity to the nasopharynx. The choanae of the two sides are separated by the posterior end of the nasal septum. [G 794; L 318; N 64; C 560, 561]
3. On the lateral wall of the nasopharynx, identify the **opening of the pharyngotympanic tube (auditory tube, eustachian tube)**.
4. Superior to the opening of the pharyngotympanic tube, identify the **torus tubarius**, which is the cartilage of the pharyngotympanic tube that is covered by mucosa (Fig. 7.70). The **salpingopharyngeal fold** extends posteroinferiorly from the torus tubarius.
5. Superior and posterior to the torus tubarius, identify the **pharyngeal recess**. The **pharyngeal tonsil (adenoid)** is located in the mucous membrane above the pharyngeal recess.

CLINICAL CORRELATION

Adenoids

Enlarged pharyngeal tonsils are called adenoids. Adenoids obstruct the flow of air from the nose through the nasopharynx, making mouth breathing necessary.

6. The **oropharynx** lies posterior to the oral cavity. It is bounded superiorly by the soft palate and extends inferiorly to the level of the epiglottis (Fig. 7.70).
7. In the oropharynx, identify the **palatoglossal fold**. The palatoglossal fold forms a dividing line between the oral cavity and the oropharynx. The transitional region between the right and left palatoglossal folds is called the **fauces**.

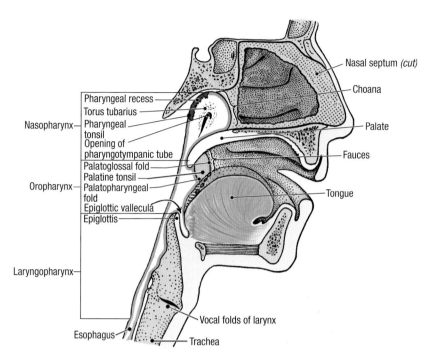

Figure 7.70. Regions of the pharynx.

8. Identify the **palatopharyngeal fold**, which is posterior to the palatoglossal fold. The palatopharyngeal fold descends along the lateral wall of the oropharynx. Between the palatoglossal fold and the palatopharyngeal fold is the **palatine tonsil**. Use a mirror to identify the palatine tonsil on yourself.
9. The **laryngopharynx** lies posterior to the larynx. This portion of the pharynx extends from the hyoid bone to the lower border of the cricoid cartilage (Fig. 7.70). [G 790; L 317, 318; N 66; R 163; C 590]
10. In the midline of the laryngopharynx, identify the **epiglottis** and the **inlet (aditus) of the larynx**. Farther inferiorly, identify the **piriform recess**, which is lateral to the midline. The borders of the piriform recess are:
    *   **Medial** – larynx
    *   **Lateral** – thyroid cartilage
    *   **Posterior** – inferior pharyngeal constrictor muscle

Dissection Review

1. Review the attachments, innervation, and action of the pharyngeal constrictor muscles.
2. Use a textbook description and the cadaver to review the pharyngeal plexus.
3. Trace each of the following cranial nerves from the posterior cranial fossa to its area of distribution: glossopharyngeal (IX), vagus (X), accessory (XI), and hypoglossal (XII).
4. Review the relationships of the contents of the carotid sheath.
5. Review the boundaries and contents of each part of the pharynx.

NOSE AND NASAL CAVITY

Dissection Overview

There are two nasal cavities: Right and left. The nostril (naris) is the anterior entrance to the nasal cavity. Posteriorly, the nasal cavity opens into the nasopharynx through the choana. The nasal cavity is lined by mucosa that is attached directly to bones and cartilages. The bones and cartilages give the walls of the nasal cavity their characteristic contours. The superior one-third of the nasal mucosa is olfactory in nature and the remainder is respiratory in nature. The nasal mucosa is highly vascular and capable of engorgement.

The order of dissection will be as follows: The nose and nasal cartilages will be studied. The nasal septum will be examined and removed. The features of the lateral nasal wall will be studied. The openings of the paranasal sinuses will be identified. The maxillary sinus will be opened and examined.

SKELETON OF THE NASAL CAVITY

In an anterior view of the skull, identify (Fig. 7.71): [G 611; L 298; N 2; R 22; C 514]

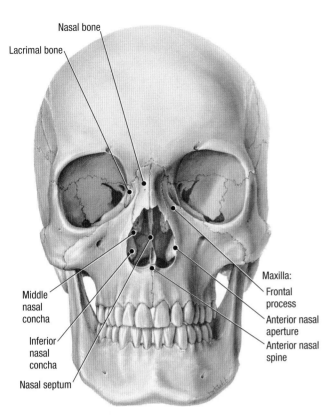

Figure 7.71. Skeleton of the nasal region.

- **Nasal bone**
- **Lacrimal bone**
- **Maxilla**
    Frontal process
    Anterior nasal aperture
    Anterior nasal spine
- **Nasal septum** – bony part
- **Middle nasal concha** – part of the ethmoid bone
- **Inferior nasal concha**

Use an illustration to identify the bony features of the lateral nasal wall (Fig. 7.72): [G 691; L 337; N 38; R 48; C 559]

- **Ethmoid bone**
    Cribriform plate
    Superior nasal concha
    Middle nasal concha
- **Lacrimal bone**
- **Inferior nasal concha**
- **Maxilla**
    Palatine process
    Incisive canal
- **Sphenoid bone**
    Opening of the sphenoidal sinus
    Sphenoidal sinus
    Body
    Medial plate of the pterygoid process
    Lateral plate of the pterygoid process
- **Palatine bone**
    Perpendicular plate
    Horizontal plate
- **Sphenopalatine foramen**

Dissection Instructions

EXTERNAL NOSE [G 690; N 36; R 49; C 558]

1. On the cadaver, palpate the nasal bone. Inferior to the nasal bone palpate the **lateral nasal cartilage** (Fig. 7.73). The lateral nasal cartilage gives shape to the bridge of the nose.
2. The lateral nasal cartilage is an extension of the **septal cartilage**. The septal cartilage separates the right and left nasal cavities and forms the anterior part of the nasal septum.

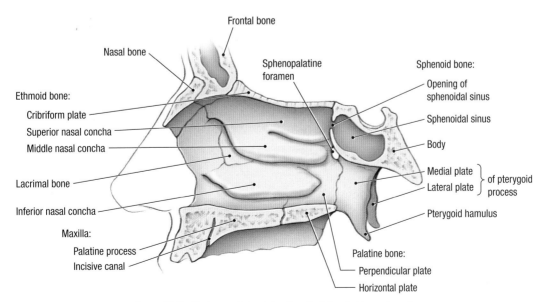

Figure 7.72. Skeleton of the lateral wall of the right nasal cavity.

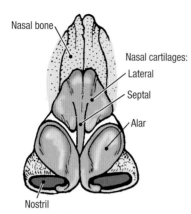

Figure 7.73. Cartilages of the external nose.

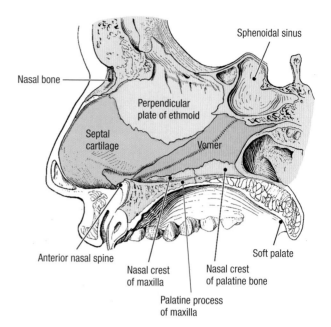

Figure 7.74. Left side of the nasal septum.

3. Lateral to the septal cartilage is the **alar cartilage** (Fig. 7.73). The alar cartilage gives shape to the nostril.

NASAL CAVITY

1. The **boundaries of the nasal cavity** are:
   - **Roof** – a narrow region bounded by the nasal septum and by parts of three other bones: nasal bone, cribriform plate of ethmoid bone, and sphenoid bone
   - **Floor** – palatine process of the maxilla and horizontal plate of the palatine bone
   - **Medial wall** – nasal septum
   - **Lateral wall** – maxilla, lacrimal bone, ethmoid bone, inferior nasal concha, and perpendicular plate of the palatine bone
2. In the cadaver, observe that the bones and cartilages of the nasal cavity are obscured by the mucosa that covers them. The vessels and nerves of the nasal cavity are contained within this mucosa.

NASAL SEPTUM [G 691; L 336, 340; N 39; R 143; C 560]

1. Examine the half of the head that contains the **nasal septum**. Strip the mucosa completely off of the nasal septum and identify the **perpendicular plate of the ethmoid bone**, **vomer**, and **septal cartilage** (Fig. 7.74).
2. Use a probe and forceps to remove the bony and cartilaginous parts of the nasal septum. Leave intact the mucosa that lines the other side of the nasal septum. In the mucosa of the nasal septum, identify the **nasopalatine nerve** and the **sphenopalatine artery** (Fig. 7.75). Note that the nasopalatine nerve and the sphenopalatine artery pass diagonally down the nasal septum from the sphenopalatine foramen to the incisive canal. In addition to the nasal septum, the nasopalatine nerve and sphenopalatine artery supply a portion of the oral mucosa that covers the hard palate.

3. Note that the mucosa near the cribriform plate is the **olfactory area** (Fig. 7.75). The olfactory area also extends down the lateral wall of the nasal cavity for a short distance.

LATERAL WALL OF THE NASAL CAVITY [G 694, 695; L 338, 340; N 37; R 144, 145; C 560]

1. Remove the mucosa and remnants of the nasal septum.
2. Inspect the **lateral wall of the nasal cavity** (Fig. 7.76). Identify:
   - **Sphenoethmoidal recess** – above the superior concha
   - **Superior concha**

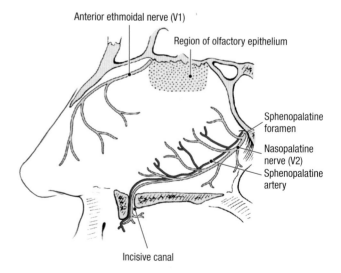

Figure 7.75. Nerve and arterial supply to the mucosa of the nasal septum. Left side of septum is shown.

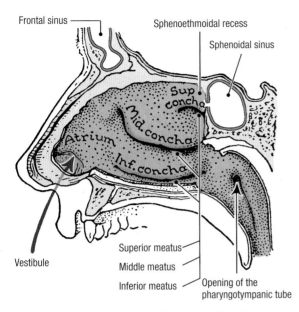

Figure 7.76. Conchae and meatuses of the lateral wall of the right nasal cavity.

- **Superior meatus** – inferior to the superior concha
- **Middle concha**
- **Middle meatus** – inferior to the middle concha
- **Inferior concha**
- **Inferior meatus** – inferior to the inferior concha
- **Vestibule** – the area superior to the nostril and anterior to the inferior meatus
- **Atrium** – the area superior to the vestibule and anterior to the middle meatus

3. Use scissors to remove the **inferior concha**. Use a probe and forceps to remove the mucosa from the lateral wall of the inferior meatus. Identify the opening of the **nasolacrimal duct** (Fig. 7.77).

4. Use scissors to remove the **middle concha**. In the middle meatus identify a curved slit, the **semilunar hiatus (hiatus semilunaris)** (Fig. 7.77). Posterior to the curvature of the semilunar hiatus, identify the **ethmoidal bulla (bulla ethmoidalis)**.

5. Within the semilunar hiatus, identify (Fig. 7.77):
   - **Opening of the frontal sinus**
   - **Opening of the anterior ethmoidal cells**
   - **Opening of the maxillary sinus**

6. Identify the **opening of the middle ethmoidal cells** on the summit of the ethmoidal bulla.

7. Identify the **opening of the posterior ethmoidal cells** in the superior meatus.

8. Identify the **opening of the sphenoidal sinus** in the sphenoethmoidal recess.

9. Examine the **sphenoidal sinus** (Fig. 7.77). The sphenoidal sinus is a paired structure that is lined by mucosa that is continuous with the mucosa of the nasal cavity. Note that the sphenoidal sinus lies directly inferior to the hypophyseal fossa and pituitary gland. [G 698; L 336; N 48; R 144; C 564]

CLINICAL CORRELATION

Sphenoidal Sinus

Surgical approaches to the pituitary gland take advantage of the fact that the sphenoidal sinus and nasal cavity provide a direct approach.

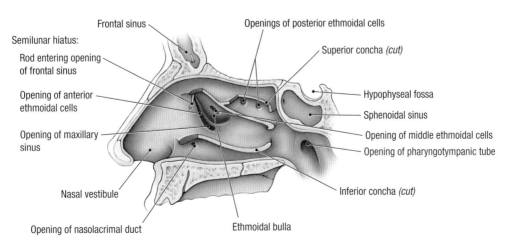

Figure 7.77. Openings in the lateral wall of the right nasal cavity.

10. Note that the **ethmoidal cells** are located between the nasal cavity and the orbit (Figs. 7.78 and 7.79). The ethmoidal cells may be observed from the superior perspective by reviewing the dissection of the orbit that was completed previously.

11. The **maxillary sinus** is a three-sided pyramid with an average adult capacity of 15 mL. Observe an illustration of a coronal section through the maxillary sinus and note the following (Fig. 7.79):
    * The roof of the maxillary sinus is the floor of the orbit and the infraorbital nerve innervates the mucosa of the sinus.
    * The floor of the maxillary sinus is the alveolar process of the maxilla.
    * The opening of the maxillary sinus is near its roof.
    * The roots of the maxillary teeth may project into the maxillary sinus.

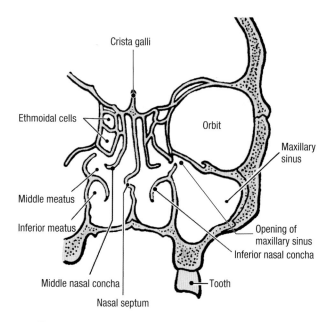

Figure 7.79. Coronal section through the maxillary sinus.

CLINICAL CORRELATION

Maxillary Sinus

When the head is in the upright position, the maxillary sinus cannot drain. If infections of the maxillary sinus persist, an opening is surgically created through the inferior meatus near the floor of the maxillary sinus to promote drainage.

When the roots of maxillary teeth project into the maxillary sinus, they are covered only by mucosa. During extraction of a maxillary molar or premolar tooth, the mucosa superior to the projecting root may be torn. As a result, a fistula may be formed between the oral cavity and the maxillary sinus.

Dissection Review

1. Use an illustration and the dissected specimen to review the features of the lateral wall of the nasal cavity.
2. Review the relationship of the paranasal sinuses to the orbit, anterior cranial fossa, and nasal cavity.
3. Review the drainage point of each paranasal sinus.

HARD PALATE AND SOFT PALATE

Dissection Overview

The palate forms the floor of the nasal cavity and the roof of the oral cavity. The palate consists of two portions: the **hard palate** forms the anterior two-thirds and the **soft palate** constitutes the posterior one-third. The palate is covered by nasal mucosa on its superior surface and oral mucosa on its inferior surface. Numerous mucous glands (**palatine glands**) are present on the oral surface of the palate.

The order of dissection will be as follows: The mucosal folds of the inner pharyngeal wall will be reviewed. The mucosa will be stripped from the inner surface of the pharynx and the muscles that constitute the inner longitudinal muscle layer will be examined. Muscles that move the soft palate will then be studied. The nerves and blood vessels of the palate will be identified. The palatine canal and pterygopalatine fossa will be dissected from the medial aspect. The pterygopalatine ganglion will be dissected. The nerves and vessels of the nasal cavity and palate will be summarized.

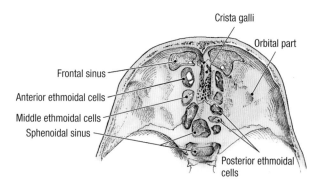

Figure 7.78. Paranasal sinuses, superior view.

SKELETON OF THE PALATE

Refer to a skull. From an inferior view, identify (Fig. 7.80): [G 682; L 301; N 8; R 45; C 582]

- **Maxilla**
  Incisive foramen
  Alveolar process
  Palatine process
- **Palatine bone**
  Horizontal plate
  Greater palatine foramen
  Lesser palatine foramina
  Posterior nasal spine
- **Sphenoid bone**
  Hamulus of the medial plate of the pterygoid process
  Medial plate of the pterygoid process
  Lateral plate of the pterygoid process
  Scaphoid fossa
  Pterygoid canal

In the infratemporal fossa, identify (Fig. 7.81): [G 665; L 327; N 4; C 541]

- **Inferior orbital fissure**
- **Sphenopalatine foramen**
- **Pterygopalatine fossa**
- **Pterygomaxillary fissure**

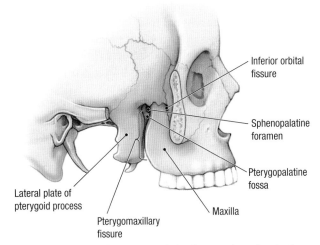

Figure 7.81. Entry to the pterygopalatine fossa and nasal cavity from the infratemporal fossa.

Dissection Instructions

SOFT PALATE

1. Review the mucosal features of the inner pharyngeal wall (Fig. 7.82): [G 794, 795; L 318, 319; N 64; R 144; C 567]
   - **Torus tubarius**
   - **Opening of the pharyngotympanic tube**
   - **Salpingopalatine fold**
   - **Torus Levatorius**
   - **Salpingopharyngeal fold**

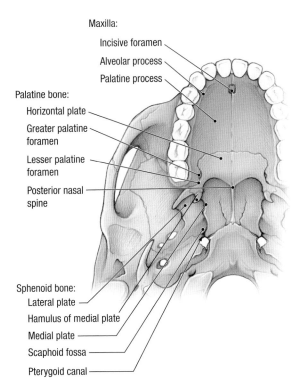

Figure 7.80. Skeleton of the palate, inferior view.

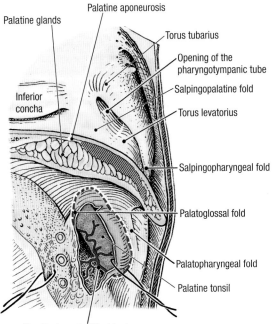

Figure 7.82. Mucosal folds in the pharynx.

- **Palatoglossal fold**
- **Palatopharyngeal fold**

2. Examine the edge of the **soft palate** where it is cut in the sagittal plane and observe (Fig. 7.82):
   - The thickness of the soft palate is partly due to the presence of palatine glands.
   - The strength of the soft palate is due to the palatine aponeurosis.
   - The mobility of the soft palate is due to muscles that attach to its posterior two-thirds.

3. Remove the mucosa from the palatopharyngeal fold and identify the **palatopharyngeus muscle** (Fig. 7.83). The superior attachments of the palatopharyngeus muscle are the hard palate and palatine aponeurosis and its inferior attachments are the thyroid cartilage and pharyngeal wall. The palatopharyngeus muscle elevates the larynx during swallowing.

4. Remove the mucosa from the salpingopharyngeal fold and identify the **salpingopharyngeus muscle** (Fig. 7.83). The superior attachment of the salpingopharyngeus muscle is the cartilage of the pharyngotympanic tube. Its distal attachments and action are the same as the palatopharyngeus muscle, with which it blends. Note that the palatopharyngeus and salpingopharyngeus

5. muscles contribute to the inner longitudinal muscle layer of the pharynx.

5. Remove the remaining mucosa from the inner surface of the nasopharynx and oropharynx. Identify the **stylopharyngeus muscle**, which enters the pharynx between the superior and middle pharyngeal constrictor muscles (Fig. 7.83). The stylopharyngeus muscle lies anterior and parallel to the palatopharyngeus and salpingopharyngeus muscles, and all three blend near their inferior ends.

6. The gap between the superior border of the superior pharyngeal constrictor muscle and the base of the skull is closed by the **pharyngobasilar fascia**. Passing through this gap are the **pharyngotympanic tube** and the **levator veli palatini muscle** (Fig. 7.83).

7. The **pharyngotympanic tube (auditory tube)** connects the nasopharynx to the tympanic cavity. The part of the pharyngotympanic tube that is closest to the pharynx is cartilaginous (approximately two-thirds of its length) and the part that is closest to the middle ear passes through the temporal bone.

8. Remove the mucosa from the **torus levatorius** and identify the **levator veli palatini muscle** (Fig. 7.83). The superior attachments of the levator veli palatini muscle are the cartilage of the pharyngotympanic tube and the adjacent part of the temporal bone. Its distal attachment is the palatine aponeurosis. The levator veli palatini muscle elevates the soft palate.

9. Remove the mucosa from the posterior border of the **medial plate of the pterygoid process** (Fig. 7.83). Identify the **tensor veli palatini muscle**, which lies lateral to the medial plate. The superior attachment of the tensor veli palatini muscle is the **scaphoid fossa**. The belly of the tensor veli palatini muscle is located between the medial and lateral plates of the pterygoid process. Its tendon turns medially around the **hamulus of the medial pterygoid plate** and forms the **palatine aponeurosis**. The tensor veli palatini muscle tenses the soft palate. Palpate the hamulus and find the tendon of the tensor veli palatini muscle.

10. Five muscles of the soft palate and pharynx are innervated by the vagus nerve (X) via the pharyngeal plexus: salpingopharyngeus, levator veli palatini, palatoglossus, palatopharyngeus, and musculus uvulae. The tensor veli palatini muscle is innervated by the mandibular division of the trigeminal nerve (V$_3$).

11. To remove the mucosa from the hard palate, use a probe to raise the mucosa on the inferior surface of the hard palate where it was cut during head bi-

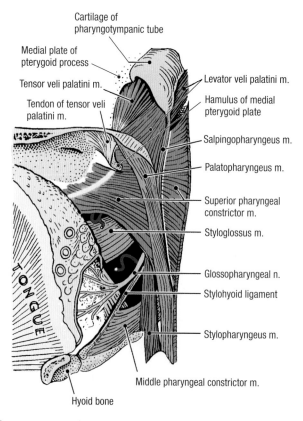

Figure 7.83. Muscles of the pharyngeal wall, internal view. Bed of the palatine tonsil.

section. Grasp the mucosa with forceps or a hemostat and use blunt dissection to peel it from medial to lateral. Detach the mucosa along the medial side of the alveolar process of the maxilla. [G 683; N 52; R 147; C 567]

12. Identify the **greater palatine nerve** and **vessels** where they emerge from the **greater palatine foramen** (Fig. 7.84). Use blunt dissection to follow the greater palatine nerve anteriorly. Note that the **nasopalatine nerve** supplies the mucosa over the anterior part of the hard palate (Fig. 7.84).

13. Posterior to the greater palatine nerve, identify the **lesser palatine nerve** and use blunt dissection to follow it to the soft palate.

TONSILLAR BED [G 796; L 318; N 64; R 147; C 567]

1. Identify the **palatine tonsil** (Fig. 7.82). In older individuals, the palatine tonsil may be inconspicuous or may have been surgically removed. When present, the palatine tonsil is located in the **tonsillar bed**. The boundaries of the tonsillar bed are:
   • Anterior – **palatoglossal fold**
   • Posterior – **palatopharyngeal fold**
   • Lateral – superior pharyngeal constrictor muscle

2. If the cadaver has a palatine tonsil, use blunt dissection to remove it (Fig. 7.82). Section the tonsil and observe the **crypts** that extend into its surface.

3. Use blunt dissection to remove the mucosa from the palatoglossal fold and identify the **palatoglossus muscle**, which lies within the fold. The superior attachment of the palatoglossus muscle is the palatine aponeurosis and its inferior attachment is the lateral side of the tongue. The palatoglossus muscle elevates the tongue and depresses the soft palate.

4. The **glossopharyngeal nerve (IX)** passes between the superior and the middle pharyngeal constrictor muscles to enter the tonsillar bed. Remove the mucosa from the tonsillar bed and observe the glossopharyngeal nerve (Fig. 7.83). The glossopharyngeal nerve innervates the mucosa of the posterior one-third of the tongue and the posterior wall of the pharynx.

SPHENOPALATINE FORAMEN AND PTERYGOPALATINE FOSSA [G 683; L 340; N 42; R 147; C 563]

1. Do not dissect the arterial network of the lateral nasal wall, but use an illustration to study the following branches of the **sphenopalatine artery**: [G 693; L 340; N 41; R 143; C 562]
   • **Posterior lateral nasal artery** – to the lateral nasal wall
   • **Posterior septal branch** – to the nasal septum

2. Remove the mucosa from the posterior part of the lateral nasal wall.

3. Use a probe to locate the **sphenopalatine foramen** (Fig. 7.85). Insert a probe into the sphenopalatine foramen and direct it inferiorly toward the greater palatine foramen. Pull the probe medially to break the medial wall of the greater palatine canal.

4. Identify the **greater palatine nerve**, the **lesser palatine nerve**, and the **descending palatine artery** in the greater palatine canal (Fig. 7.86). The

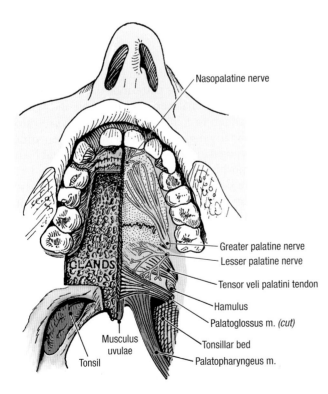

Figure 7.84. Nerves of the hard and soft palate.

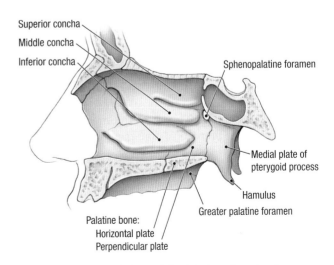

Figure 7.85. Skeleton of the right lateral nasal wall.

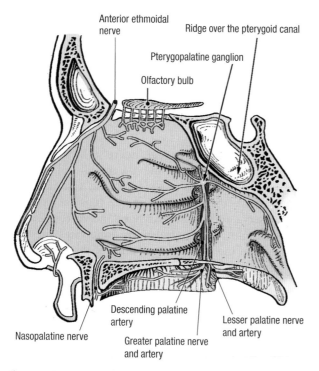

Anterior ethmoidal nerve

Ridge over the pterygoid canal

Pterygopalatine ganglion

Olfactory bulb

Descending palatine artery

Lesser palatine nerve and artery

Nasopalatine nerve

Greater palatine nerve and artery

Figure 7.86. Nerve and arterial supply to the mucosa of the lateral wall of the nasal cavity. Pterygopalatine ganglion.

descending palatine artery is one of the terminal branches of the maxillary artery.

5. At the inferior end of the greater palatine canal, use a fine probe or needle to separate the nerves and vessels. Note that the descending palatine artery divides to give rise to the **greater palatine artery** and the **lesser palatine artery** (Fig. 7.86).

6. Place the fine probe between the greater palatine nerve and the lesser palatine nerve and slide it superiorly until it stops. This is the inferior extent of the **pterygopalatine ganglion** (Fig. 7.86). The pterygopalatine ganglion is the location for synapse of preganglionic axons of the facial nerve (VII) that course first in the greater petrosal nerve and then in the nerve of the pterygoid canal. Postganglionic axons that arise in the pterygopalatine ganglion distribute with branches of the maxillary division of the trigeminal nerve (V₂). The pterygopalatine ganglion stimulates secretion from the mucosa of the nasal cavity, paranasal sinuses, nasopharynx, roof of the mouth, and soft palate. The pterygopalatine ganglion also stimulates the lacrimal gland.

7. The **nerve of the pterygoid canal** enters the pterygopalatine fossa from posteriorly. To find it, remove the mucosa from the floor of the sphenoidal sinus. Frequently a ridge in the floor of the sphenoidal sinus marks the location of the pterygoid canal (Fig. 7.86). Use a probe to break open

the pterygoid canal and identify the nerve of the pterygoid canal.

8. Follow the nerve of the pterygoid canal anteriorly toward the pterygopalatine ganglion. The nerve of the pterygoid canal contains preganglionic parasympathetic axons from the greater petrosal nerve and postganglionic sympathetic axons from the deep petrosal nerve.

9. Turn the specimen and approach it from the lateral aspect. Deep in the **infratemporal fossa,** identify: [G 669; L 330; N 69; R 80; C 512]
   - **Maxillary artery** – courses deeply toward the pterygomaxillary fissure. Near the pterygomaxillary fissure the maxillary artery gives rise to the:

     Sphenopalatine artery – passes through the pterygopalatine fossa and then through the sphenopalatine foramen to enter the nasal cavity

     Descending palatine artery – enters the greater palatine canal where it was dissected from the medial side

     Infraorbital artery – passes through the inferior orbital fissure to enter the infraorbital canal and emerge on the face at the infraorbital foramen
   - **Maxillary division of the trigeminal nerve (V₂)** – courses from the foramen rotundum to the inferior orbital fissure. The maxillary division passes through the pterygopalatine fossa and gives off pterygopalatine branches that will form the greater and lesser palatine nerves.

Dissection Review

1. Use the dissected specimen and an illustration to reconstruct the branching pattern of the maxillary division of the trigeminal nerve. Use a skull and the dissected specimen to follow the maxillary division from the trigeminal ganglion through the foramen rotundum, pterygopalatine fossa, and inferior orbital fissure to the infraorbital groove.

2. Review the distribution of the following branches of the maxillary division of the trigeminal nerve: greater palatine, lesser palatine, nasopalatine, and infraorbital nerves.

3. Return to the carotid triangle of the neck and follow the external carotid artery superiorly into the infratemporal fossa. Review the origin of the maxillary artery and its course through the infratemporal fossa. Review all branches of the maxillary artery that you dissected previously. Use an illustration to review the terminal branches of the maxillary artery (posterior superior alveolar, infraorbital, descending palatine, and sphenopalatine) and use the dissected specimen to review these branches where you have dissected them.

4. Review the muscles that move the soft palate. State their attachments and actions.

5. Review the pharyngeal wall, placing the pharyngeal constrictor muscles and the muscles of the soft palate into the correct muscle layers (inner longitudinal or outer circular).

6. Review the pharyngeal plexus on the posterior surface of the pharynx and recall its role in innervation of the pharyngeal mucosa and the muscles of the pharynx and soft palate.

7. Use the dissected specimen and an illustration to review the course of the glossopharyngeal nerve from the jugular foramen to the posterior one-third of the tongue.

ORAL REGION

Dissection Overview

The **oral region** includes the oral cavity and its contents (teeth, gums, and tongue), the palate, and the part of the oropharynx that contains the palatine tonsils. The palate and palatine tonsils have been dissected previously. The **oral cavity** consists of:

- **Oral vestibule** – bounded externally by the lips and cheeks and internally by the teeth and gums.
- **Oral cavity proper** – the area between the alveolar arches and teeth. The largest content of the oral cavity proper is the tongue.

The order of dissection will be as follows: The superficial features of the oral region will be examined on a living person. On the cadaver, the tongue will be inspected and the tongue and mandible will be bisected in the midline. The intrinsic muscles of the tongue will be inspected. The sublingual region will be studied and the dissection of the deep part of the submandibular gland will be completed. Finally, the extrinsic muscles of the tongue will be studied.

SURFACE ANATOMY OF THE ORAL VESTIBULE [L 333; N 51; C 566]

Use a mirror to examine your mouth and a clean finger to palpate the following structures through the mucosa that lines the oral vestibule:

- **Maxilla**
  Alveolar process
  Anterior surface (above the alveolar process)
  Infratemporal surface
- **Mandible**
  Alveolar process
  Coronoid process and the **tendon of the temporalis muscle**
- **Masseter muscle** – best palpated when the teeth are clenched
- **Communication between the oral vestibule and the oral cavity proper** – posterior to the third molar tooth

Turn down your lower lip and lift your upper lip. Identify the **frenulum** in the midline of each lip.

Examine the inner surface of your cheek. Identify the **opening of the parotid duct** located lateral to the second maxillary molar tooth.

SURFACE ANATOMY OF THE ORAL CAVITY PROPER

Observe the borders of your oral cavity:

- **Lateral and anterior** – the teeth and gums
- **Superior** – the hard palate
- **Inferior** – the mucosa covering the tongue and sublingual area
- **Posterior** – the palatoglossal folds (right and left)

In your oral cavity, identify:

- **Tongue**
  Body
  Apex
  Median sulcus
- **Sublingual area**
  Frenulum of the tongue (sublingual frenulum)
  Sublingual fold (plica sublingualis)
  Sublingual caruncle
  Opening of submandibular duct – on the sublingual caruncle
  Deep lingual veins – seen on either side of the frenulum of the tongue

Dissection Instructions

TONGUE [G 676; L 334; N 58; R 149; C 575]

1. Inspect the **tongue** in the cadaver specimen. Identify (Fig. 7.87):
   - **Root** – the posterior one-third
   - **Body** – the anterior two-thirds
   - **Apex**
   - **Dorsum**
     Terminal sulcus (sulcus terminalis) – divides the anterior two-thirds from the posterior one-third
     Lingual tonsil – posterior to the terminal sulcus
     Foramen cecum – in the midline at the point of the terminal sulcus
     Median sulcus
     Lingual papillae – four types: vallate, filiform, fungiform, and foliate

2. Note that the **body of the tongue** lies horizontally in the oral cavity and the **root of the tongue** lies more vertically. The root of the tongue constitutes the lower part of the anterior boundary of the oropharynx.

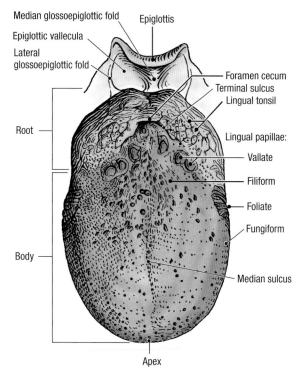

Median glossoepiglottic fold   Epiglottis
Epiglottic vallecula
Lateral glossoepiglottic fold
Root
Body
Apex

Foramen cecum
Terminal sulcus
Lingual tonsil
Lingual papillae:
— Vallate
— Filiform
— Foliate
— Fungiform
— Median sulcus

Figure 7.87. Dorsum of the tongue.

3. At the root of the tongue (Fig. 7.87), identify:
    *   **Median glossoepiglottic fold** – a midline fold of mucosa between the dorsum of the tongue and the **epiglottis**
    *   **Lateral glossoepiglottic fold** – between the dorsum of the tongue and the lateral border of the epiglottis
    *   **Epiglottic vallecula** – a depression between median and lateral glossoepiglottic folds

BISECTION OF THE MANDIBLE AND FLOOR OF THE MOUTH

1. Use a new scalpel blade. Turn the specimen to expose the submental triangle.
2. Use the scalpel to cut the **mylohyoid muscles** along their median raphe. Use a probe to separate the mylohyoid muscles from deeper structures.
3. Identify the **geniohyoid muscle**, which is deep to the mylohyoid muscle. The anterior attachment of the geniohyoid muscle is the inferior mental spine of the mandible and its posterior attachment is the body of the hyoid bone. The geniohyoid muscle pulls the hyoid bone anteriorly.
4. Use blunt dissection to separate the geniohyoid muscles in the midline. Use a saw to cut through the mandible in the median plane. Do not allow the saw to pass between the genioglossus muscles on the deep side of the mandible.
5. Do not bisect the epiglottis, the hyoid bone, or the larynx at this time. Use a scalpel to bisect the

tongue in the median plane, beginning at the apex and proceeding toward the epiglottis. Cut as far inferiorly as the hyoid bone.

SUBLINGUAL REGION [G 779; L 332; N 51; R 153; C 568]

1. On the sectioned surface of the tongue, identify the **genioglossus muscle**. The anterior attachment of the genioglossus muscle is the superior mental spine of the mandible and its posterior attachments are the hyoid bone and the tongue. The genioglossus muscle protrudes the tongue. The genioglossus muscle is innervated by the hypoglossal nerve (XII).

CLINICAL CORRELATION

Hypoglossal Nerve

The genioglossus muscle protrudes the tongue. If one genioglossus muscle does not function (hypoglossal nerve dysfunction on that side), the tongue cannot be protruded in the midline. The functional side of the tongue protrudes normally and the side with the dysfunctional nerve is protruded less or not at all. Therefore, in testing for hypoglossal nerve lesions, the protruded tongue deviates toward the side of the nerve lesion.

---

2. Use the cadaver specimen to review the sublingual features that were identified in your oral cavity:
    *   **Frenulum of the tongue**
    *   **Sublingual fold**
    *   **Sublingual caruncle**
    *   **Opening of the submandibular duct**
3. Use a scalpel carefully to incise the mucous membrane along the medial surface of the mandible. Start the incision at the frenulum of the tongue and stop near the second mandibular molar tooth. Use a probe and forceps to peel the mucosa medially.
4. Identify the **sublingual gland** immediately deep to the mucosa (Fig. 7.88). The sublingual gland rests on the mylohyoid muscle. The sublingual gland has about 12 short ducts that drain along the summit of the sublingual fold.
5. Use a probe to dissect along the medial side of the sublingual gland and find the **submandibular duct** (Fig. 7.88). Follow the submandibular duct anteriorly to its opening on the sublingual caruncle. Use a probe to trace the submandibular duct posteriorly to the **deep part of the submandibular gland**. Note that the deep part of the sub-

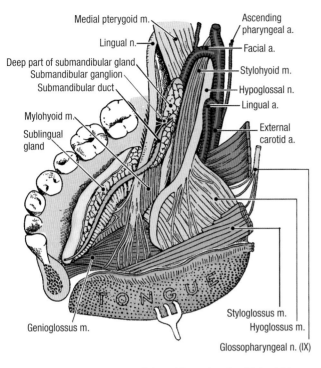

Figure 7.88. Dissection of the sublingual region (right side).

mandibular gland is located on the deep side of the mylohyoid muscle.

6. Turn the specimen to expose the infratemporal fossa. Find the **lingual nerve** and trace it into the sublingual region. Observe that the lingual nerve passes lateral, inferior, and medial to the submandibular duct (Fig. 7.88). The lingual nerve has several branches that supply the mucosa of the anterior two-thirds of the tongue with general sensation and taste fibers. [G 779; L 332; N 61; R 153; C 573]

7. Near the third mandibular molar tooth, identify the **submandibular ganglion** that is suspended below the lingual nerve. Read a textbook description of the parasympathetic function of the submandibular ganglion.

8. Turn the specimen so that the submandibular triangle is exposed. Find the **hypoglossal nerve (XII)** and use a probe to trace it into the sublingual region. Note that the hypoglossal nerve passes between the submandibular gland and the hyoglossus muscle (Fig. 7.88). Observe that both the hypoglossal nerve and the lingual nerve pass between the hyoglossus muscle and the mylohyoid muscle to enter the sublingual region. The course of the hypoglossal nerve is inferior to the course of the lingual nerve.

9. From the lateral perspective, define the attachment of the mylohyoid muscle to the hyoid bone. Use scissors to detach the mylohyoid muscle from the hyoid bone and reflect the muscle superiorly.

10. Identify the **hyoglossus muscle**, which is deep to the mylohyoid muscle (Fig. 7.89). The inferior attachments of the hyoglossus muscle are the body and greater horn of the hyoid bone and its superior attachment is the lateral side of the tongue. The hyoglossus muscle depresses and retracts the tongue.

11. Near the superior end of the hyoglossus muscle, identify the **styloglossus muscle** (Fig. 7.89). The proximal attachment of the styloglossus muscle is the styloid process and its distal attachment is the lateral side of the tongue. The styloglossus muscle retracts the tongue and draws it superiorly. [G 782; N 59]

12. On one side only, make a transverse section through the body of the tongue. On the cut surface, note the **intrinsic muscles of the tongue** consisting of **vertical**, **transverse**, **superior longitudinal**, and **inferior longitudinal groups of fibers**. [G 679; L 333; N 60; R 149; C 576]

13. Return to the carotid triangle and locate the **lingual artery** where it arises from the external carotid artery (Fig. 7.89). Follow the lingual artery until it passes medial to the hyoglossus muscle, where its name changes to **deep lingual artery**. On the cut surface of the sectioned tongue, look for the lumen of the deep lingual artery. It is usually located within 5 mm of the inferior surface of the tongue.

14. The intrinsic muscles of the tongue and the three extrinsic muscles of the tongue (styloglossus, genioglossus, and hyoglossus) are innervated by the **hypoglossal nerve (XII)**.

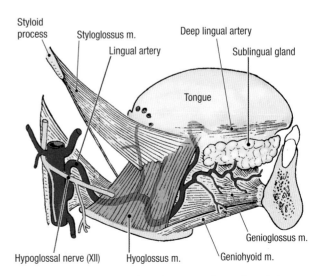

Figure 7.89. Blood supply to the tongue from a lateral view.

Dissection Review

1. Review the surface features of the tongue.
2. Review the innervation of the lingual mucosa.
3. Follow the submandibular duct from the submandibular triangle to the sublingual caruncle.
4. Trace the lingual nerve from the infratemporal fossa to the tongue. Note the relationship of the lingual nerve to the submandibular duct, hyoglossus muscle, and mylohyoid muscle.
5. Review the chorda tympani and the role that it plays in sensory innervation of the tongue and parasympathetic innervation of the submandibular and sublingual glands.
6. Locate the submandibular ganglion and state its function.
7. Trace the hypoglossal nerve from the base of the skull to the tongue, noting its relationships to arteries and muscles.
8. Organize the muscles of the tongue into extrinsic and intrinsic groups. State the attachments, innervation, and action of each extrinsic muscle.
9. Use an illustration and the dissected specimen to review the origin and course of the facial and lingual arteries.

LARYNX

Dissection Overview

The larynx is contained in the visceral compartment of the neck. The thyroid gland lies anterior to it and the pharynx posterior to it. The larynx is the entrance to the airway and it contains the **glottis**, a valve that serves the dual function of controlling the airway and producing sound during phonation. The *intrinsic* muscles of the larynx control the glottis. The *extrinsic* muscles of the larynx (infrahyoid muscles, suprahyoid muscles, and stylopharyngeus muscle) control the position of the larynx in the neck. Usually, the larynx is located at vertebral levels C3 to C6.

The order of dissection will be as follows: Illustrations and models will be used to study the cartilages of the larynx. Dissection of the larynx involves removal of the mucous membrane and identification of the underlying muscles. First, the mucosa will be removed from the posterior part of the larynx to expose two intrinsic muscles. The left lamina of the thyroid cartilage will then be reflected to expose the remaining intrinsic muscles. The larynx will be opened and the mucosal features will be studied. Finally, the nerves to the larynx will be reviewed.

SKELETON OF THE LARYNX [G 798; L 320; N 77; R 158; C 598]

The **skeleton of the larynx** is responsible for maintaining a patent airway. It consists of a series of articulating cartilages that are united by membranes. Use an illustration and a model of the larynx to study the cartilages and membranes (Fig. 7.90). Identify:

- **Epiglottic cartilage** – an unpaired, heart-shaped cartilage that lies posterior to the tongue and hyoid bone. The **stalk** of the epiglottic cartilage is attached within the angle formed by the thyroid laminae.
- **Thyrohyoid membrane** – connects the superior border of the thyroid cartilage to the hyoid bone. When the suprahyoid and infrahyoid muscles move the hyoid bone, the larynx also moves.
- **Thyroid cartilage** – formed by two **laminae** that are joined in the anterior midline to form the **laryngeal**

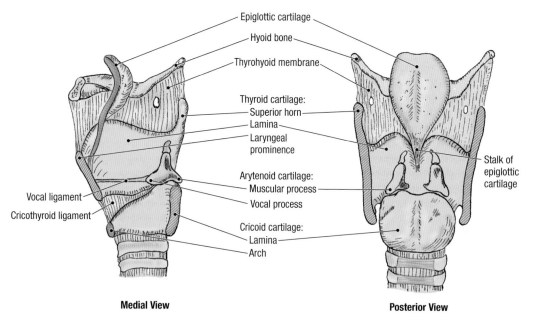

Medial View　　　　　　　　**Posterior View**

Figure 7.90. Cartilages of the larynx.

prominence. The **superior horn** of the thyroid cartilage projects superiorly. The **inferior horn** of the thyroid cartilage articulates with the cricoid cartilage through the **cricothyroid joint**.

- **Cricoid cartilage** – shaped like a ring (G. *krikos*, ring). Its **lamina** is a broad, flat area that is positioned posteriorly and its **arch** is located anteriorly.

The **arytenoid cartilages** are located on the superior border of the lamina of the cricoid cartilage. Each arytenoid cartilage is pyramid-shaped and it articulates with the cricoid cartilage through a synovial joint. Each arytenoid cartilage has a **muscular process** for attachment of intrinsic laryngeal muscles and a **vocal process** for attachment of the vocal ligament. The arytenoid cartilages are capable of several movements:

- Tilting anteriorly and posteriorly
- Sliding toward each other (adduction)
- Sliding away from each other (abduction)
- Rotation

Use an illustration to identify the **vocal ligaments** (Fig. 7.90). The posterior end of each vocal ligament is attached to the vocal process of an arytenoid cartilage. The anterior end of each vocal ligament is attached to the inner surface of the thyroid cartilage at the angle formed by the laminae.

Dissection Instructions

INTRINSIC MUSCLES OF THE LARYNX [G 802, 803; L 321–323; N 78; R 160; C 596, 597]

1. Review the external features of the larynx that have been dissected previously:
   - Infrahyoid muscles:
     Sternohyoid muscle
     Omohyoid muscle
     Sternothyroid muscle
     Thyrohyoid muscle
   - Suprahyoid muscles:
     Geniohyoid
     Mylohyoid
     Stylohyoid
     Digastric
   - Internal branch of the superior laryngeal nerve
   - Superior laryngeal artery
   - External branch of the superior laryngeal nerve
2. On the external surface of the larynx, identify the **cricothyroid muscle**. The inferior attachment of the cricothyroid muscle is the lateral surface of the cricoid cartilage and its superior attachment is the inferior margin of the thyroid cartilage. The cricothyroid muscle tilts the thyroid cartilage anteriorly, which lengthens the vocal fold. The cricothyroid muscle is innervated by the external branch of the superior laryngeal nerve.

3. To expose the posterior surface of the larynx, push the head forward and allow the chin to rest on the thoracic wall.
4. Open the posterior wall of the pharynx to expose the posterior surface of the larynx. Palpate the **lamina of the cricoid cartilage**. Lateral to the lamina identify the **piriform recess**.
5. Use blunt dissection to remove the mucosa from the piriform recess. Immediately deep to the mucosa identify the **internal branch of the superior laryngeal nerve** and the **inferior laryngeal nerve** (Fig. 7.91).
6. Use blunt dissection to strip the mucosa from the lamina of the cricoid cartilage and expose the **posterior cricoarytenoid muscle** (Fig. 7.91). The inferior attachment of the posterior cricoarytenoid muscle is the posterior surface of the lamina of the cricoid cartilage and its superior attachment is the muscular process of the arytenoid cartilage. The posterior cricoarytenoid muscle causes the arytenoid cartilage to rotate, moving the vocal process laterally (abduction of the vocal folds).
7. Superior to the posterior cricoarytenoid muscle, identify the **arytenoid muscle** (Fig. 7.91). The arytenoid muscle attaches to both arytenoid cartilages. Observe that the arytenoid muscle has **transverse fibers** and **oblique fibers**. The arytenoid muscle slides the arytenoid cartilages together (adduction of the vocal folds).
8. The **cricothyroid joint** is a synovial joint that is reinforced by short ligaments. Observe that the recurrent laryngeal nerve enters the larynx by passing posterior to the cricothyroid joint. At this location the name of the recurrent laryngeal nerve changes to **inferior laryngeal nerve**.
9. On the left side only, disarticulate the cricothyroid joint. Carefully cut the thyrohyoid membrane. Use scissors to cut the left lamina of the thyroid cartilage just to the left of the midline. Reflect the thyroid lamina inferiorly. It should remain attached to the cricoid cartilage by the cricothyroid muscle.
10. Deep to the thyroid lamina, identify the **lateral cricoarytenoid muscle** (Fig. 7.91). The inferior attachment of the lateral cricoarytenoid muscle is the arch of the cricoid cartilage and its superior attachment is the muscular process of the arytenoid cartilage. The lateral cricoarytenoid muscle causes the arytenoid cartilage to rotate, moving the vocal process medially (adduction of the vocal fold).
11. Identify the **thyroarytenoid muscle**, which is located superior to the lateral cricoarytenoid muscle (Fig. 7.91). The anterior attachment of the thyroarytenoid muscle is the inner surface of the thy-

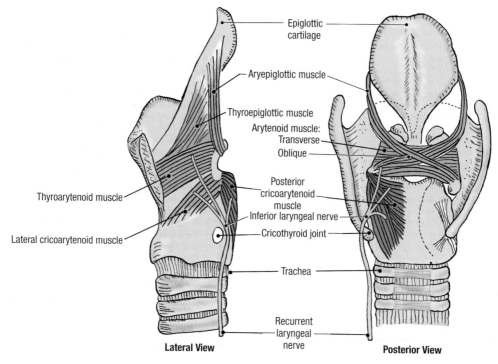

Epiglottic cartilage

Aryepiglottic muscle

Thyroepiglottic muscle

Arytenoid muscle:
Transverse
Oblique

Thyroarytenoid muscle

Posterior cricoarytenoid muscle

Inferior laryngeal nerve

Lateral cricoarytenoid muscle

Cricothyroid joint

Trachea

Recurrent laryngeal nerve

Lateral View

Posterior View

Figure 7.91. Intrinsic muscles of the larynx.

roid cartilage and its posterior attachment is the anterior surface of the arytenoid cartilage. The thyroarytenoid muscle tilts the arytenoid cartilage anteriorly, relaxing the vocal fold.

12. The **vocalis muscle** cannot be seen in dissection. The vocalis muscle is formed by the medial fibers of the thyroarytenoid muscle. The vocalis muscle is attached to the vocal ligament and it modifies the tension in localized parts of the vocal fold, modulating pitch.

13. Other delicate muscles (thyroepiglottic muscle and aryepiglottic muscle) are found superior to the thyroarytenoid muscle. Do not attempt to dissect them.

14. Observe the vocal folds from a superior view. The interval between the vocal folds is called the **rima glottidis** (L. *rima*, a cleft or crack). The rima glottidis and the vocal folds collectively are called the **glottis**.

15. Review the function of the intrinsic muscles of the larynx. **The posterior cricoarytenoid muscle is the only muscle that opens the rima glottidis.** The cricothyroid muscle tilts the thyroid cartilage anteriorly and tenses the vocal fold (higher pitch of voice). The thyroarytenoid muscle tilts the thyroid cartilage posteriorly and relaxes the vocal fold (lower pitch of voice).

Glottis

Laryngospasm is a spasmodic closure of the glottis and it is life threatening. Spasm of the intrinsic laryngeal muscles that close the glottis may be produced by irritating chemicals, by severe allergic reactions, and sometimes as a side effect of medications.

The vocal folds can be readily visualized and inspected with the aid of a mirror (indirect laryngoscopy) or with a laryngoscope (direct laryngoscopy). Persistent hoarseness is an indication for laryngoscopy. Persistent hoarseness may be caused by changes of the vocal folds or it may indicate that the recurrent laryngeal nerve is compromised in the thorax or neck.

INTERIOR OF THE LARYNX [G 801; L 318; N 63; R 161; C 600]

1. In the midline, use scissors to cut the arytenoid muscle, lamina of the cricoid cartilage, and trachea. In addition, cut the arch of the cricoid cartilage in the midline anteriorly.

2. Open the larynx and observe that the **laryngeal cavity** has three parts (Fig. 7.92):
   • **Vestibule** – superior to the vestibular folds

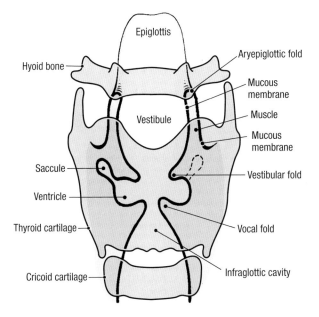

Figure 7.92. Schematic drawing of the laryngeal cavity, anterior view.

Labels in figure: Epiglottis, Aryepiglottic fold, Hyoid bone, Mucous membrane, Vestibule, Muscle, Mucous membrane, Saccule, Vestibular fold, Ventricle, Thyroid cartilage, Vocal fold, Cricoid cartilage, Infraglottic cavity

- **Ventricle** – the depression between the vestibular fold and the vocal fold
- **Infraglottic cavity** – inferior to the vocal folds and continuous with the trachea

3. Examine the **epiglottis** and note that it moves posteriorly during swallowing to close the laryngeal inlet.
4. Inspect the mucosa that lines the interior of the larynx and identify the **vestibular fold (false vocal fold)** and the **vocal fold (true vocal fold)**. The **vocal ligament** is located within the vocal fold.
5. Examine the **ventricle**. The ventricle may extend into a recess called the **saccule** (Fig. 7.92).
6. Review the **nerve supply to the larynx**:
   - **Internal branch of the superior laryngeal nerve** – provides sensory innervation to the mucosa superior to the vocal folds
   - **External branch of the superior laryngeal nerve** – innervates the cricothyroid muscle (and also the inferior pharyngeal constrictor muscle).
   - **Inferior laryngeal branch of the recurrent laryngeal nerve** – innervates all of the intrinsic muscles of the larynx except the cricothyroid muscle, and provides sensory innervation to the mucosa inferior to the vocal folds

Dissection Review

1. Replace the head and larynx in their correct anatomical positions.
2. Use a cross-sectional drawing of the neck and the dissected specimen to review the relationship of the lar-

ynx to the vertebral column, carotid sheaths, and other cervical viscera.
3. Trace the right and left vagus nerves into the thorax and follow the right and left recurrent laryngeal nerves from the thorax to the larynx. Note the differences.
4. Review the branches of the external carotid artery.
5. Follow the superior thyroid artery to the thyroid gland and review the course of the superior laryngeal artery as it passes through the thyrohyoid membrane to enter the larynx. Recall that the superior laryngeal artery courses with the internal branch of the superior laryngeal nerve.
6. Review the course of the superior laryngeal nerve from the vagus nerve to its bifurcation. Follow the external laryngeal branch to the cricothyroid muscle.
7. Use the dissected specimen to review the attachments and action of each intrinsic laryngeal muscle that was identified during dissection.
8. Review the movements of the vocal folds during phonation, quiet breathing, and rapid breathing.

EAR

Dissection Overview

The ear is composed of three parts: external ear, middle ear, and internal ear. The external ear consists of the **auricle** and the **external acoustic meatus**. The middle ear is within the **tympanic cavity of the temporal bone**. The **ossicles** (bones of the middle ear) are located in the middle ear. The **internal ear** (vestibulocochlear organ) is the neurologic part of the ear, which is contained within petrous portion of the temporal bone.

The order of dissection will be as follows: The parts of the external ear will be examined. The facial nerve will be followed from the posterior cranial fossa into the internal acoustic meatus and the roof of the tympanic cavity will be removed. The auditory ossicles will be identified and one ossicle will be removed. The temporal bone will be cut to reveal the medial and lateral walls of the tympanic cavity. The tympanic membrane will be studied. Features of the medial wall of the tympanic cavity will be examined.

TEMPORAL BONE

Refer to a skull. On the intracranial surface of the **temporal bone**, identify (Fig. 7.93): [G 709; L 362; N 9; R 30; C 531]

- **Groove for the greater petrosal nerve**
- **Tegmen tympani** – a portion of the floor of the middle cranial fossa that forms the roof of the tympanic cavity
- **Internal acoustic meatus**

On the external surface of the temporal bone, review the following: [G 617; L 362; N 8; R 32; C 536]

- **External acoustic meatus**
- **Mastoid process**

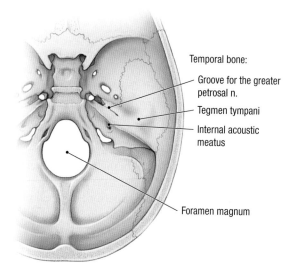

Figure 7.93. Temporal bone, superior view.

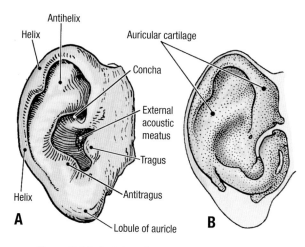

Figure 7.94. **A.** External ear **B.** Auricular cartilage.

- **Stylomastoid foramen**
- **Jugular fossa**
- **Carotid canal**
- Bony portion of the **pharyngotympanic tube**

Dissection Instructions

EXTERNAL EAR [G 703; L 361; N 93; R 124; C 602]

1. Examine the **auricle** of the cadaver and identify (Fig. 7.94A):
   - **Helix** – the rim of the auricle
   - **Antihelix** – the curved prominence anterior to the helix
   - **Concha** – the deepest part of the auricle
   - **Tragus**
   - **Antitragus**
   - **Lobule of the auricle**
2. Note that the **auricular cartilage** (Fig. 7.94B) gives the auricle its shape. There is no cartilage in the lobule. Palpate the auricular cartilage on yourself. By palpation, verify that the auricular cartilage is continuous with the cartilage of the external acoustic meatus.
3. The **external acoustic** meatus begins at the deepest part of the concha and ends at the tympanic membrane (a distance of about 2.5 cm in adults). The outer one-third of the external acoustic meatus is cartilaginous and the inner two-thirds is bony.
4. Note that the external acoustic meatus is S-shaped, first curving posterosuperiorly and then anteroinferiorly. The external acoustic meatus is straightened for examination by pulling the auricle upward, outward, and backward.

5. Study an illustration of the external surface of the tympanic membrane and relate its surface features to the structures that lie in the middle ear. [G 706; L 361; N 93; R 126; C 604]

MIDDLE EAR (TYMPANIC CAVITY) [G 708; L 360; N 97; R 130; C 612]

1. This dissection approach is intended for use on a decalcified temporal bone. It may also be used on a calcified temporal bone if the appropriate power tool is available. *Wear eye protection when cutting bone.*
2. The **tympanic cavity** is an air-filled space within the temporal bone. It is separated from the external acoustic meatus by the **tympanic membrane** and from the middle cranial fossa by the **tegmen tympani** (Fig. 7.95). The tympanic cavity will be approached by removing the tegmen tympani portion of the floor of the middle cranial fossa (Fig. 7.96).
3. Obtain a decalcified temporal bone specimen. If the dura mater is still present in the middle cranial fossa of the specimen, peel it off the superior surface of the temporal bone. Start at the superior border of the petrous part of the temporal bone and peel the dura mater in an anterior direction.
4. Look for the greater petrosal nerve in the groove for the greater petrosal nerve (Fig. 7.93). Note that the greater petrosal nerve lies between the dura mater and the bone.
5. Refer to a schematic illustration of the middle ear and orient yourself to the features of the **walls of the tympanic cavity** (Fig. 7.95): [G 708, 710, 711; L 363; N 92; R 122; C 604]
   - **Lateral** – the **tympanic membrane**

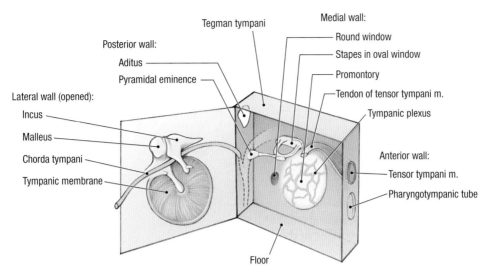

Tegman tympani

Medial wall:
— Round window
— Stapes in oval window
— Promontory
— Tendon of tensor tympani m.
— Tympanic plexus

Posterior wall:
Aditus —
Pyramidal eminence —

Lateral wall (opened):
Incus
Malleus
Chorda tympani
Tympanic membrane

Anterior wall:
— Tensor tympani m.
— Pharyngotympanic tube

Floor

Figure 7.95. Schematic drawing of the walls of the tympanic cavity. Right ear with the lateral wall opened, in anterolateral view.

- **Posterior** – the **aditus** (L. *aditus*, inlet or access), an opening into the **mastoid air cells**
- **Medial** – the **promontory** and **oval window (fenestra vestibuli)** containing the base (footplate) of the **stapes**
- **Anterior** – the opening of the **pharyngotympanic tube**
- **Superior** – tegmen tympani
- **Inferior** – the floor of the tympanic cavity,

which is closely related to the **jugular fossa** and the **jugular bulb**

6. Turn to the temporal bone specimen. In the posterior cranial fossa identify the **facial nerve (VII)** and the **vestibulocochlear nerve (VIII)** as they enter the internal acoustic meatus (Fig. 7.96).

7. Use a scalpel to remove the roof of the internal acoustic meatus and follow the **facial** and **vestibulocochlear nerves** laterally as they pass through

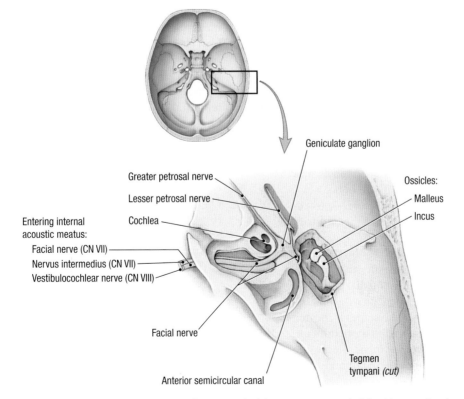

Geniculate ganglion

Greater petrosal nerve
Lesser petrosal nerve

Entering internal
acoustic meatus:
    Facial nerve (CN VII)
    Nervus intermedius (CN VII)
    Vestibulocochlear nerve (CN VIII)

Cochlea

Ossicles:
    Malleus
    Incus

Facial nerve

Tegmen
tympani *(cut)*

Anterior semicircular canal

Figure 7.96. Middle ear after removal of the tegmen tympani, right side, superior view.

the internal acoustic meatus. Remain superior to the nerves when cutting the internal acoustic meatus (Fig. 7.96). [G 709; L 362; N 94; C 612]

8. Follow the facial nerve laterally until it makes a sharp bend in the posterior direction. At this bend, identify the **geniculate ganglion** and the origin of the **greater petrosal nerve** (Fig. 7.96). The geniculate ganglion contains cell bodies of sensory neurons. The greater petrosal nerve carries preganglionic parasympathetic fibers to the pterygopalatine ganglion for innervation of the mucous membranes of the nasal and upper oral cavities, and the lacrimal gland. The preganglionic parasympathetic nerve fibers do not synapse in the geniculate ganglion.

9. The greater petrosal nerve courses anteromedially within the temporal bone and emerges on the floor of the middle cranial fossa at the **hiatus for the greater petrosal nerve**. It then passes inferiorly and medially on the surface of the temporal bone in the **groove for the greater petrosal nerve**. The greater petrosal nerve enters the carotid canal. On the surface of the internal carotid artery, the greater petrosal nerve joins the deep petrosal nerve to form the **nerve of the pterygoid canal**. The nerve of the pterygoid canal carries the preganglionic fibers of the greater petrosal nerve to the pterygopalatine ganglion.

10. Do not attempt to follow the facial nerve through the temporal bone. The facial nerve enters the facial canal at the geniculate ganglion. It travels a short distance in a posterolateral direction, then turns inferiorly and exits the skull at the stylomastoid foramen.

11. The **cochlea** lies anterior to the internal acoustic meatus in the angle formed by the facial nerve, the geniculate ganglion, and the greater petrosal nerve (Fig. 7.96). In the dissected specimen the modiolus of the cochlea may be seen, depending on the plane of cut.

12. The semicircular canals lie posterior to the internal acoustic meatus. The semicircular canals may be seen as a series of tiny holes in the bone.

13. To open the tympanic cavity, use forceps to remove the **tegmen tympani**. Observe the **auditory ossicles** within the tympanic cavity (Fig. 7.96). Note that the **malleus** is attached to the tympanic membrane, the **incus** occupies an intermediate position, and the **stapes** is the most medial of the auditory ossicles. The malleus and incus are easily seen from the superior view. The stapes is located more inferiorly, making observation more difficult.

14. Use fine forceps to remove the incus. Leave the malleus attached to the tympanic membrane (Fig. 7.97).

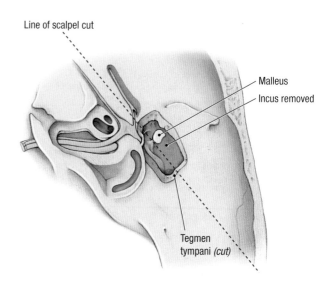

Figure 7.97. Angle of cut to separate the medial and lateral walls of the tympanic cavity.

15. Looking down from above, identify the **tympanic membrane** on the lateral wall of the tympanic cavity. Attempt to identify the tendon of the tensor tympani muscle, a thin strand of tissue that spans from the medial wall of the tympanic cavity to the handle of the malleus.

16. Insert a scalpel blade into the opening created by removing the incus (Fig. 7.97). Angle the blade parallel to the internal surface of the tympanic membrane. Make a cut that extends down the pharyngotympanic tube and divides the middle ear into medial and lateral walls (see Fig. 7.97 for correct placement of the cut). Make this cut parallel to the superior border of the petrous part of the temporal bone.

17. On the lateral wall of the tympanic cavity, observe the tympanic membrane and identify the **chorda tympani** (Fig. 7.98B). The chorda tympani passes between the malleus and the incus. [G 711; L 363; N 94; R 126; C 607]

18. On the medial wall of the tympanic cavity, identify (Fig. 7.98A): [G 710; L 363; N 94; R 126; C 608]
    - **Promontory** – an elevation on the medial wall.
    - **Stapes** – still attached to the **oval window (fenestra vestibuli)**. Look for the **stapedius tendon,** about 1 mm long, passing from the pyramidal eminence to the stapes. The stapedius muscle is innervated by the facial nerve (VII).
    - **Round window (fenestra cochleae)** – posteroinferior to the promontory.
    - **Tensor tympani muscle** – attaches to the pharyngotympanic tube and sphenoid bone

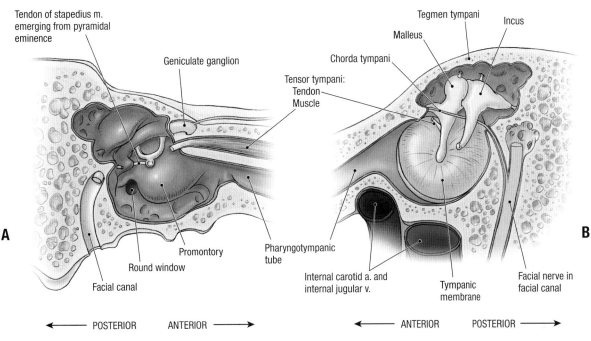

Figure 7.98. Walls of the right tympanic cavity, opened like a book. **A.** Medial wall. **B.** Lateral wall.

proximally, and to the tympanic membrane distally. Its tendon crosses the tympanic cavity. It is innervated by the mandibular division of the trigeminal nerve (V₃).

19. Note that the tympanic cavity and its associated recesses and air cells are covered with mucous membrane. The **glossopharyngeal nerve (IX)** innervates the mucous membrane of the tympanic cavity. It forms the **tympanic plexus** under the mucosa that covers the promontory.

INTERNAL EAR [G 714; L 365; N 96; R 129; C 612, 613]

The vestibulocochlear organ is best seen in sectioned histologic material. If you wish to dissect the internal ear, utilize a decalcified temporal bone. Refer to appropriate atlas illustrations and use a single-edge razor blade to cut thin slices of the temporal bone. This procedure will expose the canals, chambers, and nerve pathways of the internal ear. A dissecting microscope should be used to visualize these structures.

Dissection Review

1. Use an illustration to review the external appearance of the tympanic membrane.
2. Relate the tympanic membrane to the handle of the malleus and the chorda tympani.
3. Review the course of the facial nerve from the internal acoustic meatus to the facial muscles.
4. Review the course of the greater petrosal nerve from the geniculate ganglion to the pterygopalatine ganglion. Summarize the distribution of the postganglionic axons that arise in the pterygopalatine ganglion.
5. Review the course of the special sensory fibers contained in the chorda tympani beginning at the tongue and ending at the internal acoustic meatus. Where are the cell bodies for these sensory axons located?
6. Review the course of the preganglionic parasympathetic axons that synapse in the submandibular ganglion. Review the distribution of the postganglionic axons that arise from the submandibular ganglion.
7. Review all branches of the glossopharyngeal nerve, including those that give rise to the lesser petrosal nerve.

INDEX

Page numbers in *italics* indicate figures; those followed by a 'b' indicate boxes.